Speaking of Apraxia

Speaking of Apraxia

A Parents' Guide to Childhood Apraxia of Speech

Second Edition

Leslie A. Lindsay, R.N., B.S.N.

Woodbine House

Cataloging-in-Publication Data

Names: Lindsay, Leslie A., author.
Title: Speaking of apraxia : a parents' guide to childhood apraxia of
  speech / Leslie A. Lindsay, R.N., B.S.N.
Description: Second edition. | Bethesda : Woodbine House, [2020] | Includes
  bibliographical references and index.
Identifiers: LCCN 2020016443 (print) | LCCN 2020016444 (ebook) | ISBN
  9781606132937 (trade paperback) | ISBN 9781606132944 (ebook)
Subjects: LCSH: Speech disorders in children. | Apraxia.
Classification: LCC RJ496.S7 L55 2020 (print) | LCC RJ496.S7 (ebook) |
  DDC 618.92/855--dc23
LC record available at https://lccn.loc.gov/2020016443
LC ebook record available at https://lccn.loc.gov/2020016444

Publisher's Note: This book reflects the ideas and opinions of the author. Its purpose is to give the reader helpful information on the topics covered in the book. **It is not meant to provide health, medical, or professional evaluation, consultation, or advice. The reader is advised to consult appropriate health, medical, and other professionals for these services.** The author and publisher do not take responsibility for any personal or other risk, loss, or liability incurred as a direct or indirect consequence of application or use of information found in this book.

Manufactured in the United States of America
10 9 8 7 6 5 4 3 2 1

To Kate Riley—
my sweet, smart, and incredibly creative daughter.
Without you, I wouldn't have found my writing voice as easily.
For you, I give you a voice so that you may accomplish
whatever *your* heart desires.

To all those sweet voices yet to be heard . . .
their loving parents, grandparents,
speech-language pathologists, and teachers.

Contents

Section One

Tell Me More

The Straight Scoop on Speech Basics

Section Two

Now What?

Section Three

Helping Your Child

Section Four

Coping & Hoping

Preface

I am not an expert, but I am a mom and I am concerned. When my sweet, fun, and beautiful daughter was diagnosed with childhood apraxia of speech (CAS), I didn't even know what it was, let alone what to do about it.

What is childhood apraxia of speech? What caused it? What can we do about it? Not only did I have these questions but additional ones, too. How would this affect her social life, and how would it affect our family? I feared CAS would hold her back academically as well.

Once I got over the initial shock—after about six months or so—I hit the local library in search of resources. I'm old-school at heart and searching the internet (although an invaluable resource) just didn't appeal to me. The friendly, grandfatherly librarian found one measly resource—a chapter within a textbook that just barely touched on CAS. Instead of offering a hands-on, practical educational approach, it focused primarily on nutritional aspects of treatment. As a nurse, I wanted something more *scientific*. As a child-adolescent psychiatric nurse, I wanted something more *holistic*. As a mom, I wanted something more *sympathetic*.

When I asked my daughter's speech-language pathologist (SLP) for recommended reading, she scratched her head and said, "There's not a lot out there, but I'll look into it." Her search came up with next to nothing.

That was over a decade ago. The intervening years have brought a surge of interest in CAS—mostly for professionals who treat children with the disorder. Despite the availability of some good online resources on CAS, there's still a dearth of print materials supporting parents through the questions and obstacles typically faced. Every day, another child is diagnosed. Every day, a parent questions the same things I once did: What is childhood apraxia of speech? Will my child ever be able to speak? What can I do to help?

Parents new to the diagnosis frequently reach out to me for advice and reassurance. They come from all walks of life and all corners of the world. Australian and South American mothers have sent videos of their in-services at schools and workplaces, sharing knowledge and reducing the stigma of CAS. A grandfather—a retired physician—related that his adult daughter was in complete denial about his grandson's CAS. He pointed her in the direction of this book; she nodded with recognition, began seeking treatment. A mother in rural Appalachia emailed and said this book had been a lifesaver for her, that she no longer felt alone. A father from Quebec shared that there weren't many resources available and that this book made a huge difference in his understanding of CAS. An American SLP I spoke with said CAS does not discriminate. She has treated children with CAS who are black, white, Hispanic, Asian, and Eastern Indian, from English-speaking families and from Spanish-speaking ones too. A Scottish mother related that CAS is mostly a "hidden disorder" in the United Kingdom and that most of her comfort and support come from resources like this.

Eight years have passed since the first edition of *Speaking of Apraxia* was published; we're making strides every day in terms of diagnosis and treatment. Connections, friendships, discoveries, and celebrations happen online, at the playground, in the speech clinic, at conferences, and in colleges and universities. Children who were diagnosed in 2007, like my daughter, are now in high school. Other, older kids with a history of CAS might be heading off to college. Those parents want updates about the lingering deficits related to CAS. Some parents contact me to say, "We're making so much progress; we got this." Every so often, I get a message like this: "I was in tears twice before I reached page thirteen. Page thirteen! You are doing a wonderful job educating and supporting parents."

It's been my utmost privilege and honor to walk with you on this apraxia journey. Here, I hope to provide updated resources, books, websites, apps, and more. There's a wealth of knowledge, expertise, enthusiasm—and hope—out there.

Together, we got this.

Acknowledgments

It takes a village to raise a child and a whole city to write a book. When I think of where I was a decade ago, in the throes of writing the first edition of this book, I sometimes marvel at the tiny miracles that had to line up in perfect synchrony to get the information to you. Special thanks to Kate's first speech-language pathologist, Jennifer Usher-Carr, MS, CCC-SLP, and speech-language pathology assistant Sylvia Garland, SLPA, as well as to Teri Westra, OTR/L, who worked with Kate on "heavy work," as well as incorporating her love of movement into speech therapy sessions. I'll always be grateful for their care, support, and guidance on our apraxia journey. Special thanks to Karin Sudlow, MS, CCC-SLP, the then-clinic owner who saw a need for more education and supported the Small Talk: All About Apraxia group to be held at her clinic in suburban Chicago. Many thanks to the parents, grandparents, educators, and music therapists who attended those sessions and provided insights and challenged my knowledge on childhood apraxia of speech (CAS). You got me thinking, writing, researching, and answering your questions.

My deepest gratitude goes to my review board for this new edition: Nanette Cote, MA, CCC-SLP, Renee Mindy, MEd, and Erik X. Raj, PhD, CCC-SLP. You all brought new resources to the forefront, introduced me to additional experts in the field, and just made this second edition so much fun. Special thanks to Ayelet Marinovich, MA, CCC-SLP, and Rebecca Eisenberg, MS, CCC-SLP, for their tips and ideas on playtime, mealtime, books, and reading, and to Jennie Bjorem, MA, CCC-SLP, for her clear and easy-to-understand definition of CAS, plus her continued work with children with CAS. There are so many fabulously talented and engaging speech-language pathologists who have endless enthusiasm for this project, but also for their speech "students." You guys all rock.

I will be forever grateful for the first review board: Diane (Di) Bahr, MS, CCC-SLP, Rhonda Banford, MAT, CCC-SLP, Lisa Circelli, MEd, Morgan Holubetz, MS, CCC-SLP, and Teri Kaminski Peterson, MS, CCC-SLP. Special shout-out to Susan Oakes-Hauf and Amy Moll, mothers of older girls with resolved apraxia. Thank you to Diane Nancarrow, MA, CCC-SLP, of the Kaufman Center for reading early versions of some chapters, Tony Ebel, D.C., who took care to provide some pointers on chiropractic care, Kimberly Sena-Moore, PhD, MT-BC, for providing some "rhythm" to the music therapy section, and Emily Sevick, MSEd, MT-BC, LPC, for her assistance and willingness to attend Small Talk: All About Apraxia and provide parents hints and tips on the value of music therapy. Thanks to Larry Shriberg, PhD, who took a peek at the genetics connection to CAS. My sincerest thanks to Lloyd Wells, MD, PhD, now retired from the Mayo Clinic-Rochester Child/Adolescent Treatment Program for his review of the comorbid conditions presented in Appendix A.

Also, thanks to Ruth Stoeckel, PhD, CCC-SLP, for review of portions of this book and her willingness to respond to my many email questions, particularly in the first edition, as well as to Margaret (Dee) Fish, MS, CCC-SLP, and Kathy Jakielski, PhD, CCC-SLP, for their support and suggestions for additional resources, and responding to my email questions. You are all such an integral piece to the diagnosis and treatment of CAS, and I applaud your important work.

My understanding of CAS has been strengthened by my involvement with the now-defunct Apraxia Kids listserv and The Apraxia Connection in the Chicago area, and the connections I have made—and maintained—through these organizations. You all are amazing individuals who care so deeply for children with CAS. Thanks to Angela Grimm, the current executive director of Apraxia Kids, for providing insight and history of the organization and sharing an excerpt of the organization's mission in the networking chapter.

To the folks at Woodbine House—especially Susan Stokes—for seeing a continued need for this book. Thank you, thank you, a thousand times thank you for giving me a space to share my knowledge on CAS and desire to help others. You all do amazing work disseminating materials to parents and caregivers raising children with special needs.

To my ultra-supportive husband who suggested this book was a true need and that I was the person to write it. He was there when I wavered, when I celebrated small victories, when I ran into roadblocks. And he always, always cheered me on.

I couldn't have written this book without my precious girls, Kate and Kelly. Thank you both for the inspiration, love, and understanding when I "take too long, Mommy" at the library or coffee shop (for the first edition). Many of these chapters were written or revised in a parked minivan at soccer practice or the corner of a dance studio. I've often said, "You work on your dream, while I work on mine." You are my dreams come true.

—Leslie A. Lindsay
Chicago, Illinois

How This Book Is Organized

You're a parent. You're short on time. You want answers and encouragement. Yesterday. I know. I have been there.

The good news is, you will find some answers here. Maybe not all of them, but at least a good amount. And if you don't find the answers you thought you would, don't worry; there is a section at the end of every chapter that points you in the right direction for further study. I call it **Recommended Resources**.

But let's start at the beginning. Most chapters begin with an anecdote about one of my family experiences relevant to the chapter. The characters you will come across are real and important to me. They are Kate—redheaded and blue-eyed, spunky, and smart, and yes—she has childhood apraxia of speech (CAS). Kelly is my little precocious one, also redheaded and blue-eyed and once did express some symptoms consistent with CAS. My husband, Jim—Kate and Kelly's dad—and my rock. You may read, laugh, and cry at these introductions and completely relate to them, or you may skip them. Hopefully, they will give you a sense that I've been there too and will help you feel a little less alone on your journey to come to grips with CAS.

The Nuts and Bolts of This Chapter sections break the chapter down into tangible bullet points. You can glance over the list and see if "your" topic will be covered.

You will find sections and text boxes called

- **What's a Parent to Do?**—offering a step-by-step approach to dealing with a particular concern
- **Parents Cope**—helping you reframe a troubling moment
- **What You Can Do at Home**—giving you a quick and simple activity you can do at home to help your child with apraxia. In fact, there is an entire chapter devoted to this topic, but you will also find these suggestions in some other chapters.
- **Parents Share**—providing some insight and quotes from parents who have been right where you are now

I have talked to parents. Lots of them. Most have a child with apraxia. Some have children with other special needs. All of them love their children more than anything else in the world. They want to help you. You will find quotes from them offering *real-world advice, tips, or ideas.* There are other sections sprinkled throughout the book in the form of "Parents Ask." These are questions I have heard often in this apraxia journey. Some of them I have asked myself! Following each question is a quick-and-easy answer.

I have talked to speech-language pathologists too. Lots of them. Some are in private practice, others work within school districts, and still others are in research at universities. They know what they are talking about. Their advice and studies are peppered throughout the book.

Finally, I facilitated a support and education group in the Chicagoland area called Small Talk: All About Apraxia. Parents and grandparents came. They asked questions. I learned a lot about what is on your mind related to childhood apraxia of speech. Parents from the group were kind enough to let me use some of the information they shared in the hopes that it may help another—you!

What Should You Do with This Book?

- Skim the book and decide where you want to start.
- You don't have to start at the beginning. Feel free to pick the chapters that you feel you need most.
- Come back to the ones you don't need just yet. Someday you may.
- If you have questions, ask your SLP or pediatrician or email me at: leslie_lindsay@ hotmail.com.
- What are you waiting for? Turn the page. . . .

Tell Me More

The Straight Scoop on Speech Basics

Chapter 1

Does My Child Have Childhood Apraxia of Speech (CAS)?

At two years old, Kate was a beautiful, energetic, and happy toddler. But with the exception of one word—hi—Kate was as quiet as a mouse. We wondered if something was wrong. Even as a baby, Kate had rarely babbled and cried; she was beautiful and unique with red hair and bright blue eyes. She was, in a word, "perfect." So why were we worried? After all, she could understand everything we said, even the big words.

"Play classical music. Dance with her. Babies need that so their brains can develop," others told us. And so we did. We talked to her as if she was a little adult, making conversations even though we didn't expect answers.

"She'll talk when she's ready," my mom-friends assured me. Only their toddlers were saying words like "elephant," and when we met at the park, I cringed and rolled my lips into a tight line, sucking in a deep breath.

Was Kate stressed because of her new sibling or our impending move? No, that wasn't it. We were providing her with a loving, stable environment. So, what was it? I was confused and frustrated.

Aria, age two, was a puzzle to her parents. She was obviously quite bright and alert. She knew the names of all the birds in her Big Book of Birds and would point to the cardinal, chickadee, etc. when asked. But she struggled to say even the simplest words.

Julian was an active three-year-old who loved cause-and-effect toys, an engineer in the making. He appeared to be a typically developing child, with one exception: he was not talking. His grandmother kept saying, "Boys are late to talk—don't worry." But his parents were concerned. Could something else be going on?

Do these stories sound familiar? Does your child remind you of Kate or Aria or Julian? If so, your child could have childhood apraxia of speech (CAS). I'll admit, when I first heard of CAS, I was totally stumped. We hadn't covered *this* in nursing school! So what *is* CAS, anyway? Like you, I had a ton of questions and concerns and little time to learn about it. But most of all—my child needed help. You may be feeling the same way.

Perhaps you have already been given a diagnosis of CAS but are still searching for information to help you and your child cope with the condition. (If that's the case, feel free to skip this chapter.) Or, perhaps you are struggling to figure out exactly why your child isn't speaking in the same manner as other children her age. Perhaps you're wondering if it could be CAS.

The Nuts and Bolts of This Chapter

- A discussion of what CAS is, as outlined by the American Speech-Language-Hearing Association
- A list of symptoms and red flags related to CAS
- Terminology concerns—why are there so many names to represent one phenomenon?!
- Discussions on prevalence, intelligence, boys versus girls, the likelihood of having CAS, as well as your child's future as it relates to communication

What Is Childhood Apraxia of Speech?

Childhood speech apraxia (CAS), as most pediatric speech-language pathologists (SLPs) in the United States call it,* is best defined by what it is *not*. Historically, it's been one of the most debated disorders in the field of speech-language pathology. It took practitioners quite some time to find an easy, agreed-upon definition, list of symptoms, cause, and treatment. But they did!

If we were to define CAS in a table format, it would look something like this:

CAS IS NOT:	CAS IS:
A muscular disorder	A neurologically based motor speech *disorder*, not a delay
A cognitive disorder	A neurobehavioral disorder
A developmental delay	A *disruption* in spatiotemporal parameters of speech movement (difficulty moving articulators—lips, jaw, tongue—through space with correct timing for accurate sequencing of sounds)

---

* Elsewhere in the world, the disorder is often referred to as verbal dyspraxia.

A medical issue; there are no medical tests to diagnose CAS	Dynamic, ever changing
	Multifaceted

It's not a black-and-white answer. If this is still a bit confusing, don't lose heart.

Here is a definition provided at the 2019 SLP Summit conference by Jennie Bjorem, MA, CCC-SLP, a speech-language pathologist with advanced training and expertise in childhood apraxia of speech:

"Apraxia of speech is a speech label for difficulty with planning and programming movement for speech. Our brains plan and program the movements needed for speech including the tongue, lips, jaw, palate, vocal cords, and diaphragm. Our brains also must judge when to move, at what speed, in what direction, the distance for the movement, with how much muscle contraction . . . all at the same time. CAS is when there is a disconnect in the ability to plan out and program these movements impacting the movement for speech production and prosody."

The American Speech-Language-Hearing Association (ASHA) offers the following 2007 definition of CAS:

"A neurological childhood (pediatric) speech sound disorder in which precision and consistency of movements underlying speech are impaired in the absence of neuromuscular deficits."

Let's break this down even more:

■ Neurological refers to the nervous system (brain and spinal cord to start with).

■ Childhood/pediatric generally refers to the ages of birth to adolescence.

■ Precision and consistency refer to the accuracy of speech sounds each and every time they are spoken.

■ Movements underlying speech refers to the movements of the articulators (lips, jaw, tongue, teeth, soft palate, hard palate) in smooth, sequential, and overlapping gestures necessary for intelligible speech.

■ The oral structures of the mouth are tongue, lips, jaw, teeth, and palate.

■ Neuromuscular deficits are things like abnormal reflexes and weakness and difficulties coordinating the muscles that are controlled by the brain to produce speech movements.

In plain language, kids who have been diagnosed with "pure" CAS have completely normal facial tone and musculature. Their reflexes are *typically* normal, yet they still can't coordinate their internal thoughts, shape them into verbal communication, and produce it in a manner we can all understand. ("Pure" refers to the fact that these children have no other neurodevelopmental conditions; they are struggling with only CAS.) So, when my daughter Kate would attempt to answer a simple question about what she wanted to do for the day, *she knew what she wanted to say; she just couldn't get her mouth to cooperate with her ideas.* She would go to the back door, dangle her shoes, and point in the general direction of the park. "Eh-eh?" she would say. Our little girl couldn't say "park," even when we asked her to *and* modeled the correct word: "Oh, you want to go to the *park*. Can you say, '*park*'?" Yet, we knew what she wanted, and so did she. (Of course, every child with CAS says things uniquely. Another child might be able to say "ark" for park, thus making it much easier to piece together what she wants.)

The folks who wrote the *ASHA Technical Report on CAS* would impress upon parents that when SLPs give the diagnosis of CAS, they are *ruling out* any weakness, decreased range of motion, low muscle tone, and coordination difficulties as contributing factors to a child's CAS. These children *can* still possibly have co-occurring (in addition to) speech and language conditions such as dysarthria, phonological errors, and low tone. Children with CAS may also have developmental disabilities such as autism or Down syndrome, among others.

The problem with CAS occurs when the brain tries to tell the muscles what to do and the message gets scrambled somehow. The child typically knows what she wants to say, but her brain is not sending the correct instructions to move the mouth the way it should move. Thus, motor execution is affected. Words may or may not come out . . . and if they do, they are often unintelligible.

Generally speaking, the more a child with CAS *wants* to communicate, either to meet a need or to express something creatively, the harder it is for her. Automatic speech is easier. That is, the child hasn't stopped to think, "I want to say 'hi' when I see Grandma." She *knows* the word and *knows* it's socially polite to say hello as a greeting. She hasn't mentally planned on saying the word; it just happens that she says it at the right time. Sometimes a word or a phrase will just "pop" out, and it may never happen again. In fact, Judy Jelm, CCC-SLP, a clinician in private practice in Naperville, Illinois, coined the term *phrases out-of-the-blue* to describe this phenomenon in children with CAS. Frustrating and discouraging, yes? If *you* are feeling these emotions, then imagine how your child might be feeling.

I remember this "phrase popping" happening only once with my daughter Kate (diagnosed with CAS at the age of two and a half). It occurred when I was changing her diaper one day when she was just under two years old. In a hopeful moment of trying to teach independence and responsibility, I handed her the diaper all rolled up and asked, "What should we do with this?" I wasn't *really* expecting an answer, but she surprised me.

"Put it in the trash!" I heard it clear as day, as did Papa, who was within earshot. Little Kate toddled off, diaper in hand to the trash can. We never heard so much from her again until years down the road.

According to Dr. Kathy Jakielski, associate professor in the Department of

Communication Sciences Disorders and certified speech pathologist at Augustana College in Rock Island, Illinois: "Children with CAS live with having to think about, practice, and sequence their words. When they're speaking, they are thinking about coordinating all of those movements that require motor planning."

One mom I spoke with summed it up this way: "Having CAS is like trying to learn a foreign language." You have an idea of how things *should* sound, but you can't carry on a conversation in that language until you first master the letter sounds and basic words and *then* string them into sentences, and then—maybe even at the same time—"get" the grammar and meaning of all of the words. Only then can you become fluent in that foreign language. Of course you also need to be able to practice that language a lot with others who also speak it."

Tip: The CCC designation following a speech-language pathologist's name translates to "certificate of clinical competence" and is awarded by ASHA to speech-language pathologists (and audiologists) who have voluntarily met rigorous academic and professional standards, beyond the minimum state requirements for licensure. The CCC-SLP is a nationally recognized professional credential representing a level of excellence. These professionals have the knowledge, skills, and expertise to provide high quality clinical services and are actively engaged in ongoing professional development.

Another Way of Looking at CAS

Lots of experts and parents refer to CAS as a motor-based speech disorder, but it's crucial to recognize that it is also a developmental disorder.

A developmental disorder is defined in the Developmental Disabilities Assistance and Bill of Rights Act of 2000 as a chronic disability that is attributable to physical or mental impairment, begins in childhood, is likely to continue indefinitely, and results in the substantial functional limitations of at least three of the following: self-care, receptive and expressive language, learning, mobility, self-direction, capacity for independent living, or economic self-sufficiency.

You're probably asking, "Does it really matter what we call CAS?" It doesn't necessarily "matter," but recognizing that it's a developmental disability gives parents the appropriate perspective to implement strategies that work for childhood apraxia of speech. And if you are seeking speech-language therapy or other special services from your child's school or an early intervention program, having a developmental disability is one way to qualify for such services.

Symptoms of CAS

Many children with CAS have a history of delayed speech development. They often have a family history of speech or learning problems but may also be the first member in their family with the disorder. CAS is slightly more likely to occur in boys than girls, but it is still plenty common in girls. Below are some other warning signs or red flags to be aware of. Note that the defining characteristics will depend on the child's developmental age. The range of problems often unfolds as the child progresses. Ages presented here are meant to be general guidelines.

Warning Signs of CAS

Warning Signs in Infancy (Birth to Age 1)
☐ Decreased cooing or babbling. Others comment on what a "quiet baby" you have.

☐ May have feeding difficulties.

☐ Your baby's first words appear late (after 14 months) or not at all.

☐ If first words *do* appear, they are often "easy" sounds (phonemes) replaced with even *easier* ones. For example, "hi" might sound like "I," but is used in a greeting context.

Warning Signs in Early Childhood (Age 1 to 3)
☐ Understands most of what is said but cannot verbalize well. Large gap between receptive and expressive language.

☐ Distorts or changes sounds.

☐ Difficulty imitating words and phrases (see chapter 7 for more information on imitation).

☐ Messy and distractible eating. Requires prompts to take a bite, chew, swallow, and drink; may overstuff or "pocket" food in the cheeks. Hyper- or hyposensitivity to oral activities such as eating different textures of foods or brushing teeth; difficulty identifying an object in the mouth through touch.

☐ Prosody (melody) of speech is affected. Also may only be able to repeat a word/ sound/phrase in the context of a practiced routine; may regress or struggle with producing a word in a phrase/sentence.

☐ May have developed elaborate nonverbal or gestural communication.

☐ Struggles with speech, "searching" (groping) for the right word, but this can also be common in children who stutter.

☐ Stresses the wrong part of the word; the same word is said a number of different ways.

☐ Leaves sounds out of words (e.g., "cookie" becomes "coo-ie").

☐ The longer the phrase attempted, the less understandable the child becomes.

Warning Signs at Any Age
Neurological problems (problems that affect cognition, body mechanics, or the sensory system) may occur with a variety of childhood conditions. Those that may accompany CAS include the following:

☐ The child often gestures and grunts in lieu of oral communication.

☐ Gross motor skills (running, jumping, climbing) may also be slow in developing.

- ☐ The child appears clumsy or uncoordinated, has poor body awareness (proprioception) or difficulty with fine motor skills (holding a pencil, using scissors).
- ☐ IQ testing shows higher performance IQ (doing tasks) and lower verbal IQ (talking tasks).
- ☐ Poor sequencing (the child has difficulties putting a series of movements in order—e.g., figuring out how to get on an unfamiliar piece of playground equipment or sequencing events to relate to others).
- ☐ Poor auditory processing (listening and reacting appropriately); often needs others to repeat themselves.
- ☐ Greater difficulties in learning to read, spell, and write.
- ☐ Difficulty with a variety of components of speech (pitch, quality, rate, etc.).
- ☐ Correctly saying "difficult" words is, well . . . difficult (e.g., *butterfly*, *rocking chair*, *exercise*).
- ☐ The child can make the sound(s) of many letters when the letter is alone, but when combined in a sentence, will not be able to say it.
- ☐ Limited (correct) use of vowels and consonants.
- ☐ May have developed elaborate nonverbal and gestural communication.
- ☐ Family history of delayed language development, as well as a family propensity to have other learning difficulties.

Again, Jennie Bjorem, CCC-SLP, mentions these characteristics as consistent with childhood apraxia of speech:

1. Inconsistent productions of consonants and vowels over multiple attempts
2. Longer transitions or disrupted movements between sounds and syllables with significant difficulty in initial configuration
3. Prosody differences, making speech sound robotic (prosody differences include difficulty with intonation, rhythm, variation in pitch, controlling loudness)

This might be seen in a child who is searching for words, and once she finds them, struggles to initiate speech. Once she starts speaking, her pitch and volume varies. Her statements may sound alternatively loud and quiet, with a slight robotic, hollow-like quality to them.

For more information on the specifics of a CAS diagnosis, please refer to the section on "Childhood Apraxia of Speech" on the ASHA website (www.asha.org).

Tip: Does your child seem to have a good grasp of receptive language—understanding what is said—but still have difficulty expressing himself? SLPs often note a large gap between receptive language (speech comprehension) and expressive language (speaking) as being a "symptom" of CAS.

Different Names, Same Thing?

Historically, CAS has had many different names. But since the release of ASHA's 2007 Technical Report, the proper terminology in the United States and Canada is childhood apraxia of speech. This may be shortened to *apraxia*. In some regions, it may be referred to as *verbal apraxia, developmental apraxia of speech*, or *verbal dyspraxia*. (There are other types of apraxia as explained below, but this book's primary focus is CAS.)

The *Diagnostic and Statistical Manual of Mental Disorders, 5th Edition,* of the American Psychiatric Association (2013) uses the term *verbal dyspraxia* to describe CAS. It's discussed within the Speech Sound Disorders category. The DSM-5 indicates verbal dyspraxia as a disorder in which "other areas of motor coordination may be impaired as in developmental coordination disorder." If your child ever visits a psychologist, counselor, or other mental health professional, you may therefore see this diagnosis used.

Regardless of what term is used, the most important concept is contained within the root word *praxis*. **Praxis** can be defined as planned movement or "motor planning." **Apraxia** is the *lack* of planned movement. A **motor skill** is a highly refined pattern of movement performed automatically and no longer requiring constant attention or reminders. It just happens. Typing on a keyboard is one such example. For one reason or another, children with CAS have difficulty planning and organizing speech movements.

Sally Goddard, author of *Reflexes, Learning and Behavior,* identifies praxis as: "The brain's ability to select responses, arrange them in an appropriate order, and orient them for proper execution." Therefore, it follows that **apraxia** ("without praxia") *is the inability to select and arrange responses for proper execution, even though no motor paralysis exists.*

Tip: Does your child seem to be "searching" for the right word—pausing and thinking—while trying to communicate? This is related to planning and word retrieval, also a hallmark of CAS. Speech-language pathologists (SLPs) call this behavior *groping*.

Other Types of Apraxia

Besides CAS, which affects planning responses for speech, there are other types of apraxia. One of the more common is **Global apraxia,** often referred to as **Developmental Coordination Disorder** (DCD). Many parents report a "clumsy" or "awkward" child, who may have difficulty completing common, everyday tasks like tying shoes, zipping, or walking down stairs. Like CAS, global apraxia is due to a delay in motor skill development; there is no medical or neurological reason. According to the CanChild website, the research center affiliated with McMaster University in Ontario, Canada, 5–6 percent of all school-aged children have global apraxia or DCD.

There are also more focused types of apraxia, including the following:

■ *Limb apraxia* causes difficulty moving the arms and legs in purposeful ways. For example, a child may *want* to catch a ball, but cannot because her body and brain aren't working together.

■ *Oral apraxia* affects nonspeech movements of the lips, tongue, and jaw. For example, a child is capable of puckering, smiling, blowing bubbles, etc., but can't do so when asked.

■ *Visual/oculomotor apraxia* (OMA) is the lack of control of intentional eye movement. For example, if a child wants to look at something, she often needs to turn her entire head to see it; she has trouble moving eyes in the desired direction. More information can be found at the American Association for Pediatric Ophthalmology and Strabismus (www.aapos.org).

A child with CAS may also have these additional types of apraxia, but she may not.

As explained in chapter 3, you might see a variety of professionals when seeking a diagnosis for your child's speech difficulties. ***The only professional who can diagnose CAS is a licensed professional speech-language pathologist (SLP).*** It is out of scope for an SLP to define and diagnose limb, visual, and even global apraxia. You will need to contact another professional, starting with your child's pediatrician, if these other types are a concern.

How Do I Know If My Child Has CAS?

Just because your child has *some* of the symptoms listed above does not necessarily mean she has CAS. Many childhood conditions can cause symptoms similar to those in CAS. And there are children who have no speech or language disorder at all who may display some of the listed symptoms when they are young. Please, if you have any concerns, it is best to seek advice—and an evaluation—from a licensed speech-language pathologist.

All speech and language disorders and delays are not treated the same, which makes it essential to pinpoint what is causing your child's speech-language concerns. There are other motor-speech disorders that may look like CAS. They include the following:

■ *Dysarthria:* speech difficulties caused by central or peripheral nervous system damage resulting in weakness, paralysis, or incoordination of the speech muscles themselves. Signs include slurred speech, soft/whispery speech, slowed speech, limited tongue/jaw movement, abnormal rhythm, nasal or stuffy sounding speech.

■ *Stuttering* (officially called *childhood onset stuttering*): a temporary interruption in the forward flow of speech production that is characterized by repetitions, prolongations, or abnormal stoppages of sounds and syllables. A child may struggle to get the words out, stopping the flow of speech, and often appearing as though she has gotten "stuck." There may also be facial and body movements associated with the effort to speak and/or embarrassment, anxiety, and fear that are directly related to the act of speaking.

Or you may find that your child has one of these disorders:

- *Expressive language delay:* a delay in what a child is able to say and how it is said. It may look like you have a "shy" child who rarely initiates conversation or gives short answers to questions. She may overgeneralize names of objects (*every* furry animal is a dog; *every* drink is juice), or she may "talk in circles" (a simple retelling of a story/event is very complex), or may find it hard to put sentences together in the right order.

- *Articulation disorder:* difficulty in producing the complex motor skills required for the consistent articulation of one or more specific speech sounds because of faulty articulatory placement, timing, direction, pressure, speed, and/or integration of oral movements. For example, a child may regularly mispronounce the *r* sound at the beginning of all words by consistently producing the *w* sound instead (e.g., *rabbit* is *wabbit*).

- *Phonological disorder:* difficulty in understanding the phonologic rules that other children naturally pick up on. A child may verbally produce errors of several sounds in one word but not others. She may leave out endings to words, yet can say that sound when it occurs in the middle of the word (e.g., *book* is *booh*, but she can say *locker* or *hiking* fine). These sound errors are the result of the child simplifying certain speech sounds and sound combinations that form patterns or clusters. ***Often, kids with CAS can "graduate" into a form of phonological disorder.***

In the case of suspected CAS, the first step is to see a speech-language pathologist (CCC-SLP) for a thorough assessment, or you may even consider starting with your pediatrician. Chapter 3 explains how to get started on the road to diagnosis.

Depending on your child's age and the extent of her speech delay, you may want to seek out a professional evaluation sooner rather than later. Elaine Weitzman, MEd, SLP, the executive director of The Hanen Center, says, "We know that the window of opportunity [for language development] is greatest when a child is very young. If a toddler is late in his or her language development, parents will never regret acting early. They might, however, regret acting too late."

The bottom line: it's best to get an assessment from a licensed speech-language pathologist when you start noticing your child isn't reaching developmentally appropriate speech-language milestones.

Can CAS Occur with Other Conditions?

You may be wondering if CAS can occur with other conditions—and the answer is gray, at best. There are times where apraxia is the only concern a child has. This may be referred to as "pure" apraxia. There are also children who have CAS on top of another condition. They may have a condition that typically causes communication delays or problems, but the CAS means that they have *even more* trouble speaking than someone with that condition normally does. It can be especially difficult for these children to get a diagnosis of CAS without being told, "Oh, it's just the Down syndrome" [for example].

The most common of these other conditions are autism spectrum disorders, attention-deficit/hyperactivity disorder (ADHD), Down syndrome, and sensory processing disorders. Other, rarer genetic conditions that can include CAS symptoms are cri du chat and Prader-Willi syndrome. Please refer to Appendix A for more information.

Parents Ask

Can a smart child have apraxia?

CAS has nothing to do with intelligence. If you are dealing mostly with CAS, then your child probably does not have cognitive delays. In fact, many of these children are quite intelligent—gifted and talented in many ways! Just because you are pursuing a speech-language evaluation, it does not mean you are questioning your child's intelligence.

Sometimes CAS occurs with another condition that is associated with cognitive delays. For example, children with Down syndrome frequently have both muscle function and motor planning concerns and may be diagnosed with CAS. In this case, the CAS doesn't mean the child's intelligence will be more affected than is usual for someone with Down syndrome.

"But isn't CAS a 'special need'?" Well, yes. If your child is evaluated by the school district and it is determined that her delay in speech is significant enough to receive services (and you, the parent, consent), then your child will be labeled as having a "special need." But just because a child is receiving special education doesn't mean she is not bright. Nowadays, special education covers a wide range of services to meet a child's individual needs.

Teresa, a mother in a Chicago suburb, talks about her experience with dual diagnosis:

"My son Nick has Down syndrome, but he was also diagnosed with CAS at the age of five. His speech was quite delayed, and often it seemed like he was grasping to try to say words, like the cat got his tongue. He was definitely more behind in his speech than his peers who had Down syndrome. Once we got the CAS diagnosis, the speech therapy became tailored to address this issue. He did a lot more repetitive work along with pairing speech with motor play. So many of these disorders and their symptoms overlap, and there are certainly a lot of gray areas when deciding why a child's speech is delayed."

See chapter 6 for more information on the CAS and Down syndrome diagnosis.

If your child has CAS, recognize it early, get the appropriate help, look for ways to cope, and find resources to help your child. These topics are all covered in this book. I know you are thinking, "Easy for you to say!" Don't forget—I was once where you are too. It's anything *but* easy. **You will get through this; your child will get through it too.**

How Many Kids Have CAS?

The answer may surprise you for a variety of reasons. For one, just as with other neurobehavioral disorders such as autism spectrum disorders (ASD) and ADHD, CAS also appears to on the rise, but serious research on this trend is lacking.

One estimate suggested that CAS may occur in 1 to 2 children per 1,000. A different study cited 1–10 children per 1,000. Most researchers have found that CAS is more common among boys than girls, although estimates of the relative frequency vary.

Margaret Fish, MS, CCC-SLP, with over thirty-five years' experience in treating children with a variety of speech and language impairments, specializes in working with children with severe speech sound disorders, including CAS. She indicates that approximately 50–60 percent of the children on her caseload have a diagnosis of CAS or suspected CAS. Because of Ms. Fish's particular interest and expertise in working with children with apraxia, she treats more children with the diagnosis than speech-language pathologists with other specialties.

Tip: As a parent of a child with CAS, I was often asked by interested and well-meaning friends and family: ***"How many kids have apraxia?"***

And my answer was complicated. My initial thoughts were: A lot . . . some . . . it's rare. Almost all of those answers are correct. Let me explain:

- It may seem like a lot of children have CAS because as a parent you deal with the symptoms and logistics (going to speech therapy, home practice) of CAS every day. You likely will meet others who deal with it too (other parents, CCC-SLPs, teachers, to name a few). But when you first heard of CAS, you thought that maybe it was pretty rare. After all, you had never heard of CAS before.

- Once you started hearing more about it, you discovered it wasn't nearly as rare as you thought, but it's also not very common.

What Does CAS Mean for Your Child's Future?

I wish I could take away all of the confusion you feel right now. I wish I could ease your fears. *If I could, believe me, I would.*

There is a light at the end of the tunnel. **Children with CAS do make progress; they do get better.** But it takes hard work on everyone's part. Every child with CAS will have different symptoms and her own pattern of strengths and challenges.

> **Parents Share**
>
> *Improvements Over Time*
>
> You are probably wondering how other parents responded—and got through—the early years of CAS. You'll hear from three parents here.
>
> Ally's mom, Susan, says: "Her progress, when it started, was very fast and furious. She wanted to talk with an intensity that also took my breath away. Ally was diagnosed at 2 years, 10 months, and her speech was age appropriate by age 5. Her speech at age 7 is perfect, only breaking down slightly when she is very tired."
>
> Tanner's mom, Brandy, shares this: "It's a scary thing when your child isn't speaking [like other children his or her age]. But have faith. Our son Tanner has progressed so much over the last four years. At seven, he is—for the most part—understood by all of his friends and teachers."
>
> Diane relates these feelings regarding her son William's experience with CAS: "As a parent, I asked myself how I was going to protect [my son], how could I make him speak better? My son worked extremely hard [in speech therapy], and I am happy to report that William was dismissed from speech therapy last year. The path has been bumpy at times, but we are making our way and are beginning to see the light."

Keep in mind that CAS is a dynamic, ever-changing speech disorder. There are a lot of factors that go into making a prognosis: age at diagnosis, type and amount of therapy, at-home practice, involvement of family, school involvement, child's temperament and personality, your child's motivation, and any co-occurring condition (another diagnosis—perhaps a medical one—that may affect her progress).

So, with that in mind, ***most children with "just" CAS will make wonderful progress in being able to express themselves verbally.*** Treatment must be provided by a CCC-SLP with a background in treating and assessing CAS. That treatment must be intense and frequent, and the child needs routine home support and speech practice.

Your child with CAS won't simply "grow out of it," as some may suggest. When a child is correctly diagnosed with the condition, CAS *tendencies* typically remain throughout her life (this *does not* mean that the individual won't be able to talk). These tendencies may or may not be apparent to the waitress at the restaurant, but your child (and her close friends, her family, or a speech-language pathologist) may notice she avoids multisyllabic words or transposes words/sounds when she is especially tired or stressed.

Despite these continuing tendencies, most children who have pure CAS when young have as much chance as any other child of growing up to lead happy, successful adult lives. If a child is given proper support and treatment, CAS will likely not affect her ability to succeed in school, to pursue her interests, and to excel in music, sports, academics, or wherever her talents lie. As adults, people with CAS may choose careers in which they don't have to do much public speaking, but other than that, the sky's the limit!

The prognosis for developing effective speech when a child has CAS along with another condition such as autism or Down syndrome is not as clear cut. Whether your child will be speaking effectively depends on the child as well as the specific characteristics of her other special need(s). Your child may need to use some kind of low-tech or high-tech communication system (sign language, electronic devices, communication books, etc.) to help get her message across. But with the right kind of therapy and support, she can definitely make progress in understanding and using speech and language. See chapter 15 for more details on prognosis.

Whether you have a sneaking suspicion your child has CAS, or you know for a fact that she does, you are in good hands. This book will give you the inside scoop on everything from how to find the right help to how to navigate the school system and cope with your feelings. Childhood apraxia of speech is quite treatable if you start the journey early and stay the course.

Say That Again?! Chapter Summary

We started with a basic definition of CAS, or so it seemed. But once we got into the nitty-gritty, we learned there really is more to the disorder than meets the eye. Even SLPs grapple with the terminology and diagnostic characteristics. Warning signs for parents to keep track of were outlined, as well as discussions on prevalence, intelligence, your child's future, and co-occurring conditions.

Recommended Resources

Please take a look at the **American Speech-Language-Hearing Association's (ASHA)** webpage: www.asha.org. You can access a copy of the 2007 Technical Position Paper on CAS here: https://www.asha.org/policy/ TR2007–00278/. It might prove helpful when considering an IEP for your child (more on that in chapter 11).

Apraxia Kids™ is the largest nonprofit US organization on CAS. You'll find it's a fabulous online resource for parents and professionals and is brimming with information. Here, you can join a state-specific Facebook group, watch a webinar, locate an SLP, participate in a walk for awareness, and more. www.apraxia-kids.org.

The Hanen Centre is recognized as an international leader in early language development through parent- and educator-focused programs. For more information, visit www.hanen.org or call 877–426-3655.

It Takes Two to Talk by Elaine Weitzman (of the Hanen Centre) provides timely information for connecting speech and communication with everyday activities—getting dressed, eating lunch, driving in the car. Now in its fifth edition, this color guidebook is easy to use and evidence-based and offered as book only, DVD, or combo pack. It's available in Spanish, French, German, and Danish. Available through www.hanen.org.

Stephen Camarata, PhD, was a late talker himself and so was son. He's done extensive research in the subject and is a professor at Vanderbilt University. His book, *Late-Talking Children: A Symptom or Stage* (MIT Press, 2015), helps parents understand other reasons why their child may be late to talk.

For information on speech-language concerns in general, you may appreciate *Childhood Speech, Language, and Listening Problems: What Every Parent Should Know* by Patricia McAleer Hamaguchi (John Wiley and Sons, 2010).

ChildTalk blog by Becca Jarzynski, MS, CCC-SLP, is a parent-friendly and very helpful resource if you are looking for strategies in working with your child and gaining valuable speech-language information: www.talkingkids.org.

You may also like *I Want to Be Your Friend,* an illustrated book designed for preschoolers through early-elementary-aged children about young Emma, who has CAS. Told from Emma's point of view, the story explains that while she can't communicate as well as others, she is still just a "normal kid." Written by Emma's mother, Angela Baublitz, this is a great introduction to CAS for parents and children alike. Find your copy at Apraxia Kids: www.apraxia-kids.org.

The Something to Say series (Something to Say Press, 2017) by Eden Molineux, MS, CCC-SLP, promotes self-advocacy, understanding of speech and language differences, and embracing diversity. Each book features colorful illustrations and a relatable character with a communication difference. Look for them where books are sold or https://somethingtosay.net/.

Created by Mehreen S. Kakwan, MA, CCC-SLP, *Billy Gets Talking: A Preschooler's Journey: Overcoming Childhood Apraxia of Speech* (2018) is a fabulous resource to share with preschoolers who have a CAS diagnosis. Look for it at www.MehreenKakwan.com.

Chapter 2

Speech 101

An Introduction to Speech, Language, and Listening

Imagine if you will, a little boy who has a dream, a dream to communicate. He wishes he could answer your question so that you understand his response. He wishes he could ask for clarification when he doesn't know exactly what you want him to say or do. He wishes to connect with his friends in their verbal play, or to raise his hand in eagerness to answer his teacher. Because in his mind, he knows what he wants to say, yet he just can't get it out. Imagine this little boy is yours.

Communication is part of our everyday life. It's in the news, the radio, on television. It's on the road, in the grocery store, at school, at work. It's everywhere.

When you exchange a few words with your neighbor, you don't think much about the process of talking. In fact, it doesn't seem all *that* complicated. You have a thought, you open your mouth (insert foot—sometimes), and the thought comes out in the form of words others can usually understand. This chapter is all about talking. How it happens, why it happens, and what happens when there's a glitch in the process. Since talking also requires listening, we'll talk about that, too.

One day when my daughter Kate (now a high schooler) was in preschool, I had a brief chat with my neighbor about the weather, the past weekend, and what the kids were up to. Really, the context of what we were talking about was so simple, yet so complex to articulate, at least at a neuromuscular level.

When I mentioned my daughter's difficulty with speech, I joked and said something like, "I don't understand why she has such difficulty talking and eating . . . those happen to be two of my favorite things!" My neighbor nodded and smiled sympathetically. She knew I was concerned, she knew Kate was in speech therapy, and she could relate—her own child had received speech therapy at one time too.

But really, talking *is* complicated. There is a high-order process going on, involving speech, language, listening, and comprehension. Is it all in your mind? Yes, in fact, one important language center *is* located in the front part of your brain, in an area called the premotor cortex. This region is responsible for the planning and coordination of speech. It is primarily the left side of the brain that is "in charge" of *understanding* language. The right side is best at *detecting prosodic aspects* of language—that is, the rate, rhythm, tone, and stress of the words.

The Nuts and Bolts of This Chapter

- The "basics" of speech—definitions of common terms to get the ball rolling
- Typical childhood speech development (and a few tips on what you can do to help it along), including easy access charts
- The physiology of speech, language, and listening
- A little on the stigma and myths associated with late talkers

---

Language, Communication, and Culture

How important is the need to communicate? I would venture to say that ***the ability to develop effective communication skills is a basic need, much like the need to seek food, shelter, and comfort.*** Not only are feelings, ideas, and information all conveyed through communication, but language and communication are very much a part of the culture in which one is brought up. We use communication to pass down family stories, folklore, and experiences; record our past; and plan for our future.

Language is one of the most important skills we can develop to be successful in society. But there are things that need to line up in order for humans to have a verbal communication system. The words *speech* and *language* have similar connotations, but they are quite different, as explained below.

Speech—That's the Same Thing as Language, Right?

Well, not exactly. ***Speech refers to the sounds *that come out of your mouth and take the form of words.*** To speak, many things must happen, often at the same time, at a rate of up to fourteen sounds per second! Speech requires the coordination of more than seventy muscles and body parts. Speech is one of the most sophisticated, complex, dynamic, and highly skilled human movements.

A person first has an idea and wants to communicate it to others, and then . . .
The brain

- must formulate the idea it wants to communicate in the form of words;
- needs to send that message to the mouth;
- needs to send the correct signals to the muscles that control the tongue, lips, jaw, and palate—all structures/muscles needed to coordinate and produce speech.

The muscles in the face

- must have the strength and coordination and be symmetrical to do what the brain is asking.

The respiratory system

- must be able to orchestrate airflow into and out of the lungs;
- must use the muscles of the abdomen to drive the diaphragm;
- must direct air with enough force so the vocal cords vibrate and produce voiced sounds.
- Air must be going out—not in—for speech to occur.

The auditory system

- needs to hear correctly;
- must monitor what comes out of the mouth to make sure it's being said "correctly."

The interpersonal connection

- must be made—that is, someone else must be a part of the conversation. If no one is communicating (listening and reacting) with us, what's the point in talking?

What Is Language, Then?

Language is the content *of what is spoken, written, read, or communicated through gestures.* You've heard someone say, "I don't like your language." And that usually means "I don't like the words you're using." But language can also be in the form of body language or sign language. There are a few signs and gestures that typically mean the same thing across cultures. For example, rubbing your belly after a large meal usually means you've had enough to eat, crossing your arms across your chest might indicate that you are closed off (or simply cold—look for goose bumps). Placing your hands on your hips might signify that you are angry or showing authority (sometimes both).

In a basic sense, language is divided into two categories: *receptive and expressive.*

- *Receptive language* is the process of receiving and comprehending language. It involves a significant amount of listening and observation. If someone's receptive language does not develop properly, then the entire language system sort of stalls. In other words, people must be able to understand and correctly hear the words before they can produce (express) them.
- *Expressive language* is the process of producing (expressing) words, phrases, and sentences, along with gestures, to convey a message. Sign language is considered a form of expressive language, although no actual speech is occurring.

Tip: If the receptive language system is impaired, then you will not see progress with speech or expressive language. Children won't say or use what they don't understand.

Other important categories of language that involve both expressive and receptive language abilities include:

- *Nonverbal language* is the process by which we use body movements/postures, and gestures, tone, and facial expressions to express ourselves. Research shows that approximately 93 percent of communication is nonverbal.

- *Pragmatic/social language* refers to the use of appropriate communication in social situations (knowing what to say, how to say it, and when to say it). For example, knowing to say hello and goodbye, turn-taking in conversations, knowing the difference between talking to a baby and talking with an adult, rewording when not being understood.

According to Nanette Cote, MA, CCC-SLP, owner at Naperville Therapediatrics and author of *We Talk on Water: Guide for Developing and Orchestrating Successful Group Social Communication,* "Being aware of these other types of communication is especially important when working with—and raising—children with CAS; they must find and use other means to enhance their communication to ensure their needs are met."

In order for children to understand and use *spoken (expressive) language*, a few things need to happen:

The brain

- must have the cognitive capabilities to process and understand what is being said;
- needs to have a system of storing communicated information and be able to retrieve it later;
- needs to have a method of communicating ideas to someone else.

The muscles

- must "fire" and coordinate properly—i.e., the child must have the physical ability to speak.

The auditory system

- must have ears that "work" (or the child must learn to use a visual system such as cued speech to compensate for the lack of hearing; fitted with hearing aids if necessary);
- must be able to hear differences in tone and accents, as well as detect changes in sentence structure (such as raising the pitch of one's voice at the end of a sentence when asking a question);
- must be able to distinguish words from nonspeech sounds and extraneous stimuli.

The interpersonal connection:

- must be made by parents and significant caregivers who use and model words;
- springs from a psychological and social need to communicate with others;
- must be strengthened through listeners who are interested in what the child is saying to reinforce communication.

Are You Listening to Me?

Most parents ask their kids this all the time. But really, the act of listening is a little more complicated than it may seem. Again, a series of events must occur to hear and be heard:

- Sound waves carry sound (spoken words or other noise) to our ears.
- For the sound to travel efficiently through the outer canals of the ears, there must be nothing in the way (physical abnormality or obstruction of some kind).
- Sound vibrates the eardrum, which connects to three little bones in the middle ear. (If there is fluid in the middle ear (otitis media) due to colds, infection, or allergies, the sound will be distorted or muffled at this stage. The middle ear needs to be healthy for sounds to move through clearly.)
- Sounds move from the middle ear to inner ear; the inner ear needs to be "working" and healthy too.
- The inner ear takes sounds directly to the auditory nerve and the brain.
- The brain makes sense of it all (or tries to). A message is deciphered.

Talking Is a Two-Way Street

Communication is a two-way process. It involves a speaker and a listener. Both speaker and listener have important jobs to fulfill if they are going to communicate effectively.

I am sure you have been in the position where you have "heard" someone but weren't really listening. You didn't "get" the message they were trying to convey. The speaker may have felt misunderstood or unimportant. It's frustrating, to say the least.

Think of how your child with CAS must feel. While he is trying so hard to communicate with you, you struggle to interpret his message. He gets more frustrated, and so do you. If you are frustrated, then chances are that he is *more* frustrated; after all, he doesn't have the experience and coping skills like you do to work through such frustrations.

When Kate was younger, I facilitated a support group for parents of kids with CAS called Small Talk: All About Apraxia, and asked members to share their experience with frustration. One mother commented: "I get so frustrated sometimes trying to decipher what my son is trying to tell me. I feel bad even admitting this. He will fuss, and grunt, and point. I know he's trying really hard to tell me what he wants, but I just don't get it sometimes!"

Another mom mentioned a similar scenario when her son was trying to get her attention about a Buzz Lightyear toy [*Toy Story* character] on the top shelf of a bookcase in his bedroom: "I couldn't figure out what he wanted. This went on for a long time [his grunting and pointing]; he kept saying 'oy, oy.' I had no idea. He was in tears, and I was close to them too. Finally, it dawned on me that he wanted his Buzz Lightyear toy. 'Oy, oy' meant *toy* in his language."

Sometimes, it helps to simply say: "Whatever it is you want to tell me is really important, I can tell. I am having a hard time understanding your words, can you *show* me what you want instead?"

Parents Cope

Handling Your Child's Frustration

A child's frustration can lead to negative behaviors such as aggression, anxiety, and attention problems, and he or she may even be stereotyped as "dumb." I'll touch on stereotypes and stigma later in this chapter. If you are interested in learning more about your child's coping and socialization, look at chapter 14, which discusses a child's feelings and coping skills in greater detail.

What Causes the Glitch in Childhood Apraxia of Speech?

Ah, the million-dollar question: what is the glitch that causes CAS? There are conflicting theories; no one really knows for sure. One thing is clear, however: *Parents are not the cause of their children's CAS!*

Some folks believe that kids with CAS have difficulty creating, transmitting, and storing speech movement plans. Of course, all we "see" is a child who is frustrated because he can only produce limited or unclear speech. The reasons why are discussed more fully in chapter 6.

Myths, Feelings, and Unwanted Advice about Speech Development

I am sure you have heard your fair share of speech myths and the grandmotherly neighbor's advice along these lines:

- Einstein was a late talker.
- Some very bright children won't talk because they are bored with "baby talk."
- He'll talk when he has it all perfected in his mind.
- He just doesn't have anything to say.

- You (or big sister/brother) do all of the talking for him.
- He has all of his needs met and doesn't "need" to communicate.
- He'll talk when something really interests him, or he really wants something.

These statements can be reassuring when you first notice signs that your child's speech development is lagging. And it's true—some children "just" have a delay in speech development. A *delay*, by the way, is defined as a "slowness." Delays *could* occur in *both* receptive and expressive language *at the same time*. Everything related to speech and language could be lagging behind but generally occurring together. Then suddenly your very quiet two-year-old grows into a totally chatty three-year-old. Those things happen. Other times, they don't. Children have their own unique growth patterns with growth spurts in different areas of development at different times.

It's common for parents to second-guess themselves and wonder, "Does he have a problem, or not?" You may be quizzing your own parents about when you started talking (they likely won't remember—unless there was a problem) and whether there is a history of late talkers in your family. You might even be a teensy bit defensive. When was the last time Grandma called and asked whether her little Angel Cake was "talking," only to hear you sigh "not yet?"

What If He *Is* Just a Late Talker?

According to Becca Jarzynski, MS, CCC-SLP, a pediatric speech-language pathologist in private practice and clinical instructor at the University of Wisconsin–Eau Claire, "If a child reaches twenty-four months and isn't yet using fifty words and/or isn't yet putting two words together into short phrases (e.g., "more juice," "bye mama"), we typically recommend that [parents] talk to their pediatrician about an evaluation by a speech-language pathologist." That, however, isn't the full answer. Here are some other considerations a pediatric SLP would look at when evaluating toddlers who aren't yet speaking as much as expected:

- *Did he have difficulty nursing or bottle-feeding?* What kinds of foods does he eat now? Can he drink from an open cup or use a straw?
- *What does the child understand?* Can he follow a wide variety of directions? Find objects when Mom and Dad ask him to do so? Point to pictures in a book? Show off some body parts when they are named? Follow silly directions like "put a cup on your head?"
- *How is he communicating with gestures and facial expressions?* Is he nodding and shaking his head no? Pointing at things that he wants or that interest him? Waving hi and goodbye? Clapping with delight?
- *How is he using the words he does have?* Is he using them appropriately? Does he have inflection in the right places? Can he articulate well?

- **What kinds of sounds is he using?** Does he use his voice to get attention? Does he vocalize often throughout the day? Did he babble often as a baby? Does he use his voice in a way that sounds like he's having a conversation, even if there are no real words involved in that conversation? (At twenty-four months, for example, a child should be using a variety of sounds such as *p, b, m, n, t, d, h,* and *w*—and using them in a variety of words).

- **How is he playing?** Does he use pretend play in some very simple ways? For example, does he give a bottle to a baby or feed a stuffed bear with a spoon? Is he able to play simple rolling or fetching ball games with others and starting to imitate housework?

- **How does he imitate actions?** Will he clap when an adult does? Does he imitate stacking blocks? Will he imitate you if you do something silly and unexpected, like place a block on top of your head?

- **How is he hearing?** Is there any history of ear infections? Has an audiologist formally assessed his hearing in a soundproof setting?

Tip: Speech-language pathologist Nanette Cote says, "You would be amazed by what children pick up on visually to follow directions. Hearing may be affected by fluid with or without infections, making it hard to imitate sounds. Children can still follow through on directions or respond to a noise from another room simply because they have picked up on visual cues."

What if the child was doing everything in the list above but still wasn't talking as much as we'd expect? "Then he'd be what we call a 'late talker,'" says Becca Jarzynski. As she explains, "The benefit of getting an evaluation for a 'late talker' is that parents have a professional speech-language therapist looking specifically at all those areas and helping them to figure out what's really going on. If nothing else, this can ease a parent's mind. The SLP can also give parents some simple suggestions that can be woven into their day to increase the odds that their child will start using more words. A really good speech-language pathologist will shed light on what comes next in child development and help parents figure out how they can get their child to that next level."

Ms. Jarzynski continues, "Opinions are mixed about whether or not speech therapy is truly needed for children who are just late talkers. Some studies seem to indicate that as long as late talkers are in supportive, nurturing, and responsive families, they will catch up on their own. Other studies suggest that late talkers can potentially have lingering difficulty with reading and spelling when they enter elementary school."

"He Don't Talk Right": Dealing with Stigma

We seem to attach a stigma to folks who are quiet, reserved, or nonverbal. You think this person is dumb, stuck-up, brainy, unfriendly, a Goody Two-Shoes, an observer, shy, reclusive, reticent, introverted, indifferent, ambivalent, aloof, upset, bored/boring—you get the idea. Most of these descriptors have a negative vibe to them. Who really wants to be known as the "Unfriendly, indifferent, brainy recluse?" Um, that's right—no one.

What's a Parent to Do?

If you are dealing with some less-than-supportive folks when it comes to your child's speech concerns, you'll want to respond to them as diplomatically as possible. Try some of these "nip-it-in-the-bud" statements:

- "He's just slow to warm up."
- "We all develop at different rates."
- "Quiet and cautious, and I couldn't be more grateful."
- "He's more of an observer, like his dad/mom/you."
- "I'm glad you mentioned that. I have been meaning to ask you about it." (This works especially well if the person has a background in child development or speech-language pathology. It can also provide a great opening for digging deep into familial connections.)
- "Gosh, I don't know. What would you recommend?"
- "I appreciate your concern. Thank you."

How Communication Skills Typically Develop

As we covered in earlier sections, humans need both receptive language (the ability to comprehend what others are telling us) and expressive language (the ability to use speech or another system to transmit our messages to others) in order to communicate. The development of both receptive and expressive language is quite complex. It's easy for something to go awry in the development of either. Everything must fall "magically" into place. Let's take a quick look at the processes involved for a child to develop speech and language.

The Development of Speech (Expressive Language)

The ability to talk is developed in a gradual way. Consider this formula:

***mental growth + neuromuscular maturation
+ imitation of speech sounds = speech [talking]***

Many children are at different stages of this process, which is especially true for children with CAS. Some may move quickly through the speech development stages; others may linger or get stuck in one or more stages. Child development is an individual process. The sections below explore what is involved in each of these elements of the speech equation.

Element #1 in the Speech Equation: Mental Growth

We humans are pretty darn amazing. It is mostly because of our brain's left cortex that we are able to communicate using a complex system of words. Language itself has its own neuronal apparatus, like a computer, that evolution has inserted directly into the human brain. But it's grammar that really sets language apart from other forms of communication.

When I mention grammar, I am not referring to those boring rules you learned in middle school. Instead, you can think of grammar in this case as syntax, or the ability to arrange words and phrases into sentences that make sense in a particular situation.

Most of our speech and language abilities are housed in the left hemisphere of the brain. This is true for the majority of people, but like everything, there are always exceptions to the rule.

The left hemisphere of the human brain sorts out the sounds of the environment (the vacuum cleaner, dishwasher, and birds chirping), from the human speech noises. (Typically, the left hemisphere knows how to do this from birth.)

Wernicke's area is in charge of understanding the meaning of words and remembering and applying the rules of grammar. It is the part of the brain that is necessary for speech *comprehension.* Wernicke's area is located in the temporal lobe of the brain. Wernicke's area is where the signal is fine-tuned.

Broca's area is in charge of *speech production and the fluency of speech.* This area, located in the left frontal lobe of the brain, is anatomically a long distance from Wernicke's area, relatively speaking.

Fluid, easy communication depends on these two areas working together without much effort. For that to happen, your child needs to develop strong neural connections (pathways) between the areas. It is through listening and communication experiences that children develop strong connections between Wernicke's and Broca's areas, just as they might strengthen their biceps by lifting dumbbells.

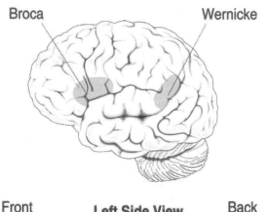

Image retrieved from the National Institute on Deafness and Other Communication Disorders

Element #2 in the Speech Equation: Neuromuscular Maturation

Learning to speak clearly and correctly is complicated. First of all, you have to have an idea you want to communicate. Then the muscles in your face, mouth, tongue, soft palate, and respiratory system must work together. You need developed pathways in your brain to "communicate" with those muscles. You also must have the right timing and coordination (which is part of motor planning) in order for your brain to orchestrate this event. All of these changes involve **neuromuscular maturation.** That is, the brain and nerves must develop in tandem with the muscles required for speech development.

To help you understand the complexity of the neuromuscular development needed for speech, consider these facts:

- **Speaking requires about 5,000 neuromuscular events per second.** These events must be coordinated in time and space to produce fluent speech.

- **There are only a few nonspeech movements that are faster than speech.** For example, your eyes move faster than you can talk. Both eye movement and speech are forms of what is called "fine motor function."

Element #3 in the Speech Equation: Imitation of Speech Sounds

You might think that developing speech is instinctive, but it's not. Without models to listen to and imitate, a baby would not learn to produce words on his own.

Kids learn to do a lot by imitation. They watch and listen and see how you do things (also known as "modeling"). For example, they watch you walk all day—to their bed, to the refrigerator, out the door. And since they are watching you do this, they naturally want to do the same thing. But there are steps (so to speak!) before that can happen, especially when you are a fifteen-pound baby lying on a quilt, happily mouthing toys. You will need to learn to roll over, sit up, crawl, pull to stand, stand alone, and then coordinate the movements to alternately move the right foot, then the left foot, and so on. It's challenging work to control all of those muscles in the feet and legs.

Of course, walking and talking are not the same, but the *idea* is the same. Talking requires a sequence of events to take place, just as walking does. To illustrate the role that imitation plays in learning to speak, let's look at how babbling typically develops.

Babies around the world—from vastly different cultures, languages, and dialects—babble similar sounds—and all right around the same age. Babies everywhere produce vowels before consonants and are sensitive to sound and tone differences. (However, the latest research suggests that there may be more differences between cultures and languages than we once thought.)

Babies begin to babble at around three to four months of age. Babies raised in English-speaking households babble in English sounds. Meanwhile, Japanese-reared babies are babbling in Japanese, and bambinos in Italy are beginning to mimic the sounds of the Italian language—all because they are imitating the speech sounds they hear in their daily lives.

For a child to be able to imitate speech sounds, the following must occur:

- He must develop the neuromuscular abilities to physically move the muscles in the precise and coordinated way needed to produce speech sounds, and also to get the message from the brain to the muscles involved.

- He needs to be able to hear well and accurately (without distortion from middle ear fluid or anything interrupting the passage and interpretation of sound from the ear to the auditory cortex in the brain). *If you are concerned about your child's hearing, have an audiologist evaluate him.*

- He must have the capability and motivation to imitate others (which can be delayed or lacking in some conditions such as autism).

  For more information on imitation, see chapter 7 on speech therapy strategies.

> **Slow and Steady**
>
> Remember, learning to communicate is a gradual process. It requires general intelligence and mental development to identify ("Yes, I know what a ball is"), associate ("Oh, the words *ball* and *roll* are related?"), remember ("Yesterday we played with the ball. I threw the ball. Yay!"), and finally, reproduce ("Ball?").

Say That Again?! Chapter Summary

This chapter was designed to be an introduction to speech, language, and listening, but all in all, it was a bit complex, wasn't it? It gets easier, I promise. This chapter provided a background on receptive and expressive language, the brain anatomy, and physiology for speech and language, and also provided some ideas to gauge your child's speech and listening development. We touched briefly on myths, stigma, and naysayers, including some tips for how to cope.

Recommended Resources

- *Let's Get Talking: A Speech-Language Therapy Companion for a Child's First Functional Words* (2019) by Mehreen S. Kakwan, MA, CCC-SLP. This colorful guide is intended for parents of children diagnosed with an expressive language delay or disorder and CAS with an emphasis on functional words (e.g., *hi*, *no*, *stop*, *help*). This title focuses on carry-over skills from speech clinic to home and includes elements of the evidence-based method of DTTC (see later chapters). Includes cut-out flashcards for on-the-go practice.

- *Nobody Ever Told Me (or My Mother) That: Everything from Bottles and Breathing and Healthy Speech Development* by Diane Bahr, an SLP with over thirty years' experience (Sensory World, 2010). This book is designed primarily for parents of typically developing kids to help keep them on track in feeding, speech, and mouth development. It gives great tips so parents can make feeding, early sound play, and the journey to better speech easier.

- Laura E. Berk, now retired, was a distinguished professor of psychology at Illinois State University, where she taught child development for many years. Her book, *Awakening Children's Minds: How Parents and Teachers Can Make a Difference* (Oxford University Press, 2004), was one of my favorites. It covers why and how children talk to themselves, classroom learning, and helping children with deficits and disabilities.

- *Thirty Million Words: Building a Child's Brain* by Dana Suskind (Dutton, 2015) demonstrates how critical early exposure to words are for children. Her tips are simple but empowering for any parent, caregiver, or teacher to implement.

- Debbie Feit's book *The Parent's Guide to Speech and Language Problems* (McGraw-Hill, 2007) is another one of my favorites. It offers real-world advice from a mom who has been there, as well as charts, tips, and advice from parents on met or missed speech milestones.

- Ayelet Marinovich, MS, CCC-SLP, distills research-based developmental information and offers simple activities to play with your baby on a week-by-week basis, guiding you through the first year of life in *Understanding Your Baby*. I love the sections on cognitive, communicative, motor/sensory, and social/emotional development as well as Ayelet's simple, no-nonsense approach to repurposing everyday objects to create play materials. There's a follow-up version, too: *Understanding Your Toddler*. Look for them at https://learnwithless.com/.

- *Baby Meets World: Suck, Smile, Touch, Toddle* (St. Martin's Griffin, 2014). Author Nicolas Day infuses these otherwise mundane infant activities with fascinating strokes of color. A mosaic of personal reflection, scientific investigation, and cross-cultural examination, plus early displays of emotion, bonding, more, all from the perspective of the baby.

- *The American Speech-Language-Hearing Association* is *the* professional organization for speech-language pathologists and audiologists in the United States. Their website offers many valuable resources for parents as well: www.asha.org.

- You may also appreciate *Speech-Language Resources for Education Professionals,* a UK online resource all about speech and language. You may find the sections on play, communication, and anatomy particularly helpful: http://www.speechlanguage-resources.com.

Chapter 3

When You Suspect Childhood Apraxia of Speech

Where to Go and What to Ask

As first-time parents, we didn't want to appear "delinquent," so when Kate was fifteen months old, *exactly*, we headed to the doctor (the same one who delivered her) for her scheduled well-child checkup. I say "we" because *both* doting parents were off work for the occasion. We came armed with our wiggly daughter, along with thoughts, questions, and toddler antics to relate to our doctor.

The Nuts and Bolts of This Chapter

- Determining the "right age" to get help for your child
- The different modes of receiving a diagnosis of CAS—from your pediatrician or your SLP—as well as a review of some of the specialists in the medical, psychological, and educational settings
- What early intervention is and is not, how to get involved, and what to expect
- How and where to look for an SLP, the qualities you'll want to seek, and the questions to ask a potential treating clinician

---

Here's Our Story

Kate was meeting all of her developmental milestones right on target. Except one: talking. She had only one word, *hi*. I was excited that she had such a friendly and outgoing first word and proud that it was the one I had predicted she'd say first. When I told others my prediction, they would all say, "You might be right—she really likes people." It seemed I had a natural extrovert (how did that happen with two self-proclaimed introvert parents?). She was smiling and saying "hi" to strangers in the grocery store, on the playground, at the library.

In the exam room, Dr. Baumgartner asked a series of questions. Is Kate doing this, doing that? Yes, yes, and yes, we nodded and smiled proudly. "Is she saying 'mama' and 'dada' and a few other words?" Nope. We held our breath, awaiting her response.

Sure, I was slightly concerned. I had friends from childbirth class whose toddlers were jabbering up a storm. As a first timer, however, I didn't want to jump the gun. Kate *was* only fifteen months old, after all. She still wore diapers, took a pacifier when distressed, and was rocked to sleep. In many ways she was still a baby, and babies don't talk, do they? Plus, I *knew* kids—through my years as a babysitter and as a child psych nurse.

We told our doctor that all Kate was saying was "hi" and that she started saying that around thirteen months. Wasn't that good enough? Our caring doctor probed a little further and eventually referred us to a local speech-language pathologist (SLP). "You can do it now, if you want to be aggressive, or wait until she is eighteen months, if you want to take a conservative approach."

I took the conservative approach. I finally made the call at eighteen months. Kate still wasn't saying "momma" and I wanted to hear my little girl call my name, instead of grunting when she needed me.

I'll admit I was skeptical of the capabilities of a speech-language pathologist at first. What could she possibly do to get my kid to talk that I couldn't? But we stayed the course—taking Kate to speech therapy weekly after the SLP determined there was a "delay."

We'll talk more about what therapy consists of in the next chapter, but in this one, you will get a good overview of how to go about getting the help you want and need. There are lots of different routes to reach the same destination: diagnosis and treatment.

Introvert versus Extrovert

Generally speaking, an introvert is someone who is more reserved and receives her energy from within. An extrovert can be described as someone who is outgoing and gets her energy from being around other people. It has little to do with speech disabilities or disorders but is more of an inborn personality trait. Says one mother of a son with CAS:

"It is soooo interesting that kids with CAS tend to be extroverted by nature! Mark always is quiet when meeting new people; he watches and waits . . . and he slips in the odd witty comment to show his nature. Then once he is confident others have accepted him, he gets more chatty. He has a fabulous vocabulary, as he is a 'reader' and this also promotes his wit to others."

"Wait a Minute—That Seemed Way Too Easy!"

I'll admit, our example does make it seem easy: you show up at a well-child appointment, and your doctor detects a delay and sends you to the right professional. You have great insurance, and there is a speech clinic down the street with no wait list. Voilà—you're in, problem solved. I am not sure if there is a "typical" sequence of events that occurs. From others I have talked with along this journey, however, I have learned that it usually takes longer to figure out what is going on. Many families seem to have a journey to diagnosis similar to this one:

> "We worried and wondered what was going on with our daughter for years. Her pediatrician thought maybe autism. She had an evaluation and it wasn't autism. My parents told me not to worry—kids talk when they want to; you can't force it. My neighbor thought it may be auditory processing disorder like her son had. The preschool was suggesting a learning disorder. I didn't know what to believe. Finally, an SLP started to rule out apraxia [CAS]. We finally received a diagnosis at 4 years and 2 months."
>
> —Small Talk: All About Apraxia Participant

Whatever your story, if you are concerned about your child's speech and language development, it is never too late to pursue a diagnosis. And whether or not you have good healthcare insurance, you're in luck: every state has some kind of early intervention (EI) program that will provide an evaluation if your child's speech concern is great enough. We'll touch more on EI later in the chapter.

The "Right Age" to Seek Help

Appendix D at the back of this book presents some typical developmental charts on childhood speech and language development. Look at the charts and highlight or mark the milestones you are concerned about. Now look over your list of concerns and determine just how concerning you think they are.

If you want a number here—an age—you aren't going to get one. Here's why: kids are developmentally unique; no one child will develop at exactly the same speed. I know that's frustrating to hear. If you are concerned that your child might have CAS, then I would aim for getting her an initial assessment at two years and three months (twenty-seven months). Okay, I fibbed. There's your number. Most SLPs won't give you a diagnosis for CAS until your child is closer to three years old. My daughter Kate was diagnosed at two years, six months, which was considered on the early side. It took just over a year to get a diagnosis for Kate after I first took her to an SLP. She had some very classic symptoms of CAS (more on that in the next chapter).

Here's something else to keep in mind: if you are concerned that a *younger* sibling may have CAS (your older one has already been diagnosed), then get an evaluation even earlier. CAS tends to run in families, so if one sibling has it and another is exhibiting similar features, then by all means, don't hesitate! (The same advice goes for anyone in the family whom you *suspect* has—or had—a speech-language issue, even if it wasn't formally diagnosed. More on that in chapter 5.)

Case in point: Kate's little sister, Kelly, wasn't saying much at her twelve-month checkup. By fifteen months, she only had three words. She was assessed by Kate's SLP, who found "characteristics consistent with CAS." At eighteen months of age, Kelly started therapy. By the time she was twenty-seven months, little Kelly no longer showed any symptoms of a motor-speech disorder. She was dismissed from speech therapy. Of course, we were thrilled. Meanwhile, Kate—who was older and perhaps had a more severe form of CAS—continued with speech therapy, much to her dismay. Try explaining *that* to a type A oldest sibling!

Why Not Wait Until School Starts?

If you wait until your child starts kindergarten to investigate the possibility of CAS, that is probably too long. Your child will likely be at a distinct disadvantage for academics and participating in classroom activities. ***Do not put off pursuing a diagnosis if you are concerned about CAS!***

Here are some reasons to convince you to get early and aggressive treatment:

- School at this age is all about the group setting. Kids are expected to sit still, listen, have a good memory for spoken language and a decent attention span, and be able to articulate their basic needs, such as "May I use the bathroom?"

- Kindergartners learn to sound out sounds, associate sounds with letters, and understand that sounds make up words. In "fancy" talk, this is called phonological awareness. Chapter 12 is devoted completely to phonological awareness and CAS.

- Another skill that emerges in kindergarten is the ability to tell and retell stories. Sequencing becomes a big theme in the classroom. Your child will need to describe *in words* what comes first, middle, and last in a story.

- Finally, for a child to explain something as simple as what she brought in for show and tell, she needs the ability to put words together and communicate them intelligibly to others.

I remember our goal for Kate was to have her ready for kindergarten. We wanted her to be on par with her peers by then, in hopes that no one would ever know she had CAS. And Kate attended full-day kindergarten in a neurotypical classroom setting and did fantastic verbally.

But I need to throw in this monkey wrench: ***getting help before kindergarten does not guarantee a trouble-free school experience.*** Kids with CAS often have other academic concerns that could pop up in later school years (difficulties with reading, sequencing, executive functioning, even math and science). Chapters 11 and 12 discuss these concerns step by step. However, the earlier you start getting your child the appropriate help for CAS, the sooner you will see positive results.

Doctors and Specialists

Let's jump right in with descriptions of those professionals who could point you in the right direction when you are seeking a diagnosis.

Pediatrician/Family Practice Physician (MD)

Just as in our situation, your child's treating physician could detect a concern and give you a referral to an SLP (more on this later). If you do get a referral, call the member services number on your insurance card to verify coverage and amount of benefit. Your child's doctor won't and can't treat CAS; that's the role of a speech-language pathologist. If there are other concerns, your doctor may give you a referral to a pediatric neurologist (see below)

If your pediatrician doesn't think there's anything to be concerned about, follow your gut instinct. Please, be an advocate for yourself and your child. You can always ask your pediatrician for a second opinion or a recommendation to see a specialist. Try saying it this way, "I know you treat many children and you'd tell me if there was a problem. But I am still feeling uneasy about my child's speech development. Do you know of another physician, speech-language pathologist, or organization who may be able to give me another opinion?"

> **Parents Share**
>
> **Pediatricians**
>
> We saw a wonderful pediatrician who agreed with almost everything I said, was impressed with the research articles I brought along, and told me that I was doing a great job being a parent. You don't get that every day.

Pediatric Neurologist (MD)

A medical doctor by education, a pediatric neurologist typically spends two additional years gaining general experience treating children and then three *more* years training in child neurology. That's nine years of post-college specialization.

Pediatric neurologists can rule out other causes of speech delay through medical exams such as CT scans, EMGs (electromyography—determines muscle disease), and EEGs. Take your child to a pediatric neurologist if she has a serious neurological history such as seizures, hydrocephalus (unusual amount of fluid in the ventricles of the brain), or progressive muscle weakness.

On occasion, a neurologist will suggest brain-imaging studies such as an MRI. This test is typically done for children who have "focal" neurologic findings (like weakness on just one side of the body, loss of coordination, and speech/language difficulties among others).

An EEG (electroencephalography) may be ordered if your child has a history of seizures, episodes of "zoning out," autistic-like symptoms, or a regression in language skills. An EEG measures the tiny electrical currents generated by brain activity. It's possible to analyze these findings to determine which is responsible for certain cognitive tasks—like talking and understanding speech.

All of these scans are painless but can be anxiety producing. But it's not all about imaging scans. There are some laboratory tests than can rule out metabolic diseases that can occur in children with a speech delay or hypotonia. Tests may include the following:

- ■ *Chromosome analysis for fragile X syndrome,* which is an inherited disorder seen almost exclusively in boys. It generally causes intellectual disabilities and sometimes autistic features, as well as speech and language delays and differences. Women and girls who are "carriers" and don't have the disorder themselves can also have some speech differences.

- ■ *CPK,* which is a muscle enzyme that is increased in instances of muscular dystrophy. If muscles aren't firing correctly, it can be difficult to produce intelligible speech.

- ■ *Lead screening,* which will likely be done to determine if increased blood lead levels have resulted in behaviors that look like autism or developmental (speech) delays.

Parents Share

Neurologists

One mother of a daughter with CAS shares her experience with a pediatric neurologist:

"I was so disappointed in my appointment with the [pediatric] neurologist. I had this appointment on the calendar for four months. I wanted to have my daughter evaluated. We went right after the holidays. I was frazzled. All [the doctor] did was confirm that my daughter had CAS. I was hoping for more, especially after that long wait."

Not all experiences with a pediatric neurologist end like this. Like everything, there are some experiences that are better than others:

"We had a great experience with a pediatric neurologist. We took our son because we wanted to have another look [at his CAS]. Owen responded well to the doctor's bedside manner, and we left the appointment feeling hopeful. He told us, 'A child that has no other delays outside of CAS and is able to comprehend what others are communicating has a high probability of developing normal speech communication.'"

Developmental Pediatrician (MD)

A pediatrician who has completed four years of medical school, two years in a pediatric residency program, and then an additional year in developmental-behavioral postgraduate training is a developmental pediatrician. A children's hospital in your area should be able to help you find a developmental pediatrician. They are known best for looking at the "whole" child within the context of the family. They can provide guidance on development, behavior, eating, and sleeping. These professionals are able to diagnose ADHD and learning disabilities and may be able to advocate for your child at the school level. Of course, it goes without saying that you should consult one who has interest and experience in childhood speech issues.

Some SLPs believe that developmental pediatricians and pediatric neurologists give the diagnosis of CAS when the child is making no attempt to talk whatsoever. Not attempting to talk is *not* a criterion for the diagnosis of CAS. *Typically, kids with CAS want to communicate and try to do so.* Please keep in mind that while some developmental pediatricians are well-versed in childhood speech-language problems, the diagnosis of CAS is in the scope of practicing SLPs. *Always have a diagnosis confirmed by a speech-language pathologist.*

Pediatric Physiatrist (MD)

Not a psychiatrist, but a *physiatrist* . . . a *what*?! This doctor is usually board certified in pediatrics and physical medicine and rehabilitation (physiatry). These docs work closely with occupational therapists, physical therapists, and speech-language therapists. Because a good number of pediatric physiatrists specialize in motor disabilities such as CAS and feeding issues, you may find some treatment options here. Look for a qualified professional through a rehab facility or a major university hospital.

Neuropsychologist (PhD, PsyD)

A psychologist who has received further training in brain-behavior relationships is a neuropsychologist. These professionals typically have an intense background in psychology and neurology. "Brain-behavior relationships" is simply how the brain and body connect, such as when learning and forming memories, and not "bad behavior."

A neuropsychologist is helpful if you want to determine your child's areas of weakness as well as strengths. He or she can provide a detailed profile of brain functioning related to language, spatial skills, memory, attention, executive functioning skills (organization), and problem solving, to name a few. This might help in terms of determining your child's best ways of learning in a school setting. For example, assessments may be able to determine if your child learns best by seeing, hearing, doing, or reading.

Interestingly, learning and behavior styles of children can affect kids' academic achievement, behavior, and social adjustment. The assessment and evaluation provided by a neuropsychologist is typically more in-depth than that of an educational psychologist.

Why it's important if your child has CAS: Often kids with CAS have difficulty with academic achievement, attention, and organizational skills. A neuropsychologist can provide information to help optimize these day-to-day functions at home and school. See chapter 10 for more discussion on how a neuropsychologist can be beneficial.

We took Kate to a neuropsychologist when she was exhibiting more and more symptoms of what looked like ADHD in addition to her already confirmed CAS diagnosis. The doctor was fantastic with Kate! When the comprehensive testing period was all over (a total of six hours over three weeks), our neuropsychologist sat down with my husband and me for a full hour and reviewed her findings and recommendations. She provided a wonderful written report for us to pass along to the school to help Kate focus and also supported us through the diagnosis. Now fourteen and doing remarkably well, Kate was prescribed medication for her ADHD at seven years. Results were immediate. She was better able to attend to her surroundings and didn't move as frenetically; everyone experienced a new kind of calm. Plus, I think her speech and language also improved.

Educational Psychologist or "School Psychologist" (MEd, PhD, PsyD)

These professionals focus mainly on how students learn in educational settings. They study student attributes, instructional processes directly related to the classroom, how effective that education is, and the psychology of teaching. They might act as a consultant to a teacher who is directly responsible for your child's education. Further, educational psychologists commonly administer IQ tests, as well as achievement tests and can diagnose ADHD, executive function problems, and learning disabilities, as well as autism. They can figure out whether a child's academic struggles are due to a disability, and whether difficulties communicating are due to cognitive problems. You may encounter this professional when your child is being evaluated for EI or special education.

An educational psychologist may also be referred to as a school psychologist and employed by your school system. Although some psychologists employed by schools have master's degrees, if you are hiring someone to do a private evaluation of your child, you will probably want to look for someone with a PhD and experience working with students with speech-language disorders. They can choose different tests (that require little or no verbal response) for your child if she can't answer the questions verbally.

Another caveat: if you suspect a problem, consider getting an "outside" or third-party evaluation rather than one within the school system. This way, your school—and you—can be objective about the results. Same thing goes if the school does testing on your child; you would be a good consumer if you got a second opinion. Keep in mind, however, that schools often like to do their own evaluations, as they often have different standards than private practice clinicians.

Child Psychologist (PhD, PsyD)

A child psychologist can help you and your child cope with the diagnosis, as well as work with her on social issues, frustration, impulsiveness, anxiety, and aggression—all of which may be related to CAS. He or she may or may not also do testing for cognitive and behavioral disorders such as ADHD, learning disabilities, autism, or mood disorders. However, a psychologist cannot diagnosis a child with CAS.

Child and Adolescent Psychiatrist (MD)

A psychiatrist is a medical doctor who has received specialized training in child/adolescent development, behavior, and mental health. He or she can be a great resource if your child has a co-occurring behavioral or mental health concern such as ADHD, an anxiety disorder, or obsessive-compulsive disorder (OCD), among others. Unlike a psychologist, a child/adolescent psychiatrist can prescribe medications to treat certain conditions. As far as *diagnosing* CAS, child/adolescent psychiatrists aren't the "go-to" professionals. They may, however, understand what it is and be able to help you understand how to cope with it.

Speech-Language Pathology

The "gold standard" to getting your child diagnosed and treated for CAS is an evaluation by a speech-language pathologist (SLP), according to the 2007 Position Statement from the American Speech-Language-Hearing Association (ASHA). Please keep in mind that if you live outside of the United States, your therapist may have a different professional title than SLP. This section will help you understand the process of referrals and selecting a SLP and will give you some encouragement on taking that first leap to your first appointment.

Getting to a Speech-Language Pathologist (SLP)

If you are lucky enough to have a doctor who catches a concern on a well-child visit, consider yourself blessed. If not, you may contact your doctor's office and explain that you are interested in having your doctor make a referral to a SLP because your little pumpkin isn't progressing like you think she should. If your doctor knows and remembers you and your child well, he or she might just go ahead and make that referral without troubling you to come in for an office visit. Most likely, though, you will have to make an appointment.

The appointment will probably go something like this: The doctor will look at your child and say, "Your mom tells me that you are having trouble talking—is that right?" Your child will nod and smile and won't say anything when prompted (as most kids do when they are in a new/unfamiliar setting).

Your child's doctor will likely ask you to describe your child's *attempts at communication* (sounds and gestures commonly used). If they seem remarkable, you'll get a referral to a SLP.

But, what should you do if your doc doesn't think a referral to a SLP is in order?
Be polite but persistent. Come with some research or a list of symptoms of CAS; present them to your doctor. Remember, you know your child better than anyone else. If you feel there is something more going on, be proactive. You do not necessarily need a referral from your doctor to take your child to an SLP (unless your insurance requires it or you want to see an SLP whom your pediatrician especially trusts and respects). You can find lists of SLPs on the ASHA website: https://find.asha.org/ and can search by keyword to include your state or your child's suspected diagnosis. Worst case scenario: you go to the SLP only to hear nothing is wrong. It's better to be safe than sorry!

What *Is* a Speech-Language Pathologist (SLP), Anyway?

Simply put, the SLP is the key player in helping your child make progress with speech skills and a sounding board for you. He or she is also a professional with a master's degree (some may have a PhD) with a background in communication disorders. SLPs complete a practicum—usually a year in length—following their graduate program. SLPs are required to be licensed in the state in which they practice and must complete continuing education criteria to maintain their licensure. They are also accredited by the American-Speech-Language-Hearing Association (ASHA). They perform evaluations, deliver a diagnosis, carry out therapy, and recommend "homework" for you. They are also there to field questions and concerns and give you resources for additional information.

By the way, ***SLPs are the only professionals qualified to* treat CAS.** And while this is a subjective piece of information, you may also hear that an SLP's diagnosis of CAS is more respected than that of another professional. SLPs work hard with your child to model and support developmentally appropriate communication. It takes patience, persistence, humor, and creativity, along with organization and good interpersonal skills to be an effective child SLP .

Qualities and Qualifications to Look for in Your Child's SLP

If you are fortunate enough to be able to choose your therapist, consider yourself lucky. Not all SLPs are created equal, and you are going to want the one who meshes best with you and your family, has flexible (accommodating) hours, and is very knowledgeable about CAS. Here's a list of qualities and characteristics you'll want to look for:

- Educational background should include at least a master's degree.
- Certification by ASHA, indicated by "CCC" (Certificate of Clinical Competence) after the SLP's name is important. This shows that the SLP has met a minimum level of training and has agreed to ASHA's code of conduct and ethics and has committed to continuing education. This is similar to being a "board-certified" physician, but for speech-language pathologists.

- Years of experience is a bit of a gray zone. Some may think that the more experience, the better. But, that's not always the case. Some seasoned therapists may be set in their ways, lack excitement and passion, or be a little too "old school" for your taste. On the other hand, a new graduate may not have the necessary experience; however, new graduates have the most up-to-date information on CAS, especially in terms of newer evaluations and therapeutic approaches.

- Your therapist should like working with children. Does she have experience working with kids in your child's age group? Does she have experience with CAS? Not all therapists are trained in pediatrics.

- The therapist should have experience working with children with CAS. Ask directly, "How many children with CAS have you worked with?" The more, the better. Also, inquire about the therapist's continuing education in regards to CAS and overall level of comfort in providing treatment for children with CAS.

- Parents should be an integral part of therapy. Will you be in the room or observing from a one-way mirror or sitting in the waiting room? Therapy is most effective when parents and therapists work as a team. In the beginning, it is ideal if you are in the room. This way you can see what the SLP is doing and how your child is responding, and you will be able to ask questions. It is also helpful if your child is not used to being away from you.

- When we first started therapy, I sat in with Kate. I felt more confident and eager to replicate some of the techniques she was using in therapy. On the other hand, your child may be less likely to perform with you in the room; you might be a distraction. Your therapist may ask that you not sit in the room. If this is the case, ask if you can at least sit outside the door (leave it open slightly) and listen in.

- The SLP should provide regular updates. Ask if you will get a blow-by-blow account of the session and your child's performance. Will she do routine reevaluations? How often will you know if and when your child has reached a goal set by the therapist? Can you help to set goals? Will you get regular written reports? As Kate progressed, she happily toddled off with her SLP to do her "speech work." I sat in the waiting room. Her SLP always followed up in person at the end of their session—what they did and how Kate responded. She often gave me ideas for things to work on at home.

- Your therapist should give you "homework" and instruct you on how to do it with your child. Simply handing you a piece of paper and telling you to work on it for the next week isn't very beneficial. You'll want to reinforce whatever your child is doing with the therapist.

- You should feel accepted, valued, and respected by the SLP.

- The setting where therapy is provided may make a difference. Does the therapist work from an office or come to your home? Pros of the office: it's a new environment; work feels "important." Cons of the office: it may be too far away; may feel too clinical. Pros of at-home therapist: you and your child are comfortable in your own setting; no driving. Cons of the at-home therapist: "Too comfortable" can prevent progress (therapy no longer feels important) and can be too distracting (toys, TV, dog, siblings, phone). What do you prefer?

■ Billing and payment issues should be clearly explained. Don't be afraid to ask how much the SLP charges for therapy. How is billing done: expected at time of service, once a month, billed through insurance? How are copays handled? Some SLPs only take checks or cash. Know your financial facts before moving forward.

Tip: Parents and caregivers can help devise a functional vocabulary list for addressing speech. What words are important to your child? What are his favorite activities, games, books, foods, sibling names? For help compiling a list, consider *Let's Get Talking: A Speech-Language Therapy Companion for a Child's First Functional Words* (2019) by Mehreen S. Kakwan, MA, CCC-SLP.

A Speech-Language Pathologist's View on Selecting an SLP

"In addition to providing a warm and supportive environment for children, one of the best things that families can do for a child with CAS is to locate a therapist who understands the unique needs of children with motor-speech challenges. Request that your SLP explain the goals and methods, as well as the types of things you can do at home to support your child's communication skill development. It is encouraging as I travel around the county to meet so many SLPs who are interested in learning more about helping children on their caseloads with CAS. I am hopeful that increasing knowledge and supporting new research will serve to improve communication outcomes for children with motor speech challenges."—*Margaret (Dee) Fish, MS, CCC-SLP, author of Here's How to Treat Childhood Apraxia of Speech*

If you have choices when it comes to selecting the best speech-language pathologist for your child, don't waste any time in finding one. Be systematic and efficient, and don't be afraid to change therapists if you feel like your child isn't progressing, isn't happy, or it just isn't a good fit for your family. If you don't have choices (perhaps because you don't have insurance that will pay for speech therapy), see the section on early intervention, below. Remember, a "good" therapist is flexible (adjusts to the needs of the child), eager to learn and research better ways to help *your* child, attends continuing education events and conferences, and is able to admit that she or he "doesn't know" but is willing to help find an answer.

"Cheat Sheet" for Interviewing a Potential SLP

Consider asking the following questions:

1. Tell me about your areas of interest in the field of speech pathology.
2. What types of kids do you usually see: Their ages? Their diagnoses?
3. Have you worked with many kids with CAS?
4. What can you tell me about CAS? How is it diagnosed? How is it treated?
5. What can you tell me about your specialized skills, knowledge, and experience related to CAS?

The ASHA strongly recommends that SLPs working with children with CAS have special knowledge in CAS, motor learning theory, and differential diagnosis, and experience with a variety of intervention techniques—so a good answer to the last question will include a high number of patients with CAS and lots of continuing education classes with a strong emphasis on evidence-based research and treatment modalities, which are the only proven approaches in treating CAS.

Parents Share

Reevaluating Your Child's Progress and SLP
Amy, the mother of a daughter with CAS, says this:

"Basically, it's a constant reevaluation process. Consider asking yourself these questions, "Is the therapist a good fit for my child? Does she or he have the experience necessary to treat my child? Is my child responding and making progress? Are there other factors—financial, educational, insurance-related, family status—that require us to change SLPs?"

"[My daughter] Brooke is getting ready to switch for the fourth time total. We've jumped ship for a variety of reasons: the SLP didn't have the right experience, not a good fit for my child's personality, transitioning to an educational setting, and pending family move."

Where SLPs Work

The *best* way to find a qualified SLP is to ask for a recommendation. Talk to your friends with kids or your child's pediatrician. You'll find that SLPs work in a variety of settings. Here are other places where you may find an SLP:

- *University Clinic:* Some universities provide students with an extensive training ground and give you reduced fees in return. But the "therapist" is a student. This can be a good thing—he or she is energetic and motivated and eager to please. Most students are closely monitored by a seasoned SLP (but not always) and will almost always "rotate off" your child's case, whether or not therapy is "done."

- *Hospital Outpatient Clinic:* Hospitals that accept your insurance will submit claims on your behalf, which is like heaven to a stressed parent. If your child has additional medical needs or requires physical therapy (PT) or occupational therapy (OT), this is ideal. Hospitals have high hiring standards, so you are likely getting a really good therapist as well. However, hospitals can feel cold and clinical and have that "hospital smell." If this bothers you (or your child), this isn't the place for you.

- *Private Therapy:* If flexibility and personal service have a good ring to your ears, you may want to go this route. SLPs in private practice offer one-on-one therapy (sometimes group therapy), may have accommodating hours so you can get there after work if need be, and offer continuity through the whole year—not just the school year. You can also work directly with your therapist to determine how long and how often you should bring your child to therapy. But all of this comes at a price. Private clinics can charge $100 and up an hour. Multiply this by two or three (or five!) sessions a week, and you've got a hefty bill. Most health insurance will pay for therapy through a private clinic, but your insurance will likely cap off at some point. *How* speech-language pathologists work (provide therapy) is covered in chapter 7.

- *Early Intervention (EI):* You may have heard of **IDEA** (Individuals with Disabilities Education Act). It is a federal law in the United States that allows kids with disabilities (including speech and language impairments such as CAS) to have free special education services from birth to age twenty-one (referred to as **F**ree **A**ppropriate **P**ublic **E**ducation, FAPE). Early Intervention (EI) is designed for kids up to age three (see below).

Tip: A good place to get recommendations of SLPs is in parenting groups on Facebook and other social media. Try asking members about their experiences with local providers.

Early Intervention 101

There's a lot to know about early intervention. In fact, I could probably dedicate an entire chapter to the topic. I'll give you a brief overview of the processes involved, some first-hand experiences, and resources, if this is a route you'd like to pursue.

Your first step is to determine whether your child qualifies for early intervention. Under the law, early intervention is only available to infants and young children who are found to have delays in development or who are diagnosed with a disability that is likely to cause delays in development. (The amount of delay that qualifies a child for services varies from program to program and state to state.)

To find out whether your child qualifies, contact your local early intervention office. You can find a state-by-state guide for locating an EI office in your area on the website of the Early Childhood Technical Assistance Center (ECTA): http://

ectacenter.org/contact/ptccoord.asp. You'll be referred to an early intervention coordinator (sometimes referred to as an intake coordinator), who will coordinate the evaluation and become your contact person. All of this coordinating takes time, so try to be patient.

Resources on Early Intervention

For more information on what is involved in early intervention, consider visiting these websites, even if they are outside of your state.

- Missouri's program is called First Steps: www.mofirststeps.com/
- California has First Five: www.ccfc.ca.gov
- In Pennsylvania, it's Achieva Early Intervention: www.achieva.info/early-intervention
- The National Center for infants, toddlers, and families is called Zero to Three: www.zerotothree.org

---

The coordinator will likely come to your home at a prescheduled time. You'll get the chance to chat, and he or she will meet your child, take some notes, and leave you with a mountain of paperwork to complete.

Next, a speech-language pathologist will probably come to your home to evaluate your child. In some cases, your child might be evaluated by another professional, such as an early intervention specialist or infant educator, or you may be asked to bring your child to an office or center for an evaluation. Don't be surprised if your coordinator recommends additional evaluations from the EI staff: physical therapist (PT), occupational therapist (OT), or psychologist. You may be put on a waiting list for your child to get an evaluation. Also, be prepared for the possibility that you may initially be assigned a developmental educator if an SLP is not readily available.

Once the evaluation is complete, you will be notified as to whether your child qualifies for early intervention services. If so, the next step will generally be to meet with all of the professionals who will be on your child's early intervention "team." There you will develop something called an Individualized Family Service Plan (IFSP). The IFSP is a legal document that sets out the following:

- Your child's present level of performance (results of tests detailing her strengths and needs)
- The goals that you and your child's team want her to work toward (for a child with CAS, these may include being able to say a targeted sound/word/phrase, make approximations for commonly used words, or learn sign language until she can use speech to communicate her needs)
- Whether your child needs any assistive technology (low-tech or high-tech equipment such as a communication book, special software, or an electronic communication device)

- The services that will be provided to help your child meet her needs (such as speech therapy or OT)
- The setting where the services will be provided (in your home, at your child's day-care or nursery school, at a center)
- The amount of time anticipated for the process, including when reevaluations might occur

Be aware that the evaluating SLP may not be the *treating* SLP. After your child's evaluation is completed, it may take some time for her to be assigned to an SLP or other therapists/educators.

Other plus-sides to early intervention:

- It's free or reduced cost. This will depend on several factors: your state, your income (some states provide services on a sliding-fee scale), and how your EI office operates (some services may be offered free of charge; others may not).
- The service providers almost always come to your home or to your child's daycare or preschool, if that is more convenient for you.
- They are there to help you, the parent, understand the disorder and learn to become your child's advocate, as well as teaching you positive coping skills.
- They will become very familiar with you, your child, and your family.
- They help you navigate the transition between the early intervention program and the next steps of sending your child to preschool (around age three).

Parents Share

Experiences with Early Intervention

"We love our early intervention [SLP]! She comes to our home first thing on Wednesday mornings. I don't have to rush around getting myself and my son ready to go out—in fact, sometimes we do speech therapy in our pajamas! Marcus is happy to be in his own home where he is comfortable with the environment, and I like the fact that it's free."—*Mom to Marcus, 2.6 years with suspected CAS*

"I am nervous about when Henry turns three [and we no longer qualify for services]. I hope the therapist walks me through the next steps. We've had a hard time coordinating schedules. At first she came at 8:00. That was too early. Now she's coming at 11:30, which isn't working well either. Henry is getting hungry and cranky at that time. But, really, he has made some progress."—*Mom to Henry, 2.6 years with 1-year speech delay.*

"I got the sense that the therapist [speech pathologist] wasn't really doing any therapy with my son. She was teaching me how to do it while my son just sort of sat there. I wanted her to work directly with my son. I felt guilty when she came back next week and asked me if I did any of the things she suggested and I told her I simply hadn't had the time."—*Mother of a son with CAS who has outgrown EI*

What Are the Downsides to Early Intervention?

Programs vary by state and sometimes also by county, so look into what's available in your area. As with anything, there are downsides. Here are the few I uncovered:

▪ You have to "catch the wave" early in order to qualify for EI before your child is too old for it. Some parents (especially first-time parents) aren't sure what to look for, or they deny that their child is exhibiting any problems with speech. You could miss the boat as we did (see text box). If you find yourself in this situation, you might consider special education services instead (see chapter 11).

▪ Chances are, if school is out for summer break, your child will be out of therapy. We already know that frequent and intense therapy is crucial to success in CAS—so you'll want to find out if you can secure therapy for summers and holiday breaks, either through special allowances through the early intervention program or privately. You'll also want to take costs into consideration—expect to pay out-of-pocket or higher rates for *intensive* summer therapy or day camp style programs (but SLPs should not increase their rates for traditional therapy simply because it is summer).

▪ Another potential downside is heavy caseloads for SLPs. There is a huge demand for speech therapy in early intervention programs, which equates to decreased time and attention you may desire.

▪ Unlike with private therapy, you probably won't be able to pick your therapist. One will likely be assigned to your child.

There are many merits to an early intervention program. Don't overlook them.

Tip: To reiterate, EI follows a transdisciplinary model, meaning SLPs are considered EI providers who can implement motor, social, and language enrichment. Some families may be assigned developmental specialists rather than SLPs; you may see this as a plus or a minus. ***Families may opt to do both EI and private therapy.***

Our Experience with Early Intervention

When my family first started down this CAS path, I looked into our local EI program. We had the coordinator come to our home and I was inundated with papers and forms and acronyms—at the same time I was dealing with a clingy ten-month-old and an indifferent toddler. My head was spinning when she left. Plus, I was discouraged to hear that there was a waiting list for a SLP. Then I learned that Kate would "age out" of their services in six months—she was two and a half at the time. (Typically, when kids turn three, the school district takes over.) We went the private route instead.

Say That Again?! Chapter Summary

As parents, we are the ultimate experts on our kids. While there are lots of good specialists out there, you'll want to stick with a certified speech-language pathologist to evaluate, treat, and diagnose CAS. If you have the resources or insurance coverage to hire a private SLP, it's your job to find a qualified speech pathologist who meshes well with your child's personality.

Your therapist will likely be your hero once your child reaches some developmental verbal milestones with her help. She will become your friend, your support, and your child's cheerleader. Pick him or her wisely. And don't be afraid to switch if you are no longer feeling the vibe.

This chapter also covered the basics of early intervention programs. Please find out about the services in your county or area if this is a route you'd like to pursue.

Recommended Resources

- When *selecting a speech pathologist* to treat your child for CAS, you may want to look to the Apraxia Kids website. They have a list of qualified SLPs by region: www. apraxia-kids.org.

- Also, consider the PROMPT Institute for *trained therapists*, whose focus is on a dynamic, tactile approach to treating CAS: https://promptinstitute.com/. From there, go to "families," and then from the drop-down menu, select "Find a PROMPT SLP."

- Laura Baskall Smith, MA, CCC-SLP, is a practicing speech-language therapist in the Denver area specializing in CAS. Her book, *Overcoming Apraxia* (Bowker, 2019), may be helpful on your journey.

- *Let's Get Talking: A Speech-Language Therapy Companion for a Child's First Functional Words* (2019) by Mehreen S. Kakwan, MA, CCC-SLP. A guide intended for parents of children diagnosed with an expressive language delay or disorder and CAS with an emphasis on functional words.

- *Parents' Guide to Speech and Language Problems* (McGraw-Hill, 2007), by Debbie Feit, a journalist and mother of two children with CAS (now resolved), has done a great job of compiling information on related speech disorders in an easy-to-use guide, complete with tips for finding a speech-language pathologist.

- *Childhood Speech, Language & Listening Problems: What Every Parent Should Know* by Patricia McAleer Hamaguchi (Wiley, 2010) offers a good overview of basic questions about where to go and what to ask, understanding IEP jargon, and common speech-language problems.

- *My Brother Is Very Special* by Amy May (Trafford Publishing, 2004) is a picture book designed to help kids understand the need for speech therapy. Ms. May, a nurse and "apraxia mom," wrote the book to help her daughter understand why her little brother was going to speech therapy.

■ If you are looking for a book about the speech therapy process in general to share with your child, consider the fully illustrated *Speech Class Rules* by SLP Ronda M. Wojcicki, MS (The Speech Place Publishing, 2007).

■ *The Mouth with a Mind of Its Own* (Speaking of Speech Publishers, 2014), written by a speech-language pathologist, Patricia L. Mervine, MA, CCC, is about Matthew, whose mouth "has a mind of its own." His brain thinks one thing, but his mouth says another. He can't participate in class discussions. He can't ask the other kids to play with him at recess. He can't even say his own name. Relatable and empowering.

■ *The Early Intervention Guidebook for Families and Professionals: Partnering for Success* by Bonnie Keitty (Teachers College Press, 2014) provides a good overview of what early intervention is all about.

■ I also really like *Early Intervention Every Day: Embedding Activities in Daily Routines for Young Children and Their Families* by Merle J. Crawford and Barbara Weber. It uses everyday activities to work with your child on a variety of skills, including behavior regulation and expressive and receptive language plus gross motor, fine motor, and self-care/adaptive skills (Brooks Publishing, 2014).

■ *Working with Families of Young Children with Special Needs,* edited by R. A. McWilliam (Guilford Press, 2010), is a user-friendly guide designed for professionals, but can give parents an inside view of the early intervention model. Expert contributors, tools, and checklists included for kids ages birth to six years.

Chapter 4

Your First Appointment with a Speech-Language Pathologist

S o the day had rolled around. We were scheduled to be at the SLP's office in just fifteen minutes. I really had no idea what to expect, but I imagined it would be no big deal. As a nurse, I was used to assessing kids and being in a clinical setting. I knew that the more nervous I felt and acted, the more Kate would think this *was* a big deal. I wanted her to be relaxed and happy, like usual, so I tried very hard to be natural and at ease, but in reality, I was feeling a little unsure myself.

The Nuts and Bolts of This Chapter

- The continuation of our story of working with a speech-language pathologist (SLP) for the first time
- Everything you can expect to discuss with the SLP at the initial appointment—demographics, family history, medical concerns, prenatal and birth history, social history
- How your SLP will get to work with your child, assessing things like receptive and expressive language, pragmatics, gestures, behavior, play skills, and oral-motor and feeding skills
- Tips on how to read your child's first speech report—because these things can be pretty dense!

Our Assessment Story Continues

I gently tapped on the sliding glass partition between the waiting room and the receptionist's office, signed in, and showed her our insurance card. Meanwhile, Kate made her way to the child-sized table and chairs—and reached for a crayon. I was amazed and impressed that at only nineteen months old she was eager to create something artistic. Immediately, I engaged with her—partly because I wanted to—and partly because I wanted the SLP, or the receptionist—*anyone*—to hear that I really *was* a good mom and that yes, I *did* work with my child to help coax out the sounds and words.

It appeared as though my tactic worked, at least to some degree. I sensed the SLP "spying" on our interactions from the hallway. She invited Kate and me back to her office with a nod and smile, and I found that she was quite friendly and pretty good with kids, even though I knew she had none of her own.

Her cramped office was stuffed with books, toys, and a computer. Kate was impressed with the dry erase board and I was impressed with the vast assortment of toys. I crammed my very pregnant self into a desk chair and searched for a stool to prop up my swollen feet.

The SLP asked about Kate's developmental history—my pregnancy, her birth, medical concerns, and illnesses. I mentioned that I fell on the ice when I was about six months pregnant and required oxygen during labor, as Kate's heart rate decelerated when I pushed. Neither seemed to raise an eyebrow, although I considered both occurrences "remarkable."

The SLP leaned her body back as she searched for something on her overstuffed bookshelf. Flip charts. My heart raced a bit, because this definitely felt like Kate was being "tested."

Kate was asked to point to simple animals and objects like pig, cup, and house. She did so perfectly. I smiled, thinking, *She doesn't really have a problem, does she?*

A shiny red toy barn appeared from under the desk. Kate found the cow first, picked it up, and inspected it. She presented it to the SLP as a sort of peace offering.

"Moo," the SLP said. "The cow goes 'moo.'"

Silence from Kate.

I began to feel nervous. *Come on, kiddo, you can do it,* I cheered in my mind.

"Can you say *moo*?" she asked. Silence again. And then Kate lost interest in the cow and gravitated back to the dry erase board.

Together, Kate and the SLP tried blowing bubbles and saying *bubble* and *pop*. The big grin on her face told me that Kate enjoyed blowing bubbles, yet she didn't have a single thing to say about them! *Why not? Come on, Kate, I want you to talk.*

The SLP asked Kate to find a toy and "take it to Mommy." She did. I clapped and smiled and praised her up the wazoo.

The SLP asked, "Who's that?" and pointed to me. I so badly wanted to hear Kate call me Mommy, but nothing. I choked back tears. I didn't expect this strong sense of emotion to overcome me. I felt Baby Kelly kick from inside of me and tried to chalk it up to pregnancy hormones. But, no—these feelings were real and painful. It was as though I was "hearing" for the first time that my sweet little girl *couldn't* talk.

For the next twenty or thirty minutes, we continued with toys and prompts while the SLP crouched on hands and knees trying to elicit a sound or a word from my daughter. Kate couldn't care less, although she *was* interested in mouthing the toys and showing me what she had discovered with her customary "eh?"

I feigned interest with bright eyes while saying, "Oh! Wow. A truck." But in reality, I was tired. I was scared. I was not comfortable with my pregnant body crammed into a tiny room. And most of all, I was fearful of what the speech-language pathologist was going to tell me. I was beginning to see that Kate's language—or lack thereof—was concerning.

The SLP caught my eye and pulled her lips into a tight line as she nodded. "Well," she began, "Kate definitely has a delay. It's hard to say if there is anything more at this point. She's probably three or four months behind her peers. We could do therapy once a week or so, if you want to."

I sucked in a deep breath and let my eyes wander around the room. I bit my lower lip and then looked down at Kate. I nodded ever so slightly.

When my husband heard there was a "delay," he thought an hour of speech therapy a week couldn't hurt. And that's when he 'fessed up that *he* had been a "late talker." His first word was "clop-clop" for *helicopter*, and that wasn't until he was *three*! I had known about his trouble saying *s* words and his experience with speech therapy through third grade, but *late talking*—this was something he hadn't shared during those "tell me about your childhood" date discussions.

After I mulled over my husband's late-talking "confession," I followed up with our pediatrician, who said, "Leslie, really, what can it hurt? I know you want the best for Kate."

It took some time, but I warmed up to the idea that Kate did need speech therapy. But I was skeptical that playing with toys could *really* get her to talk. After all, she played with toys all the time at home, at playgroups, and in the daycare at the gym— and this was *structured* play, often with me at the center of it all. The only utterances we were hearing were "eh?" and "hi." *(Later I learned that play-based therapy is very good for kids; it taps into their innate need to discover and manipulate objects).*

Needless to say, we went back. On visit 2 or 3, The SLP told me that motion activates the vestibular system—which is responsible for the body's balance and coordination—and suggested that movement might get Kate to say more. So we tried the large swing in the clinic's "gym." After about fifteen minutes of swinging and repeating the words over and over, something resembling "mama" popped out of Kate's mouth.

You'd think I'd grin from ear to ear as my eyes welled up, but actually it was a bit anticlimactic, "Did she really just call me 'mama' or was that what I *thought* I heard?" But the SLP was convinced Kate was saying 'mama' all because of the swing.

Swinging Kate as often as possible—with prompts to make sounds and say words—was strongly recommended on our departure from the clinic that day. But this was November in Minnesota, too cold for the playground.

"Hang a plastic swing from a rafter in your basement," the SLP chirped on several occasions. We considered her suggestion, but with a finished basement, decided against it.

We eventually heard Kate say "mama," "dada," and "ball" over the course of the next six weeks. *Six long weeks.* Of course, I was pleased, but I couldn't help but be worried. "Is this normal for it to take *so long and feel so hard*—on both Kate and us [parents]?"

The SLP made no formal diagnosis besides a "delay." With Christmas around the corner and a baby sister due in three weeks, Kate was released from therapy with a promise of a follow-up phone call in January. The call never came, and neither did any more words.

But, baby sister Kelly did, and so did a job offer for Dad—out-of-state. The house went on the market, the boxes got packed, and speech therapy went on hold.

Bear in mind that our first experience with an SLP was not the "one and only" we worked with throughout our journey. We started in Minnesota—where we learned Kate had a "delay." Then we moved to Illinois—where the formal diagnosis occurred and therapy followed. While we were at the *same* clinic in the Chicago suburbs, we had three different SLPs. Changes happen for a variety of reasons (job change, maternity/paternity leave, back to school, staffing needs, etc.).

Parents Share

My Resistance to Speech-Language Therapy

To be honest, I really didn't want to take my daughter to speech therapy, at least not at first. I wondered why it would do Kate any good to sit in a small office jam-packed with toys for a pricey hour of therapy (granted, insurance paid for it) when we could easily do the same thing in the comfort of our own home for free and no appointment to disrupt our tidy routine? Later, I learned that in order for Kate to be a typically speaking child by the time she entered kindergarten (a goal we had established early on based on her severity, attention span, willingness to engage), I really needed to get her to speech therapy as often as possible. Kids with CAS respond and make the most progress when they receive frequent, intense therapy and plenty of home practice.

Forms, Forms, and More Forms!

At this point, there may be an SLP you have done a bit of homework on. You know a bit about his or her experience, philosophy, and background. Or, maybe you were like me: you knew nothing and just showed up at your appointment.

Every clinic and every SLP is going to have a different approach. But there is a general recipe all SLPs follow.

After you have made your appointment (perhaps weeks or even months out, depending on the availability of SLPs in your area), you will likely receive a stack of paperwork from the evaluating clinic.

These forms will ask you to detail everything about your little one from the moment of conception (well, not quite—but almost)!

- *General information* will include demographics, insurance, and your occupations.

- ***Overall language problem*** is *your* description of why you are bringing your child to an SLP: what you believe the concern/diagnosis is, what caused it, what helps, and what makes it worse.

- ***Family history*** will be covered—speech, language, and academic difficulties. Pay close attention to relatives you may have never met but have heard about through other family members. For example, Uncle Pete used to stutter or Great-Grandma Effie struggled with finding the right word. Perhaps there is a history of learning disabilities or late-talking children. Make sure you note any and all relatives who may have contributed to your child's genetic makeup.

- Another section will cover ***medical concerns*** such as surgeries, major accidents, hospitalizations, medications your child is currently taking (include vitamins, supplements, and anything over-the-counter and be sure to mention if your child has any negative reaction to medications.

- There will likely be a section on ***prenatal and birth history***—covering things like mom's general health during pregnancy (illness, accidents, medications) and how long the pregnancy lasted. Mention everything you can think of: the fall on the ice in your fifth month counts, as does your diet and exercise routine. You will need to note how long you were in labor and if there were any complications. Be sure to note the use of oxygen, forceps, whether a C-section was necessary (these concerns could indicate a child in distress). Your SLP may also ask for your child's birth weight. In addition, you'll want to make special note of any complications your child had immediately after birth. Please don't panic as you read this—just because these things were part of your child's birth does not indicate they caused your child to have CAS—they're just worth mentioning.

- Your ***child's developmental history*** will be detailed in yet another section. Dust off—or find—that baby book. When did he crawl, sit, stand, and walk? What about feeding himself, dressing himself, and using the toilet? When did he first use a single word? What are the words or approximations he attempts? Does he use gestures to communicate his needs or wants? What are they?

- ***Social history*** will cover things like shy versus outgoing, your child's general level of cooperation, whom he spends most of his time with, his preferred style of inter-action, and whether he goes to preschool or daycare.

- ***"Anything else you would like to share"*** will come last. Try not to overlook this section. Your SLP will know what to do with this information. Here are some examples:
  - "Jayce loves his pacifier. He won't go or do anything without it."
  - "Paisley loves her baby blankie. I hope you won't mind if she brings it to therapy."

- "Anthony is very afraid of dogs. Talking about or playing with them will not be effective."

- "Nora has separation concerns right now. It's probably just a phase, but if I could stay in the room, it will make things much smoother for all."

- "Josiah's great-grandmother died recently. They were pretty close."

> **What If Your Child Was Adopted?**
> If your child was adopted, it will no doubt be challenging to complete these forms. Every adoption, like every child, is unique. If you know the answers to some of these questions, then great. If not, do what you can. If you have just partial knowledge of the birth mother and her family, indicate what you do know.

After you have filled out this tedious paperwork, you'll have a major case of writer's cramp and need a breather. Go ahead and indulge in something that makes you feel better. You need to take care of yourself too.

When we completed this paperwork, it was just that—paper. And lots of it. However, you may be able to complete much of this via an online portal. Whatever the case, make sure it gets delivered to your treating SLP prior to the first meeting.

At the Appointment

You might be excited, nervous, indifferent, or in complete denial. Depending on the type of SLP you have—and how she or he prefers to work—you'll likely see a combination approach to formal and informal testing at your first appointment. If your SLP is completely informal, you may wonder, *How can playing with Play-Doh and blowing bubbles really help?*

Your SLP should have enough toys to hold your child's attention for a good hour or so. You'll *want* to feel like you just walked into a toy superstore. But on another note, it should be organized and well-maintained, and not too overwhelming. A good SLP will know this and perhaps only bring out a few items at a time.

Besides developing trust and rapport and assessing your child's behavior, your SLP is busy evaluating. Remember how your child's job is to play? Well, your SLP's "play" *is* her work. Here are some components of a typical speech-language evaluation:

- **Behavioral Observations:** How your child engages in play, whether his play style is developmentally appropriate (similar to play of other kids his age), alertness/attentiveness/excitability. Be sure to tell your therapist if the behavior is an accurate representation of your child's abilities.

- **Pragmatics:** Your SLP is evaluating how your child uses language to communicate with others in his environment. Examples of pragmatics include responding to other's vocalizations, pointing to/showing/giving objects, making eye contact, responding to greetings, and controlling behavior.

- **Gesture:** How does your child uses gesture to express thought and intent without spoken language? Examples of gestures include taking on/off articles of clothing when asked, "dancing" to music, pushing a stroller/shopping cart.

- **Play:** This piece of the evaluation actually determines your child's development of representational thought. This is really a fancy way of saying your child's ability to think in analogies; to understand symbols and infer meaning. Can he show how to play with a toy in different ways? Hand a toy to an adult for assistance? Group objects together? Use two toys together? Put toys away when asked? This is also an opportunity to see your child's temperament and personality; important for planning future speech sessions.

- **Language Comprehension (Receptive Language):** Determines how well your child attends to, processes, understands, retains, and integrates spoken language with and without linguistic cues. This may be tested by asking your child to pick just one object from a group, follow two-step commands, identify body parts/clothing items on himself, and perhaps follow novel commands.

- **Language Expression (Expressive Language):** Examines how easily your child can put words together to express himself verbally to others. If your child is able to sign certain concepts such as "more" or "thank you," it's still considered expressive language, though not verbal. Your SLP is looking to see if your child can shake his head yes/no, name an object, say several meaningful words, consistently identify five to seven familiar objects when asked, or use single words correctly and frequently. (See chapter 2 for more information about receptive and expressive language.)

- **Speech and Articulation:** What speech sounds are in your child's repertoire, and how accurately and meaningfully does he produce them? Does "down" sound like "done?" If so, he is unable to differentiate his speech. Does your child have one word that represents several different concepts? (Kate's word was "nanni." It meant "Grandma," "pacifier," and "blanket.") Does your child appear to be looking for the right word, but come up empty-handed (groping)? Does he grunt, squeal, and scream to get his needs met?

- **Motor-Speech Examination (MSE):** An essential tool for speech pathologists faced with diagnosing CAS is the MSE. The child is asked to imitate utterances of increasing length and complexity. Your SLP is looking to see if your child can make the same sounds in different contexts. When the SLP makes modifications to the MSE by slowing down the rate or by giving the child cues (by touch or gesture), she can begin to determine severity, and even get clues for determining the prognosis.

- **Oral Motor Skills:** Do your child's tongue, lips, jaw, and facial muscles work together to formulate words? Are facial and oral features symmetrical? Can he smile, frown, and press his lips together? Your SLP might use a flavored tongue depressor and gloves (mention if your child has a latex allergy) to examine his mouth. This can be tricky—some kids hate having someone's gloved hand in their mouth and some kids are painfully reminded of the dentist or doctor. Your SLP should ask you and your child if this is acceptable. Some SLPs will allow your child to play with the instruments used for this examination.

- **Feeding:** Your child may be asked to eat something like a cracker or cookie and take a drink of water (or juice). This will assess whether your child has any difficulty drinking, swallowing, chewing, or aspirating (drawing in air and liquid at the same time—choking). Your SLP will also ask if you have observed any eating difficulties at home. Pay close attention to the texture of foods that your child eats well and those he doesn't (does he hate applesauce but eat yogurt in earnest?). Mention these foods to the SLP, as well as any food allergies or insensitivities your child may have.

Impression and Initial Comments

At the end of your child's evaluation, the SLP will likely give you his or her impression and initial comments. You may even receive a diagnosis. But keep in mind that most SLPs will need some time to look over the results of the standardized testing (if used) and review their notes from the session.

Others may hesitate to give a diagnosis until they have worked with your child for a length of time. Perhaps they will suggest therapy once a week to rule out CAS. They may give a *suspected* or *working* diagnosis of CAS. This will ensure that the diagnosis is accurate. ***It is worth noting that CAS cannot be diagnosed if your child is completely nonverbal.*** Once your child attempts to communicate verbally, the SLP will be looking for any inconsistencies and patterns in your child's speech that may indicate he has CAS.

Many SLPs may be reluctant to give a formal diagnosis of CAS until your child's third birthday. Some parents and SLPs feel that waiting until three is too long. Others may tell you that a diagnosis prior to three years sets you up for an emotional roller coaster. What if you worry and curse and cry, lose sleep, spend hours online, and then learn it wasn't CAS after all? This happened to one of my blog readers:

We were told that Ryan had CAS when he was just about 27 months. I was a wreck. I didn't know what to make of it. He started a special preschool and they couldn't get him to talk for a long time, either. Finally, they told me they thought Ryan had autism and some other neurological issues. It wasn't CAS, after all. I felt cheated. I took him to this school, read so many books, spent hours on the internet. I want that time back.

Parents Ask

Isn't there a simple test for CAS?

The evaluation consists of several components: clinical observation by an SLP, your observations as a parent, and some test batteries. However, for these tests to "work," children need to be able to talk; that is, they need to be able to repeat words, phrases, or sentences and use spontaneous conversational speech. If your child can't, then the evaluation depends on just observation. Here are some tests that may be used:

- **The Apraxia Profile.** Two versions exist: the Preschool and School-Age Profile. Both include an oral motor exam and assess words, phrases, and sentences and connected speech. A checklist of common CAS characteristics is used. The Preschool Profile is shorter and less complex. The School-Age Profile includes rhymes, counting, and sentences with a rhyme.
- **The Kaufman Speech Praxis Test for Children (KSPT).** A standardized test that can be used for initial evaluation and reevaluation. This test includes subsets for oral movements, syllables, vowel sounds, and conversational speech.
- **Dynamic Evaluation of Motor Speech Skill (DEMSS).** A criterion-referenced assessment designed to help facilitate, confirm, or rule out a diagnosis of CAS. It might also be used to determine the severity of the disorder and the prognosis. It is used with children over the age of three years (often with very limited or no verbal communication skills). The DEMSS was developed by one of the leading experts on CAS, Dr. Edythe Strand.

A Label? I Don't Want My Child to Have a Label!

Another concern I am sure you have is the label: childhood apraxia of speech. Perhaps the idea that your child has a "problem" is worrisome, or you just can't stand the idea of your child being labeled. Or perhaps you have a completely different concern. Hang tight—I'll be sure to touch on some of your concerns. For now, having a label means you know what you're dealing with, you'll learn about ways to help your child, the label may qualify your child for early intervention or other special help through the school, and it helps in terms of insurance reimbursement (more on that in Appendix B).

Experiences with Learning the CAS Diagnosis

As you can see from the mothers' comments below, when and how children receive the official diagnosis of CAS varies. SLPs, children, and parents are all unique individuals. It is often this combination of uniqueness that determines how and when you get a diagnosis.

- "Our SLP didn't come right out and say that Marcus had CAS. It wasn't like it was a secret; it just was never really discussed. I continued to take him to therapy knowing that things were improving [with his speech], but I never really knew what to call it until she mentioned it casually to me one day."

- "I was mad when our SLP told me that she had been treating Finley for CAS all along. Never once was this brought up to me. Finley has other issues as well [cri du chat syndrome] and everything is delayed. But when our SLP said she codes for CAS, I was dumbfounded."

- "We didn't know at first. Our early intervention therapist was calling it a 'delay' for a long time. I was okay with that. As soon as she called it child-hood apraxia of speech, I went bonkers. Somehow 'delay' felt safe and fixable.

- "Our daughter wasn't diagnosed until kind of late. She was seven. She has some other issues, too, and we just thought her communication skills—or lack thereof—were related. It was all sort of a hoax about how and when she was diagnosed."

You may actually be pleasantly surprised by what happens after you get a label, as Amy of St. Louis was:

> As the months tick by since Brooke was officially diagnosed with CAS (she was 2 years, 3 months at diagnosis), one thing that I have routinely noticed throughout all of our doctor visits, therapy appointments, and developmental evaluations is that they were all hesitant to label a child. Which is really outstanding for so many reasons!
>
> One of our biggest fears when we first noticed Brooke had developmental delays was that she was going to be labeled—correctly or incorrectly—and that it would "stick" and forever change the way people see her. It has been nothing short of amazing to see that the exact opposite has happened. Labels are not slapped on without significant thought, and even when they are applied, it does not impact how people treat her.

Other than needing a formal diagnosis to secure services or insurance funding, a label doesn't really matter. What matters is that each child is getting the right amount and type of support to help them reach their greatest potential.

Don't worry about the label; instead ask yourself, *"Is there anything else my child needs to be successful?"*

After the Evaluation

Whether or not your SLP gives you a diagnosis immediately after the evaluation, you should most definitely be advised *on what type of therapy* would best serve your child and how often he'll need it. I hope you are offered some resources such as contacts for parent support groups, website guidance, or this book!

You should receive a written evaluation from your SLP in the next several weeks. Please remember, speech clinics are busy. You may have to place a follow-up call to ensure you will be receiving a written report. Consider asking for it to also be mailed to you electronically. That way you always have a backup if your paper copy is misplaced.

> **Parents Share**
>
> Remember where you keep your paper copies. You'll need to access them from time to time—when your child goes to preschool or when working with insurance. (Refer to chapter 11 for tips and hints on organizing all that paperwork.)

How to Read That Report

The report of a speech-language evaluation is exciting in some ways, hard-to-hear in others, and sometimes excruciatingly boring and cumbersome. The written report will likely be long—5 to 7 pages—and very detailed. You will come across words and phrases you probably aren't familiar with and many of them may cause you some alarm, question, or anxiety.

Reading about your child's problems described in black and white by a "stranger" who is also a professional is often a wake-up call. Brace yourself. You may choose to hold on to the report—unopened—until your spouse or significant other can be there with you. Even if you already suspect CAS and are looking for validation and justification from a professional, it's not easy. No parent wants to be faced with the fact that their child is struggling.

Here are some tips that may help you make heads or tails of the report:

- *Remind yourself: I am the parent.* "I am concerned about my child's developing speech. I want to help my child, and so does this SLP."

- *Take turns reading the report out loud to your spouse, partner, or trusted friend.* This sort of depersonalizes the words. At the end of each section, pause to ask questions, clarify, make notes, etc.

- *When making notes about the report, refrain from writing directly on the report.* You never know when you'll need to provide a copy of the report to the school or a medical provider. Keep your originals clean. Use a Post-It note instead.

- *If you don't understand a word, phrase, or some terminology specific to speech pathology, make a note of it and look it up later.* You will likely see lots of words you aren't familiar with. (Refer to the glossary located in Appendix E if you'd like.)

- *If you notice something inaccurate in the report, bring it to your SLP's attention immediately.* Give her a call or send an email and explain your concern in a diplomatic manner. You may not agree with everything your SLP observed during your child's evaluation; if you feel a particular observation is not a true representation of your child, kindly ask if your SLP can add a statement to the report indicating something along those lines. For example, "Mother indicates it is not typical for Kate to drool during speech." (Kate really *did* drool during her evaluation, and I was sure to tell the SLP that it wasn't typical.)

- *Take time to digest the information.* You've learned a great deal about your child's communication difficulties. You need time to absorb it all.

- *Do what you need to do to cope with it.* Reading the report is going to dredge up some feelings you may or may not be ready to accept. You may be in denial, you may be angry, you may seek to receive a second opinion, or you may just want to cry. Go ahead and let it out. Do something proactive, though. What have you done in the past to cope with unpleasant news? Do it now.

- *When you're ready, begin sharing the results with those who love, support, and encourage you and your child.* You will need to pull from various sources as you and your child cope with CAS.

What's a Treatment Plan?

A treatment plan ("Tx plan") is typically about a paragraph or two of detailed recommendations for therapy generally printed at the end of your report. It may include a target date for a re-screen or reevaluation. Your SLP will list *specific initial goals*, along with possible recommendations for additional therapy (OT, PT), and suggestions for family and educational professionals.

When I practiced as a Child and Adolescent Psychiatric R.N., we often used this acronym for setting treatment goals: **S**pecific, **M**easurable, **A**ttainable, **R**ealistic, and **T**oward dismissal [from speech therapy]. Keeping this acronym in mind can give you a quick and easy way to remember ways to create goals and keep tabs on your child's treatment place. The acronym also works for speech-language therapy, with one addition. SLPs always need to keep the reason for the goal in mind, whether or not they include it in the written goal. The following sample illustrates how SLPs may write their goals with SMART in mind:

- **S**(pecific): To improve articulation, Josh will produce target CVCV [consonant-vowel-consonant-vowel], CV, and VC syllables with correct articulation in structured therapy.

- **M**(easurable): 80% accuracy on target words, even if he needs visual cues, and during therapy time, not necessarily in his spontaneous speech.

- **A**(ttainable): An SLP will likely describe the circumstances under which Josh was expected to produce the targets (for instance, during structured therapy in which notes are being taken).

- **R(ealistic):** "To be realistic, I would never take a child who couldn't do CVCV, CV, and VC syllables and expect him to be producing three-syllable words in spontaneous speech in a year's time," says Rhonda Banford, MAT, CCC-SLP. "Of course, if the child made quick progress, I would adjust my goals to reflect higher level skills. If the child truly has CAS, however, we have to be cognizant of the fact that it may take him quite a while to truly establish basic motor movements with consistency. As he progresses and internalizes new motor movements, I would anticipate his therapy to start moving along with greater speed."

- **T(oward dismissal):** Remember that CAS is a dynamic disorder, meaning it changes over time, so it is challenging to pinpoint a specific date for the expected end of speech therapy. SLPs often have time constraints imposed upon them, particularly when they work in hospitals and schools. Many children with CAS will be seen for therapy in the schools. School IEPs typically cover a period of one year, so goals must be attainable in that period of time (in effect, until children are dismissed for summer break).

- [**Reason:** To improve articulation.]

You likely won't see your child's goals written out next to the SMART acronym. Instead, you will see all the elements combined into a paragraph, as in these examples:

- In order to improve articulation, Josh will produce early developing consonant phonemes /p, b, m, t, d, n, w, h/ in target CVCV, CV, VC, and CVC words during structured conversation, with 80% accuracy over 3 data days.

- In order to improve expressive language, Emily will produce target CVC words with correct articulation in four carrier phrases (I want ___, I have ___, I see ___, I need) during structured therapy, with 80% accuracy over 3 data days.

The treatment plan is something you will hear mentioned often. Know it well. Ask for revisions if you find that things aren't progressing as they should, your child has reached some goals, or a new concern has cropped up.

Say That Again?! Chapter Summary

This chapter presented you with an initial-speech-pathologist-visit-in-a-nutshell scenario. Do your homework ahead of time by filling out the appropriate forms and getting them to the speech clinic before your first visit. As you read the report from the SLP, it's important to remember that he or she is there to help your child. Reading that first report is never easy. No parent wants to admit that his or her child has a concern that is best dealt with by someone else. Reach out to supportive and helpful individuals as you make sense of the treatment plan and the recommendations of the speech-language pathologist.

Bottom line: if you *suspect* there is a *potential* diagnosis of CAS, get your kiddo to an SLP ASAP.

Recommended Resources

Tip: Textbook-type resources can be pricey. Please don't feel you have to run out and spend good money on them. Amazon and Barnes & Noble allow you to rent textbooks for a fraction of the purchase price. We borrowed some from our speech clinic's lending library, and our SLP had a few textbooks from grad school she was willing to share. I checked out many books from college and university libraries through an interlibrary loan (ILL). You might check whether your local library can obtain materials in this manner. Finally, hit up your local used bookstore. You can often find copies of the same books there. Even ones with older copyright dates are generally okay because communication skills and assessment and evaluation processes and skills don't change too much over time.

- You may appreciate Speech Therapy Information and Resources (STIR), a UK online resource that's all about speech and language. You may find the sections on play, communication, and anatomy particularly helpful: http://www.speechlanguage-resources.com/.

- *Assessment of Speech-Language Disorders in Children* by Rebecca McCauley (Psychology Press, 2006) is a great resource, although it's not exactly written for parents. You may find it tough going because it's so comprehensive—and designed mostly for a professional or graduate student audience.

- At 800 pages, this is a huge volume of information, but you will find plenty of examples, assessment styles, and treatment plans in *Language Disorders from Infancy through Adolescence: Assessment and Intervention* by Rhea Paul, PhD, CCC-SLP (Mosby, 2006). Most definitely a textbook or desk reference for speech-language pathologists, this text can be found (or requested) through your public library, as can the book listed above. Also, purchasing a used copy for a fraction of the price may not be a bad idea.

- *Parent's Guide to Speech and Language Problems* (McGraw-Hill, 2007) by Debbie Feit, a journalist and mother of two children with CAS (now resolved), does a great job of compiling related speech disorders in an easy-to-use guide, complete with tips for finding a speech pathologist, as well as assessment and intervention.

- *Here's How to Treat Childhood Apraxia of Speech* by Margaret (Dee) Fish (Plural Publishing, 2015) is mostly written as a textbook, but is readable for motivated parents as well. It covers a substantial amount of information about assessment but is mostly concerned with treatment.

- *Dynamic Evaluation of Motor Speech Skill (DEMSS)* by Edythe A. Strand, PhD, CCC-SLP, and Rebecca J. McCauley, PhD, CCC-SLP (Brookes Publishing, 2019). This resource is intended for clinicians in practice and is not meant to be used by lay individuals. Referencing here just in case you wish to learn more.

Now What?

Chapter 5

Getting the CAS Diagnosis

Initial Reactions

"Well," she began, "I think she has childhood apraxia of speech." I sat there looking at Kate and then at the speech language-pathologist who had just completed the intense hour and fifteen-minute assessment.

"OK," I thought, "At least we know what to call it." But just what exactly *is* childhood apraxia of speech? The only words I caught in the SLP's answer were "neurologically based" and "motor-speech disorder." It was clear as mud. I was stumped and had questions—lots of them.

I was tempted to just scoop up my children and our belongings and hustle on to the next stop: the craft store. You may think I wasn't taking this seriously. Rest assured that wasn't the case. At the time, I wasn't sure what to make of this information. I was tired and drained after the evaluation. I had been entertaining a wiggly baby in a new environment. And there were plenty of things floating around on my mental to-do list.

I had no knowledge and no past experience with speech disorders, so I asked the SLP if she had any handouts or pamphlets on the diagnosis she had just handed my daughter. She didn't. But she did recommend a few websites.

Speech therapy was recommended twice weekly for one hour until Kate reached "age-appropriate speech milestones." I had no idea what that meant either. The SLP said she would provide a full report, complete with therapy goals.

I told my husband how the evaluation went as he flipped through the mail and kissed his family. "It's called childhood apraxia of speech. That's why Kate isn't talking yet," I informed him. He had questions similar to mine: What does that mean? What caused it? What can we do about it? What's the prognosis?

After the girls were off in dreamland, I pulled out my laptop and did some research. Not a lot. Just enough to get a few of my most pressing questions answered. I still needed time to digest all of this information.

It may sound as though I was taking this news about Kate's CAS all in stride. In reality, I was confused, yet relieved that we finally had something to call "it." I was worried yet trying to remain hopeful for her sake and mine. I screamed at my dad, my husband, anyone who would listen, "My daughter can't talk—this is a *big* problem!"

The story that I relate above really did happen pretty much as I tell it here. It took time and energy to muster up the courage to learn more about CAS. Once I did, I realized just how serious it was.

> ### The Nuts and Bolts of This Chapter
>
> - You're on an emotional rollercoaster—we'll talk about that
> - A trip back in time to 1891, when we *believe* the first case of CAS was identified
> - Information on prognosis, or the likelihood that your child's CAS will resolve

Learning the Diagnosis

You may have been searching for years for the reason why your child isn't talking like every other child. Perhaps you weren't that concerned in the first place but took your child to a SLP because your friends, your mother, or a concerned neighbor or teacher urged you to. In either case, you now have a term to describe the phenomenon: childhood apraxia of speech. What's next?

Common Reactions

If it took you a while to arrive at a diagnosis, you may be feeling like your competence as a parent has been challenged.

> *"Gosh, I knew there was something wrong.*
> *Why wouldn't (or couldn't) anyone tell me what it was?!"*

You may feel some resentment toward any professionals you consulted who shooed you away, assuring you everything was "fine."

> *"I knew I was right! Those doctors were so incompetent.*
> *Their lack of competency and time wasted really irks me!"*

You might feel like I did: relieved.

> *"Now I know what to call this thing that was preventing*
> *my little one from saying much more than 'eh?'"*

But you could also feel discouraged, as I did.

> *"What now? What does this mean for my child?*
> *Will he ever be able to talk? Where do I go from here?"*

Case in point: One of my playgroup mom friends said, "Oh, CAS. . . that's a tough one. I was so glad when Jackson didn't have it after all. Call me if you want to talk." I didn't. Not to her, anyway. If Jackson didn't really have CAS, I didn't want to get stuck talking with someone who would make it sound like the end of the world. Plus, I wanted to believe that it would be an easy fix.

Another mom friend of mine—who also has a daughter with CAS—indicated she felt naïve when she first got the diagnosis: "I just didn't know what to think. Maybe one or two months of therapy and then she'd be talking normally."

Really, the "fix" is somewhere in the middle. Receiving a diagnosis of CAS *is* pretty serious, but it's not the end of the world, and it's certainly not a quick fix. We'll cover therapy approaches in chapter 7.

Here are some ***other feelings and emotions you might be experiencing*** after learning the diagnosis of CAS:

- disbelief /uncertainty
- confusion
- denial
- information overload
- numbness
- isolation
- loss
- shock
- anger
- guilt
- sadness

Yet you may also feel acceptance, and even a proactive sense of duty.

Here's an excerpt from my journal at the time, expressing my mishmash of feelings:

I am feeling a bit dumbfounded about Kate's diagnosis. I used to be in speech & debate [club]. I wrote and performed an oratory at a competition level; how could I possibly have a daughter who couldn't talk?!

Some folks have a more positive reaction from the outset. They may even say they feel "blessed" or as though they were "chosen" to have a child with such a diagnosis. For example, here's how one mother I spoke to came to terms with her child's diagnosis:

I'm a nurse in a neuro-rehab unit. We see a lot of patients who are suffering from brain injuries, stroke, and such. I know CAS isn't really the same, but there are a lot of similarities. I have a good knowledge base of neurological issues, so learning about CAS isn't so out of my comfort zone.

For now, sit tight with your feelings about your child's diagnosis. Listen to them, accept them, and talk them over with someone such as a friend, your spouse, or your child's SLP.

Parents Share

Early Feelings after the Diagnosis

"It is a funny thing, CAS. It just CONSUMES you as a parent when you are at the worst of it. I can remember wondering what Allison's voice even sounded like. And wondering what she would say when she started talking. Would she talk? I remember when a friend's son, who was a year younger, started talking precociously and—I hate to admit it—it filled me with despair that took my breath away."—*Susan, mother of Ally*

More on Denial

Chapter 2 covered some common remarks that others may make to explain your child's speech delays. For example: *You do all the talking for her, so she doesn't need to talk. She'll talk when something really interests her.* Sometimes when parents get the diagnosis of CAS, they don't believe it and may actually wonder if the comments that others made to them are true.

Along those lines, you or your spouse may wonder, "Is she just shy?" In reality, there is a big difference between having a speech disorder like CAS and "just being shy." A shy child might have genetic tendencies to be more introverted (that's perfectly okay) or might not have developed the social skills, confidence, or maturity to speak up in uncertain or new situations. Some kids (and adults) need time to "warm up" before they feel comfortable conversing with others—even those they know well. Shy kids *can* talk; they just prefer not to—at least at that moment.

At the time, I was absolutely convinced Kate was an extrovert at heart and that her mouth simply couldn't keep up with her extroverted thoughts and modes of relating to others.

Having CAS—while not exactly a good thing—can be corrected with early, frequent, and intense intervention. Although feelings of denial are common after the diagnosis of CAS in a child, remember: Before you are given the diagnosis of CAS, everything else that it *could* be should have been ruled out through the process of *differential diagnosis.*

What Is a Differential Diagnosis?

You might hear folks refer to the "differential diagnosis." What this means is the process that professionals use to tease out other disorders or factors that may be contributing to what *looks like* CAS. "It is difficult for SLPs to diagnose CAS when a child has little or no speech because many of the characteristics of CAS *involve* speech," explains Di Bahr, MS, CCC-SLP, and author of *Nobody Ever Told Me or My Mother That!* "For example," she says, "kids with CAS often leave sounds out in words or make the same [consistent] speech errors in spontaneous speech but make different [inconsistent] errors when *asked* to imitate. In order to observe these characteristics of CAS, the child must have some speech."

Also, SLPs will consider whether your child may actually have word-finding problems, an autism spectrum disorder (ASD), social anxiety (shyness taken to an extreme), hearing loss, auditory processing disorder, or something else.

To use the CAS label with utmost confidence, the practitioner(s) must find evidence that the child has the symptoms characteristic of children with CAS that are listed on pages 6–7 in Chapter 1.

Are verbal apraxia (CAS) and oral apraxia the same thing?

No. While these two disorders sound like they are similar, they are actually quite different.

Oral apraxia is the impaired ability to voluntarily perform nonspeech tasks with the mouth and tongue, such as kissing, puckering, puffing out cheeks, licking lips, sticking out the tongue. To clarify further, a child might be able to lick an ice cream cone without any problem, but when asked to stick out her tongue, she might be unable to. If asked by her SLP to "pucker your lips like you are going to give someone a kiss," she might not be able to, but she might be able to kiss her mother good night without any delay. These children may be late talkers, but can often speak normally, if they don't also have CAS.

CAS (sometimes referred to as "verbal apraxia") is the impaired ability to voluntarily perform speech tasks with the mouth and tongue. The child may have no problem imitating or producing nonspeech mouth movements (sticking out tongue, puckering, etc.) on command, but sometimes a child has both CAS and oral apraxia.

However, verbal and oral apraxia are not the same thing. Apraxia of any kind is a motor programming problem, not a muscle function problem. For more information on the other types of apraxia, see Appendix A.

Coping with Bad News

We all deal with bad news in a uniquely predictable manner. As I came to terms with my daughter's CAS, I recalled my clinical experience in hospice care with the grief process. One of the best-known theories as to how people cope with loss comes from Elsabeth Kübler-Ross, the author of *On Death & Dying*, published in 1969. Her theory is a continuum that looks something like this:

→ **Denial** → **Bargaining** → **Anger** → **Fear** → **Acceptance**→

She indicates that individuals who are confronting the loss of a loved one can vacillate between the stages, finally ending at acceptance at some point.

Although Kübler-Ross developed her theory to explain how people manage the loss of a loved one, her theory has been extrapolated to explain how people cope with other types of bad news as well. When it comes to parents dealing with grief related to a child's disability, it's a similar, yet different route, mostly because that child is alive and with us every day. As a parent, you won't neatly arrive at the final level of acceptance after going through the prescribed stages above. Instead, CAS feels like a roller coaster—perhaps feeling "up" about the diagnosis, then feeling "down" about it, and finally coming to terms with it as the ride nears its completion. The discussion about the completion of this process (resolving CAS) is found in chapter 15.

Another take that may help you understand the adjustment process comes from Holly Olmsted-Hickey, former parent leader and moderator of The Apraxia Connection (whose teenage son has struggled with CAS):

There are three ways I've described the process of learning about a child's development:

1. *Peeling an onion: discovering something new with each peeled layer. Like an onion, sometimes those new discoveries make you cry.*

2. *Playing a game of whack-a-mole: with great fervor and determination, whacking at the mole only to discover something new popping up in the process.*

3. *Wandering in a dark, underground maze with a candle and a key to a door: sometimes your candle goes out and your key doesn't fit the door, but you always find someone on your path to light your candle and point you in a new direction.*

What's a Parent to Do?

We all cope in unique ways. I am sure you have a few "favorite" coping techniques you can pull from. This list may get you started:

- Get support by seeking out an online support group. Apraxia Kids offers an official, moderated Facebook group of over 25,000 members (www.apraxia-kids.org). This group is private (closed) and offers many valuable resources and tips curated by the organization. If you're interested in joining, pop over to www.facebook.com/groups/apraxia.kids.group/.

- Apraxia Kids also offers a state-by-state guide for finding local in-person support groups. Go to apraxia-kids.org, click on the "community" drop-down menu, and select "support groups."

- You might also want to explore The Apraxia Connection (serving areas of suburban Chicago, NW Indiana, SE Wisconsin, and Eastern Iowa), if they are in your region. Even if they're not, you may still glean some valuable information.

- CHERAB Foundation is a worldwide nonprofit organization working to improve the communication skills and education of all children with speech and language delays and disorders. Their emphasis is on autism, CAS, and oral apraxia. Visit them at www.cherabfoundation.org.

- Try to connect with others in your community with a similar diagnosis. A good starting point is to ask your child's SLP or school for contacts.

- Seek out other information you need to feel empowered to help your child. You may find other books, magazines/newsletters, or online resources/social media helpful.

- Express and acknowledge your emotions, whether in a journal, blog, social media outlet, talking with friends, spouse, family members, your child's SLP, a counselor, or clergy.

- Balance all of this with a healthy diet and exercise. Sometimes, a quick jog can clear your mind and help you feel empowered.

Tip: When weighing pros and cons of various organizations, styles of treatment, and coping methods, it's best to stick with evidence-based research by qualified professionals. Not all organizations are evidence-based. Choose wisely.

Parents Share

Coping Advice

I interviewed "apraxia mom" and music therapist Katie Eshelman and asked, "What would you tell parents just learning their child's diagnosis of apraxia." Here's her response:

"Personally, I just needed time. Time to process, time to cry, time to share, and finally time to make a plan. I also needed to remember that [my daughter] was the same mischievous, sweet, funny little girl regardless of the CAS. Therefore, when the diagnosis comes up, I tell them I have a daughter with CAS, not an 'apraxic daughter.'"

Of course, since Ms. Eshelman is also a music therapist, I had to ask her if her career choice was a natural extension of helping her daughter communicate:

"Although my education and experience in the field [of music therapy] gave me some of the technical knowledge and theory to support my musical techniques, there is such an emotional component to working with your own child. I often tell people I am the kind of music therapist I am because I am a mom and I am the type of mom I am because I am a music therapist." (You'll find more references to music and music therapy in chapters 7 and 8.)

If you look for coincidences like these in your own life, you just might see how you are the best parent for your child with apraxia of speech, too.

My Feelings Are All Over the Place!

If you feel like you might need a little extra time or TLC to absorb all this information, you are not alone. Consider seeking out a counselor or psychological therapist. It's not wrong or bad if you feel the need for professional help. Remember, it's a *process* of accepting and coming to terms with a diagnosis. It's not supposed to happen overnight, and everyone deals with it in their own unique way.

Families perceive and adjust to a diagnosis of CAS in different ways. It depends on the family's cultural background, resources (financial, insurance coverage), religious beliefs, social supports, and temperaments of individuals within the family. Your response may be different than your spouse's and your mother's. Just because someone isn't responding in the manner you think they should, it doesn't mean they aren't affected.

Your Child's Prognosis

Probably one of the first questions you had after you learned your child's diagnosis was something along these lines: "Will she ever be cured?" "Will she have speech problems her whole life?" In other words, you wanted to know your child's prognosis—or the likelihood of her getting better.

Unfortunately, that is not something that anyone knows at diagnosis. At most, your SLP may describe your child's CAS as mild, moderate, severe, or profound. Of course, you probably want to know what these degrees of CAS mean.

"The terms 'mild, moderate, severe, and profound' are related to a scale of goodness," according to SLP Di Bahr. As she explains, "A scale of goodness has to do with the percentage of characteristics exhibited by the child. If a child has few characteristics of a disorder, the child has a mild disorder. If the child has many characteristics of a disorder, the child may have a severe to profound disorder. Disorders like CAS (where there is a list of behavioral characteristics) are often evaluated with a scale of goodness."

At present, there are no commonly accepted definitions of the various degrees of impairment in CAS. As Rhonda Banford, MAT, CCC-SLP, explains, the use of the terms mild, moderate, severe, or profound is a subjective decision made by the SLP:

"If a child has an extraordinary number of speech errors and is almost entirely unintelligible, I would probably characterize him or her as having profound difficulty. If she is largely unintelligible but is able to say a few things correctly, I would characterize her speech as severely impaired. If she is intelligible about half of the time, I would call her speech moderately impaired, and if she only has a few difficulties, I would use the mild designation. The terms are rather arbitrary.

"A child who has a profound speech problem has just as good a chance of becoming intelligible as a child who has a lesser speech problem. It will just take her longer to get there, especially if she has CAS, and it will take therapy with an SLP who has a good understanding of her speech concerns and the most effective ways to address them. This is assuming that she has good cognition, adequate receptive language, appropriate attention and task focus, etc. If she does not have these precursors to good speech, it will be difficult for her to attain the same level of proficiency."

The authors of *Developmental Apraxia of Speech: Theory and Clinical Practice* concur that severity ratings of CAS are quite subjective. They note that some SLPs base it on only one observation, while others may predict severity with improvement over time. So, if a child is progressing quickly, her CAS may be judged as "not as severe" as that of another child who doesn't progress as quickly. However, one characteristic that differentiates CAS from other speech disorders is *relatively* slow progress in speech treatment. Here are some other factors that authors Penny Hall, Linda Jordan, and Donald Robin take into account when assessing the severity of CAS:

- Does the child's speech get worse with longer words? (If so, it is more severe.)
- Does the child have the ability to control the environment through speech? (If so, less severe.)
- What is the child's developmental lag (usually given in months)? (Less lag = less severe.)
- How well can a listener understand what the child is saying (intelligibility)? (Better intelligibility = less severe.)
- Finally, there is the impact of co-occurring problems. (Additional concerns/diagnoses = more severe.)

Although nobody can predict today what your child's speech will be like when she is older, a variety of factors can affect how well and how quickly she is able to overcome her speech difficulties. I have summarized an article by Lori Hickman, MA, CCC-SLP, "What Does the Future Hold," for you to follow as you track·the variables considered in the prognosis of apraxia:

Factors That Affect Prognosis

Cause of the Child's Apraxia (often called "etiology," the fancy way of saying "cause" or "origin")	Is the cause of your child's speech problem primarily motor or linguistic? The cause of apraxia is unknown, as is the prognosis. The difficulty for the SLP lies in the differential diagnosis of CAS vs. other types of speech disorders. (A "motor problem" can be due to a muscle function problem or a motor programming issue, sometimes both. Phonological disorders are "linguistic problems." **CAS is a motor-speech disorder**). See chapter 6.
Family History	When other family members have a similar speech history, it is likely the child's long-term outcome/prognosis may be similar to that family member's outcome (providing, of course, that their causes are truly the same). See chapter 6.
Severity of Apraxia	In general, the more severe a child's apraxia is, the longer treatment is needed.

Verbal Apraxia (CAS) with or without Oral Apraxia	Children who exhibit *oral apraxia* (difficulty puffing cheeks, licking lips, sticking out tongue on command) *in addition* to CAS often require treatment longer than children who have only CAS. ***Remember, oral apraxia and CAS are not the same thing.***
Overall Health	Children whose overall health is good are more available to speech therapy than kids who have periods of time when they are less "learning available" due to illness (middle ear infections, upper respiratory infections, etc.).
Cognitive Skills/General Intelligence	Children who score in the average to above average range in intelligence testing have a better prognosis than children with cognitive and intellectual delays.
Attention & Ability to Focus	Children with concerns such as attention-deficit/hyperactivity disorder (ADHD) often require intervention for longer periods than children without these concerns, as attention, focus, and concentration are *required* for motor learning. The SLP can focus on the child's sound productions rather than working to maintain her attention. Children with attentional concerns tend to have more difficulty monitoring their own speech.
Child's Reaction to His or Her Intelligibility Deficit	Children who seem unaware of—or less bothered by—the difficulty other people have understanding them often require longer treatment. See chapter 14 for information on coping skills.
Ability to Self-Monitor	Children who are able to monitor their own speech tend to progress more quickly. Children who are unable to "self-monitor" continue to need their SLP or others to comment on their speech. Self-monitoring occurs when the child begins to "hear" her own speech and "edits" it as necessary. If a child doesn't "hear" an error, it will be nearly impossible for her to correct it.
Age at Which Intervention (Treatment/Therapy) Begins	The younger the child is when treatment begins, the better the long-term prognosis.
Appropriateness of Therapy	The therapeutic approach used in treatment ought to be tailored to each child individually. **A "one-size-fits-all" approach does not work for children with CAS.** The child's SLP needs to be able to adjust sessions according to the child's needs.

Frequency of Therapy	The more frequently the child receives appropriate therapy, the better the long-term prognosis.
Comorbidity (other diagnoses that *may* occur along with CAS, co-occurring).	Children who have other disorders in addition to CAS (dysarthria, autism, ADHD, Down syndrome, etc.) generally have a poorer prognosis than children whose primary disorder/delay is CAS. See Appendix A.
Motivation	A child who is happy and enjoys working with an SLP has a better outcome than a child who is resistant or indifferent toward therapy.
Parent Involvement, Education, and Support	Informed parents can encourage a child's communication skills. They are also much better equipped to advocate, network, and seek out additional resources.

Information taken from "Prognosis for Apraxia: What Does the Future Hold?" by Lori Hickman, MA, CCC-SLP. Adapted with permission from Apraxia Kids, www.apraxia-kids.org.

Generally, when children are neurologically different in one area (as is the case of CAS), other neurological conditions/concerns (such as learning, motor, or behavior issues in other areas of development) are usually part of the overall "package."

Parents Ask

Is there any research about the prognosis of CAS?
There are no definitive studies on the outcome of children with CAS. Since there is a lack of agreement/identification of this group of children, it is hard to design studies that would measure their prognosis. Kids with CAS vary quite a bit in terms of their apraxic characteristics. Therefore, it is nearly impossible to establish a control group to determine efficacy and results of long-term speech therapy.

In a nutshell, the prognosis for the average child with CAS is that she will likely learn to use speech as the primary method of communication and will eventually be able to communicate in complete, grammatically correct sentences. Most people will not even realize that she ever had a speech disorder when she was younger. But this will take time, regular speech therapy, and plenty of practice at home. Each child with CAS progresses at a different rate, but you can probably count on at least one year of speech therapy. Kids with more severe CAS or additional disabilities may continue to receive speech therapy through adolescence. Please defer to your SLP for a more specific range for *your* child.

If you are interested in learning more about resolving/recovering CAS, stay tuned. It will be covered in chapter 15.

Cultural and Social History of Childhood Apraxia of Speech

Have you ever wondered what would have happened to your child if she had been born with CAS-like symptoms a hundred years ago? Would she have been labeled as "dumb and mute?" Would she have been institutionalized? Would she have "outgrown" it? Well, I did a little historical research. History buffs, rejoice!

The first case of CAS published in the medical literature was not called CAS but was referred to as "aphemia." This case was reported in 1891 by English physician W. B. Hadden. Dr. Hadden made a house call to see eleven-year-old Charles M. to assess his lack of intelligible speech (intelligible meaning "understandable," not a reflection of one's intelligence). Young Charles hadn't attempted speech sounds until he was three years old. His older sister was the only one in the family who could understand him, thus becoming his interpreter. After some work with Dr. Hadden, Charles was able to produce short, automatic words and phrases better than he produced longer, more spontaneous speech. Today we recognize this as a symptom of CAS.

An 1897 edition of *The Lancet* included an article by neurologist H. C. Bastian. His conclusions about the disorder were more organic in nature than Dr. Hadden's. He wrote, "Speech has now become a truly automatic act for human beings . . . and if children do not speak at birth . . . its main cause is due to the fact that their nervous systems are too immature." His century-old statement reflects present-day thinking that CAS is a delay or inadequate development of those neurological pathways required for speech and not a result of a cortical (brain) lesion.

A progressive woman by the name of Muriel Morley first described the condition of CAS in the late 1950s. She didn't call it CAS at the time, but instead referred to it as "defective articulation" and also "developmental apraxia/aphasia." Children began to be labeled with these diagnoses sometime in the 1960s, most likely in response to the most severe cases. However, today we know that CAS occurs on a continuum from mild to moderate to severe to profound.

I was curious enough to do a little biographical research on Dr. Muriel Morley. I invite you to join me as we travel through speech pathology history. Muriel was born in 1899 in Halifax, England. She studied physics and biology and taught at a girls' school for ten years. In 1932, she answered a newspaper ad from a plastic surgeon looking for an "educated woman" to assess the speech of children before and after an innovative surgery to correct cleft palate. For the next five years, Muriel read all she could about cleft palates and speech. She began studying speech-language pathology by working with colleagues in Liverpool and London. In 1938, she received a certificate from the British Society of Speech Therapists.

Muriel founded The College of Speech Therapy in 1945. She insisted that speech and language be studied and taught at universities and that it should include studies of pathology based on normal developmental behavior. She also insisted that students complete a clinical rotation with supervision. It wasn't until 1955 that speech-language pathology was recognized as a college major.

Even before Muriel published her work in the 1957 edition of *The Development and Disorders of Speech in Childhood,* the subject of apraxia (adult apraxia and acquired apraxia, *not just* CAS) had been controversial for over 130 years. The characteristics, the explanations underlying the disorder, and the very label itself have been debated for a very long time.

More about Muriel Morley's Theories

Dr. Morley concluded that kids with the disorder she called "developmental apraxia/aphasia" failed to develop the central processes of speech to begin with. In other words, the child has never had normal speech and therefore has not "lost" it somewhere along the lines as brain injured (aphasic) adults have.

Here you'll find a list of Muriel Morley's findings/symptoms from her study conducted in 1947 (published in 1957). Children with Developmental Apraxia/Aphasia:

- [have] poor expressive language (delayed neurological maturation for motor processes in verbal expression)
- can understand others' speech with no problem (good/normal receptive language)
- [are]friendly and cooperative; making every effort to communicate with others, but unable to do so through speech
- [have] little or no interest in imitation of sounds of speech, even making animal sounds like "moo" and "baa" is difficult
- [have] little or no vocal play or babbling as a baby
- [are] quiet children—they rarely use sound and voice
- may show signs of frustration when they can't make requests known
- rely mostly on gesture to achieve needs/wants
- [may have] one or two isolated words that may be used during the first two to three years of life (ages twenty-four to thirty-six months)
- Have a slowly developing vocabulary
- Have a sudden growth in vocabulary around 4+ years of age

As I read Morley's list of symptoms, I thought, "This is it! This is exactly what my daughter has . . . and this is the woman who identified it. Amazing." If your child has CAS, you will also probably feel as if this list of symptoms describes your child well. Your child may not have *all* of these traits, but she will probably have most of them.

Today, SLPs and researchers continue to tweak the diagnostic criteria for CAS. Perhaps a few traits that are missing from Ms. Morley's early criteria are the following:

- saying words out of the blue,

- difficulty following sequenced directions (e.g., "Put your shoes on and then grab your backpack before going outside"),
- errors with vowel usage, and
- decreased intelligibility as phrases get longer.

Some Advice for the Road

Here are some important points to keep in mind as you set about your journey:

- *CAS is dynamic and can change over time.* Most kids with CAS have difficulty making sounds. As these children get older, their motor planning improves. Yet they will still have difficulty making the *correct* sounds, even though—in theory—they are able to. It may *appear* as though a child previously diagnosed with CAS now has a phonological delay, but in reality she just has a more sophisticated version of CAS. (A phonological delay/disorder is a language-based disorder. It has to do with difficulties underlying the sound system of a given language, not the neuromotor connection, as in CAS). *Keep in mind that not all features will be present at the same time; some may not be present at all. CAS is complex and individual.*

- *If there is a "problem area" or a breakdown in your child's speech output, it's important to begin to understand where in the system that breakdown is occurring.* A child could have a breakdown in the retrieval system, for example. Think of it this way—your Golden Retriever can locate the stick you threw into the lake and bring it back to you for another round of fetch without any problem. But your child with CAS . . . well, she's no retriever. You throw a word out to the lake and she can't plan the path to find/form it. She *knows* the word, but she just can't find it when she wants to use it. Please refer to chapter 7 on speech therapy for more information on this.

- *Another little snag your child with CAS may encounter is difficulty producing certain speech sounds and sound patterns.* Let's face it, some sounds are just harder to produce. What can we do? Practice, practice, practice! I don't want to sound patronizing, but that practice piece of it is the hardest part of CAS (more on that in chapter 9: What You Can Do at Home).

- *Speech learning can be interrupted as the brain learns new things and tries to figure them out and make sense of new knowledge—be it cognitive or motor.* I am sure you have heard this theory on child development before: "Your baby isn't babbling because she is working really hard at learning to roll over or sit up or crawl. Once she masters that motor skill, she'll get back to babbling." One thing at a time, right? Well, there is some truth to that, but don't latch onto this as the one and only reason your child isn't talking yet.

- *Once your child with CAS does start talking more, she may mumble, stutter, self-practice, or grope for words.* (Self-practice simply means that she is working on speech sounds on her own, without any suggestion or direction to do so. It may sound as though your child is babbling, but this is a very important step to being a more effective communicator.) Don't lose heart—She may just be learning a new aspect of speech production, developing a word retrieval system, or learning to combine words into sentences. It might look like a regression in her speech-language skills, but in reality, it's probably just your child's brain working faster than it can produce the sounds. This may become more apparent as your child gets older.

Help! I Need a Dictionary!

No doubt you will continue to come across new words on your quest to learn about CAS. Please refer to the glossary (Appendix E) for more detailed definitions and additional words and phrases you may come across along your CAS journey. No worries—there won't be a test!

Say That Again?! Chapter Summary

You may have never heard of childhood apraxia of speech. Don't despair. Reading this book is a great first step. Applaud yourself for seeking out resources and information. Your feelings and emotions will change once you learn the diagnosis. There is no right or wrong way to feel. Seek therapy from a professional who has experience with disabilities if you feel like it's too much to adjust to.

This chapter also presented a history of early accounts of CAS (or suspected CAS). The idea of CAS has been controversial for nearly two hundred years.

Finally, rest assured that *children with CAS can and* do *get better.* As a parent, the best thing you can do is to provide your children with frequent and intense therapy at an early age.

Recommended Resources

- If it's truly CAS your child is struggling with, it's unlikely she'll "outgrow" it. Instead, your child will need the professional services of a speech-language pathologist. Check out this educational/informational video by Teri Peterson, MS, CCC/SLP: www.youtube.com/user/ChatterboxBooks#p/u/0/7C6NAXvljpw.

- *Reflexes. Learning, and Behavior: A Window into the Child's Mind, a Non-Invasive Approach to Solving Learning and Behavior Problems,* by Sally Goddard (Fern Ridge Press, 2005).

- For more guidance and support in your CAS journey, try ***You Will Dream New Dreams: Inspiring Personal Stories by Parents of Children with Disabilities*** by Stanley D. Klein and Kim Schive (Kensington, 2001). It includes inspiring personal stories collected from parents around the US. It's like "a support group in a book."

- ***Shut Up about Your Perfect Kid: A Survival Guide for Ordinary Parents of Special Children*** by sisters Gina Gallagher and Patricia Konjoian (Three Rivers Press, 2010) is another great resource—funny, too—in which you will see these parents' frustration, sadness, and battles with stigma as they share frank accounts of raising children with special needs.

- ***A Different Kind of Perfect: Writings by Parents on Raising a Child with Special Needs*** by Cindy Dowling (Trumpeter, 2006) includes fifty personal essays written by parents of children with special needs. Here, you'll find heartbreaking honesty as these parents grapple with grief and despair to gratitude and laughter.

- Speech-language pathologist Dr. Edythe Strand, emeritus consultant in the division of Speech Pathology at the Mayo Clinic, recorded a fabulous YouTube video, ***Treatment of Childhood Apraxia of Speech***, at New York University in December 2016. It's mostly geared toward practitioners and covers motor-learning principles, treatment, and Q&As. At three hours, it's intense. You might want to skip to sections you are most interested in: https://www.youtube.com/watch?v=ML7Jx-JbGxWI.

- There are many videos on YouTube about CAS. Look for those produced by reputable hospitals, universities, or organizations as well as those featuring speech-language pathologists with CCC (Certificate of Clinical Competence) after their name. In addition to Dr. Strand, above, I also recommend Dr. Ruth Stoeckel.

Chapter 6

So What Caused All of This?

Theories and Medical Diagnoses Related to CAS

You'd like to blame someone, *anyone,* for the misfortunate combination of luck and biology that led to your child having childhood apraxia of speech. But chances are, there is nothing or no one who can take the blame. There is a lot of conflicting information out there about what causes CAS. To date, the professionals can't agree on a cause—but there are lots of theories. I am certainly no expert in CAS theory, so if you really have an interest in this topic, I urge you to seek out additional resources.

Of course, you are wondering why *your* little one has CAS. As mentioned before, CAS is a relatively new diagnosis (not used for children until the 1960s) and much research is still going on. In fact, some practitioners and researchers say that we are still at square one in identifying this disorder. ***There are no clear-cut answers as to what caused your child to have CAS.***

But there are theories—several of them. Some theorists believe that CAS is based on underlying language issues. Others believe that the brain isn't formulating and sending the correct message to the muscles involved in speech. Still others think that children with CAS have problems listening to and interpreting speech. Genetic experts point out that CAS seems to runs in families—that members may have a history of apraxia, another speech concern (late-talking or stuttering for example), or other learning differences. Recent research findings point toward this genetic perspective.

The Nuts and Bolts of This Chapter

- A review of the ASHA 2007 *Ad Hoc Technical Document on Childhood Apraxia of Speech,* which summarized what is known about CAS and advanced three theories about its causes
- Familial factors, infectious diseases, and medically based diagnoses that may be involved with a CAS diagnosis
- Some theories about causes proposed by parents, including traumatic birth experiences and environmental toxins
- A discussion on the possibility of an "apraxia gene"

Starting at Square One: The ASHA Technical Report

We already know that it is hard to define CAS. If it's hard to define, then it's hard to identify its cause. CAS has been defined mostly by its characteristics, which has led to theories about its cause.

In 1994, SLPs Edythe Strand and Shelley Velleman suggested that CAS is a disorder of the "hierarchical organization of elements of the language/speech system into larger organized patterns." To put this into my own words, this means that children with CAS may be able to say some isolated speech sounds, but the more difficult words and phrases become, the harder it is for children to articulate what they want to say.

Velleman and Strand also asserted that kids with CAS may be impaired in their ability to organize and analyze information from their sensory, motor, and linguistic systems for spoken language. That is, kids with CAS may mentally receive and store information, yet they don't have the skills to organize and sequence that information into movements needed to make words and phrases. Much of what Velleman and Strand suggested in 1994 is still considered true today. But a lot has happened in the world of speech-language pathology since then—perhaps most importantly, the publication of the 2007 ASHA *Technical Report on Childhood Apraxia of Speech.*

In terms of the "discussion of apraxia," 2007 marked a pivotal point for the SLP community. ASHA convened a committee of highly respected SLPs to study the available information on CAS. ASHA's technical report was an important matter to the members of the committee and the SLP community at large. It is now a respected go-to document for caregivers, SLPs, and other healthcare professionals who need detailed information on childhood apraxia. If you have specific questions, concerns, or need more direction than provided here, please ask your child's SLP.

The definition of CAS proposed by the ASHA Ad Hoc Committee in the technical report was this:

> *Childhood apraxia of speech (CAS) is a neurological childhood speech sound disorder in which the precision and consistency of movements underlying speech are impaired in the absence of neurological deficits. . . . CAS may occur as a result of neurological impairment, in association with complex neurobehavioral disorders of known and unknown origin, or as an idiopathic neurogenic speech sound disorder. . . . The core impairment in planning and/or programming spatiotemporal parameters of movement sequences results in errors in speech sound production and prosody [under the link "definition" of the on-line report].*

Possible Causes of CAS Addressed in the ASHA Technical Report

With the exception of cases of *acquired apraxia of speech*—in which a child has a specific damage to the motor programming area of the brain (e.g., stroke, brain injury)—CAS typically does not show up on common brain scans. Therefore, the possible causes of CAS are mostly theoretical. The ASHA Ad Hoc Committee that studied CAS suggested three theoretical perspectives: 1) suprasegmental, 2) sensorimotor, and 3) auditory processing. As discussed below, all three perspectives take into account that the timing and coordination of speech is "out of whack."

Suprasegmental Perspective on Childhood Apraxia

Suprasegmental refers to the way in which a word is formed, the syllables involved, and the rate, rhythm, and stress [of the syllables] of the word. Most theorists agree that *both* syllables *and* prosody are affected in "more profound, distinctive ways in CAS" than they are in other speech problems. (See the link "Theories of CAS" in the ASHA technical document.)

As a parent, you may describe suprasegmental issues like this:

"My child seems to really struggle to find the right sounds when he speaks; when he finally 'gets it out,' his message sounds choppy." ("Choppiness" is part of prosody, as are rate, rhythm, stress, and intonation.)

Or perhaps you might say:

"He can say simple things just fine, but when he learns new, bigger words, it's really hard for him to say them." (Bigger words have more syllables = harder to communicate.)

Perhaps the "cause" in this perspective is an unidentified glitch underlying the motor-linguistic system that results in difficulties putting syllables together and producing them smoothly.

Sensorimotor Perspective on Childhood Apraxia

You may be wondering if apraxia is *just* sensory or *just* motor, or could it be a combination of both—*sensorimotor*? Well, the ASHA Ad Hoc committee had similar questions. They suggested that the core problem of CAS is in the relationship between perception (sensory processing) *and* some part of motor processing.

In 2002, Dr. Ben Maassen suggested that kids with CAS may have "poor sensorimotor learning," which can lead to weak "auditory mappings," which make talking more difficult. ASHA's 2007 technical document says, "A sensorimotor deficit could also underlie proposed difficulties in automating motor programs, such that each word production needs to be planned anew." In other words, children with CAS may have difficulties finding the "mental map" or "program" to say the word.

As a parent, you may recognize this as you think, "He really struggles to find the right sounds in words when he is talking."

Auditory Processing Perspective on Childhood Apraxia

While many children with CAS have "normal" results on hearing tests, they may have *some* subtle hearing/listening (auditory) deficits. If that's the case, then it could be that kids with apraxia aren't able to correctly detect and encode speech sounds from conversational speech, as Maggie Snowling and Elizabeth Bridgeman found in

1988. And ASHA's 2007 technical document says, "A few studies have addressed the hypothesis that children suspected to have CAS have deficits in auditory perception, auditory discrimination, and/or auditory memory." (For additional information on this theory, see the link "Speech Perception Characteristics" in the AHSA technical document)

As a parent, you might note a problem along these lines if you observe, "Even when I model the word correctly, it's as though he doesn't hear me right."

Parents Ask

Did I do something to cause my child to have apraxia?

The short answer is probably not. It's a completely natural and normal reaction to blame yourself, however. Parents I spoke with who shared their speculation and feelings about where their child's apraxia came from offered these theories about possible causes:

The top of the list included "traumatic birth." Moms mentioned umbilical cords being wrapped around their babies' necks (thus decreasing oxygen to the brain), emergency C-sections, low muscle tone noted at birth, and decreased heart rates during labor and delivery as potential concerns. One mother shared that her baby was born with poor suck reflexes, paralyzed vocal cords, and a need for tube feedings.

Others mentioned premature birth followed by a stay in the NICU. Some had babies with jaundice and wondered if that had anything to do with CAS. Other families mentioned that their child with CAS had chronic ear infections as an infant.

Many mothers were concerned that a glass of wine or a fall while they were pregnant did something to the developing neurological system of the embryo.

Finally, some theories from "apraxia moms" had to do with the environment and the food we consume. A mother in one of my Small Talk: All About Apraxia groups commented: "There's got to be some environmental connection here . . . pesticides or processed foods and preservatives that we are consuming as a nation."

While some of these factors might contribute to CAS, theorists agree that we simply don't know the cause. Eventually researchers will probably have a better idea of the causes, but for now, try not to blame yourself. Focus on helping and loving your child instead.

Genetic Disorders

A genetic disorder is one that is caused by a *difference* in the child's genes or chromosomes. Some genetic disorders are inherited (passed on from parent to child), while others occur spontaneously or randomly during conception or pregnancy. There are several noninherited and inherited conditions that are sometimes associated with CAS or CAS-type symptoms. If you are concerned that your child may have one of these genetic disorders, you should visit a geneticist. Genetic testing might be warranted.

Galactosemia

One group of CAS researchers—Donald Nelson and colleagues—found some connection between kids with CAS and a condition called galactosemia. It's an autosomal recessive inborn error of metabolism. *Autosomal recessive* means that it's an inherited genetic condition that is passed on through a particular type of chromosome (an autosome; not a sex chromosome) and that both parents have to have the gene for the disorder in order to pass it along to their offspring. Approximately 1 in every 60,000 kids in the United States have this condition. Basically it's when the body has a deficiency in the milk enzyme that converts galactose to glucose.

These researchers did a study of twenty-four kids and found that 54 percent had some characteristics of CAS, specifically syntax and word retrieval problems requiring extensive therapy.

If you suspect your child might have galactosemia, it's best to get the professional guidance of a physician and dietician. In the meantime, be sure to mention to your SLP any dietary issues such as milk intolerances. For more information, see that 2007 ASHA online report on CAS under the link "CAS Research in Complex Neurobehavioral Disorders."

Fragile X Syndrome

Fragile X syndrome is another inherited genetic disorder that can be accompanied by CAS. It is the second-most common cause of intellectual disabilities.

For some unknown reason, these individuals—usually males—have a "fragile" long arm of the X chromosome. (The X chromosome is one of two chromosomes that determine an individual's sex. Girls are born with two X chromosomes; boys have one X and one Y chromosome.) When there is damage to this area of the X chromosome, the child usually has some degree of intellectual disability. They also may have large ears and testes, an elongated jaw, prominent forehead, double-jointed joints, autistic-like behavior, heart defects, and speech delays. Girls and women "carry" the genetic material that cause fragile X-syndrome (they can pass it along to their sons), but do not often have symptoms themselves. Sometimes, though, they have difficulties with speech and language, anxiety, or learning disabilities.

By no means all kids who have CAS also have fragile X syndrome. And not all kids with fragile X have CAS—there is just a correlation.

For more information on fragile X, please visit the National Fragile X Foundation at https://fragilex.org/. The organization offers support for families and sponsors research toward improved treatments and possible cures.

Parents Share

"[My son] has fragile X syndrome but has never been officially diagnosed with apraxia. But the things I have read about it indicate we're also dealing with apraxia. Even his SLPs have said that he has it. He seems to understand what is said to him but he is unable to express verbally what he wants to say. And the few words he does say aren't very clear, or it may just be the beginning of a word."—Beth, mother of a child with fragile X syndrome

Down Syndrome

Almost every child with Down syndrome has some speech and language delays and difficulties, but there is a subset of children who have bona fide CAS symptoms on top of the usual speech and language delays in Down syndrome. Often the diagnosis is missed because SLPs will say, "Oh, it's just the Down syndrome [low muscle tone]." But children who have Down syndrome *plus* apraxia need different treatment than those who have Down syndrome alone.

One mother of a child with Down syndrome shared this: "Lily's therapist has always said she has 'motor planning issues' but blamed it on decreased tone. That makes it tricky—is the motor planning a result of the hypotonia or a disconnect with the brain?"

Lily's mother isn't the only person who has wondered about motor planning issues in children with Down syndrome. In 2003, Dr. Libby Kumin, CCC-SLP, completed a survey study in an effort to determine whether CAS was a widespread problem for children with Down syndrome. Over 1,500 families completed her survey.

Dr. Kumin found that 16 percent of the children with Down syndrome in her study had either been diagnosed with CAS or had been told that their child had difficulties with oral motor skills. Even when parents *had not* been given a diagnosis of apraxia, survey respondents often said their children were experiencing many symptoms consistent with CAS (most notably: more difficulty being understood than their peers with Down syndrome, sound reversals, and sound errors). The survey also showed that children with Down syndrome and apraxia tend to begin speaking at a later age—around five years—than kids with "just" Down syndrome.

Yet children with Down syndrome historically have not been identified as having childhood apraxia of speech. That's because early studies describing and identifying CAS were of children who had "normal" intelligence, as well as hearing within normal limits, and absence of muscle weakness (or paralysis).

If you have a child with Down syndrome and suspect CAS, please look for an SLP who has knowledge and experience in both disorders. One test an SLP can administer to a child with Down syndrome who has *some* verbal ability is the Kaufman Speech Praxis Test (KSPT). If the child cannot imitate words, CAS is often assessed with pictures such as those in the Kaufman Speech Praxis Treatment Kit (Basic Level) and a CAS characteristic checklist. At home, consider reading predictable books with your child, "singing" daily routines, using scripts and phrases repeated throughout the day ("Hi. How are you? What are you doing? See you later"). Picture clues to enhance communication can also help. These techniques can give your child with CAS and Down syndrome some experiences of success.

Prader-Willi Syndrome

Prader-Willi syndrome (PWS) was first discovered by Andrea Prader and Henrich Willi in 1956. It's a rare genetic (inherited) condition in which seven genes on chromosome 15 (q11–13) are missing or unexpressed ("switched off"). These children have a whole host of concerns, including the following: often a breech presentation resulting in a C-section birth, lethargy and low tone at birth, and, nearly always, decreased muscular tone, decreased suck reflex (feeding issues in infancy) leading to failure to thrive as an infant, delays in reaching childhood milestones, crossed-eyes/wandering eyes (strabismus), and intellectual delays. Children with PWS also have *speech delays, perhaps presenting as dysarthria and CAS.* As these children get older, they seem to "overcome" their infant feeding problems and become obese because they develop insatiable appetites. You can learn more about PWS at the International Prader-Willi Syndrome Organization by visiting https://www.pwsausa.org/international/.

Potocki-Lupski Syndrome (PTLS)

PTLS is a "contiguous" gene syndrome—meaning that there is an abnormality of two or more genes located next to each other on the same chromosome, thus carrying an extra copy of a tiny portion of a chromosome (in this case, it's a part of chromosome number 17). The condition is not inherited; it's due to an error in the formation of egg or sperm and cannot be prevented. PTLC is a recently discovered syndrome—the first case study appeared in 1996, and a detailed clinical description was published in 2007 by Drs. Lorraine Potocki and James Lupski of Baylor College of Medicine. As of this writing, about one thousand individuals have been described as being diagnosed with PTLS in the medical literature. However, it's predicted to occur in 1 out of 20,000.

One of the many symptoms present in this condition is CAS. Other symptoms include low muscle tone, poor feeding, failure to thrive as an infant, delayed development of verbal and motor milestones, mild intellectual disabilities, autistic-like behavior, ADHD, heart defects, sleep apnea, and possible crowding of teeth. For more information, visit the website of the PTLS Outreach Organization, http://ptls-foundation.org/.

Familial-Genetic Theories

Many children with CAS do not have one of the named genetic disorders discussed above. And yet there may still be a genetic component to their speech and language difficulties. That is, speech-language problems seem to run in some families. The idea that families may pass along the predisposition to have CAS is known as the familial-genetic theory.

In fact, science backs up this idea. In various studies conducted between 1957 and 1990, researchers found that there is a frequency and severity of speech problems within families of kids with CAS, at least according to Penny Hall's 1993 text, *Developmental Apraxia of Speech*. And in 2003, a study of family pedigrees of children with suspected CAS was published in the *Journal of Communication Disorders*. This study determined that speech-sound and language disorders tend to run in families with CAS (this is referred to as the "affection rate"). However, this study couldn't distinguish between environmental and genetic influences, nor could it ignore the fact that our historical memory can fail. ("Was it Aunt Mimi who had a stuttering problem, or Aunt Molly? Did Uncle Pete always have problems finding the right words—or was it just after he had that stroke?") The section "An Apraxia Gene?" on page 93 summarizes some more scientific studies on the family link.

Could a Genetic Problem Run in Your Family?

Without being too intrusive, take a look at your relatives—immediate and extended. You might want to refer to family photographs or just notice the next time you are all together at a family event. Is there a physical trait that everyone seems to have? Maybe they all have similarly spaced eyes or maybe all of the folks who have red hair also have a speech issue? Is there a family history of heart defects?

Look at any "odd" behavior(s) they may share. Do all of the women blink their eyes when they are trying to think of a word to complete their thoughts? Does everyone over a certain age have a noticeable shake in their hands or face? Is anyone in the family particularly restless to the point of being hyperactive?

Of course, you are not applying a formal scientific method to this homemade experiment. But you may find that your observations add up to something meaningful for you. If so, you might mention your observations to your child's doctor or SLP.

The Missing Link

Have you thought about the family members—extended and immediate—who may have had a speech disorder? I hadn't thought much about this until my husband told me that he had a lisp as a kid, "Everyone used to think it was cute, but I was sort of embarrassed by it, especially as I got older." I learned he received speech therapy through the third grade. And then I began asking more: Did your parents have a speech disorder? How about your grandparents?

Of course, it's hard to bring this up in an everyday situation. Ever had a Thanksgiving conversation in which you shoot the breeze, talk about the weather, politics, *and* religion and *then* ask, "So which one of you lovely relatives gave my kid childhood apraxia of speech?"

My Daughters' Genetic Legacy

I was more than curious. I was downright nosy. I asked my in-laws about the apraxia connection in our family. Here's what I learned:

Aside from **my husband's** lisp, he reportedly didn't talk until he was three years old. He has no idea if he started speaking in full, complete sentences at this time or if he just started with a few words. Unfortunately, his mother has passed away, and his dad just doesn't recall. My husband will tell you that he believes he had apraxia as a child, but this was never formally diagnosed. He would have been three—the typical age for a CAS diagnosis—in 1973, and we know that was a bit early in the development of diagnosing CAS. At best, he had a speech delay. Today, he's still introverted, but he can speak quite intelligently when he needs to.

And so I probed a bit deeper. I wanted to know about **his mother's speech history.** He told me that he felt his mom often had difficulties finding the right word (*dysnomia*) and confirmed that his maternal aunts also sometimes groped for words. Interestingly, two of these sisters are very extroverted, while the other is quite reserved. I would assume that if they truly have trouble finding words, they have adapted quite well. (CAS and word-finding problems are often confused. One SLP I talked with treated a bright child who had been unsuccessfully treated for word-finding. She actually had moderate to severe CAS. Keep in mind that there are separate tests for these disorders).

As for my **father-in-law**—well, he's a man of few words. Smart, yes. He worked for the Army Corp of Engineers his entire adult life—he can build a great dam, crunch some mathematical formulas—but communicating verbally is not one of his strong suits. To this day, he's the quiet one listening and soaking up family trivia at the Thanksgiving table. He's an only child, so no siblings to compare. He did mention, however, that he had a cousin who stuttered.

My outgoing **brother-in-law** seems to have no problems whatsoever with his speech. He loves to talk and make jokes and has the most contagious chuckle you've ever heard. He doesn't have biological kids, so it's hard to tell if he would have passed along an "apraxia gene."

At our last family gathering I learned that my **husband's cousin's children** had been treated for speech problems (though not CAS). Pieces of the puzzle were starting to come together! The cousins are the same generation as my girls . . . wonder what the connection is? Perhaps those maternal genes were coming into play?

OK, I'll be brief with my side of the family. **My dad** is a friendly, outgoing sort of guy who can play a game of golf with a stranger. But he would identify himself as an introvert. **His two brothers** have no problems communicating, although they all have a bit of a southern drawl thanks to their wholesome upbringing in southern Missouri. **His mother** had difficulty finding the words to communicate. As did **his father**—everything was a "whatcha-call-it" or a "thingamajig." My father would say this was because they weren't very educated and just didn't know the proper names of certain objects. Perhaps he's right, or maybe there's more to it.

On **my mom's side** there was a late-talking cousin, who we believed received speech therapy in the 1960s.

No apparent problems with **my younger sister.** She spoke on time and was a bit precocious. She did see a SLP at the urging of her orthodontist; apparently she needed training to know where to rest her tongue when it wasn't busy talking!

Me—well, I was a shy kid, but I could talk when I wanted to without any problems. I said my first words when I was supposed to but generally was a quiet child—engaging in my own creative world of art and literature. When I was in high school, I was active in speech and debate. But I can't carry a tune in a bucket.

Learn about Your Own Family

I give you this background so that you may begin the process of learning more about your family. It may give you an excuse for bringing the topic up: "I was reading this book about CAS, and the author mentioned several relatives with speech issues within her own family, including two daughters with CAS. What can you tell me about our family?"

When you do ask, keep in mind that there are lots of speech and language disorders to consider. Here's a list, though not exhaustive:

- late to talk
- stuttering
- stammering
- selective mutism (choosing not to speak in certain social situations)
- trouble finding the right words (groping and silent posturing)
- lisp
- trouble with certain sounds (e.g., words with the *r* sound)
- unintelligible and imprecise speech (others cannot understand his or her speech)
- volume of voice
- quality of voice (whispery, high-pitched, grating, hoarse, nasal)
- unusual rhythm to voice
- mumbling
- chewing/swallowing/eating difficulties
- learning disability
- writing/reading disability
- dyslexia

Remember, accidents from traumatic brain injuries, paralysis, or stroke causing some kind of speech impediment are not "passed down" and should not be considered in this equation.

What You Can Do at Home

Keep track of your "family speech pedigree"—that is, individuals in your child's family who may have had a speech-language or learning concern. Remember, this is not a diagnostic tool. It's just interesting to you and your child's speech pathologist to see whether there is a family connection. It does not indicate that there is a clear genetic cause for CAS, but it may show a *tendency* for speech problems for your family.

An Apraxia Gene?

You may be wondering, Aren't there any *real* genetic studies done on CAS? Yes, there are. We will end with a heady discussion on such matters. Please bear in mind that just as I am not a neurologist, I am not a geneticist. But I can help you understand what these two disciplines have to say about the possibility of an "apraxia gene."

In the early 1990s, a group of folks wanted to know if there really is an apraxia gene. Lo and behold, they found a mutation of a gene on chromosome 7 that they believe is strongly linked to CAS in one family—the "KE family" of London, England.

Researchers call this gene the *FOXP2* gene. There is still a good amount of research currently going on to better understand the role of *FOXP2* in childhood apraxia. Generally, the family members mentioned in this often-cited study had other differences as well: learning and academic disorders, sensory issues, linguistic and craniofacial (head-face) involvement that is not seen typically with kids who have *idiopathic* (no known cause) CAS. So, this means that although *FOXP2* may be involved in *some* cases of CAS, it's likely not involved in *all* cases.

Needless to say, findings from the KE family stirred many researchers into action. The London-Oxford group studied the KE family for over fifteen years and found that *FOXP2* genes were expressed widely in the cells throughout the brain. That is, the cognitive, speech, and language centers were affected. In fact, they found that the gene mutation affects *both* sides of the brain, which would explain why individuals with CAS tend to have *some* trouble with CAS-like characteristics beyond childhood (finding the "right" speech sounds for words when stressed, for example, or having difficulty saying larger words).

Other case studies have also recognized that there is a specific gene region on chromosome 7—and perhaps some other chromosomes—that appears to be connected with severe speech delay and CAS. For example, a 2005 research group in the United States headed up by Dr. Larry Shriberg found that CAS and dysarthria appeared in a mother and daughter with a chromosome "flip-flopping" (translocating) in a region affecting *FOXP2*. In Canada, researchers have identified a *FOXP2* deficit in a child who reportedly has CAS, as well as a craniofacial difference. However, it's really hard to say whether or not there are other genetic influences at play.

So, yes—it *does* look as if there are one or more CAS genes out there. We just need to be patient and let the genetic folks do what they do best: discover more. Again, more information on this topic can be accessed online via the 2007 AHSA Technical Report on CAS under the link "CAS Research in the KE Family."

Point to Ponder: Some researchers believe there are different factors (familial, genetic, neurological) that contribute to CAS, which would mean that there are subtypes of CAS. This could explain why every child with apraxia shows unique characteristics.

Parents Share

Talking about Possible Causes of CAS

One mother in a Small Talk: All About Apraxia group volunteered:

"I agree that it must be genetic. It shows up in my father's side of the family. My parental grandfather did not speak until he was five, and my dad is very hard to understand in either of the two languages he speaks fluently (English and Spanish). All of my sisters had speech therapy but are fine now. I never did myself, but I do have trouble pronouncing certain words for some reason. I somehow work around those hard words. My oldest daughter has no problems with speech; my middle daughter has severe verbal apraxia [CAS]. We noticed it at age one but were in denial. She was diagnosed when she was four. My youngest daughter is only twenty months old. She has some symptoms similar to her older sister, but not as severe. I guess it is genetic but doesn't affect all children in a family."

A mother of a son with apraxia added:

"I agree that a look into your family might help understand where CAS came from. There is a family connection to my son's apraxia. Now as an adult, I realize that I probably had CAS and so did my uncle, who received therapy in the 1930s. Once I had a child with apraxia, I began to understand why I had problems pronouncing words the same as my peers, in childhood and even adulthood."

Another parent stated: "My sons represent the fourth generation of speech disorders on my husband's side of the family, with each generation getting more severe."

A grandmother who contacted me said: "I was just at a family reunion. The subject of the grandkids came up, and I just learned my nephew was diagnosed with apraxia some twenty years ago. Makes sense now that my grandson has it [apraxia] too. I worry I've passed something on."

Finally, I once attended a meeting of The Apraxia Connection in the Chicago area and learned that every attendee had at least one family member who had a speech impediment or a strong suspicion that someone in the family had undiagnosed CAS!

"I Feel So Responsible . . . and Guilty"

Looking too hard at yourself or your family or analyzing everything about your pregnancy (or your partner's) can lead to guilty feelings. ***But there is nothing you could have done to have prevented this condition!*** If you knew without a doubt what caused your child to have CAS, would you suddenly feel relieved? Most likely, the answer is no.

But you still have questions and concerns. I bet they sound similar to these:

- How can I (the parent) help?
- What will my child's future academic life be like?
- Will it go away . . . and how?

All of these concerns will be discussed in later chapters.

Although it's interesting to think about possible causes, it's important not to dwell on them for too long. Believe me, I've been there. To this day, I *still* wonder why Kate had apraxia. I wonder if it was something I did when I was pregnant, or if I failed to use enough "mother-ese" when talking with her. Eventually, I got to the point where I said, "It doesn't really matter. It is what it is. I love her regardless. I will do whatever it takes to help her become a better communicator."

Your next step is helping your child be as successful and happy as possible!

It's clear we need more research into causes. Not to fear—plenty of researchers are hard at work trying to make sense of this complex disorder. You are doing your part by questioning and reading about it. Below is a list of more tips and ideas to support research related to the causes of CAS:

- ***Consider getting an appointment with a geneticist.*** Seeing a geneticist is not entirely necessary in order get a diagnosis of CAS. Genetic testing may be recommended, however, if your child has other features or delays (poor motor skills or auditory processing or cognitive problems) that may indicate a genetic condition. Talk to your pediatrician first and then your insurance company to get the green light to enter the "genetic district."
- Remember, if you had ***amniocentesis or CVS*** (chorionic villis sampling), that counts as genetic testing. Review those results before pursuing major genetic studies.
- ***Read and research what others have done (or are doing)*** to help the discipline of childhood speech and language disorders. Consider making a donation to such organizations.
- ***Help advocate for your child.*** Having a genetic diagnosis can open some doors to services such as therapies and educational support through an early intervention program or the public school.

- *Don't beat yourself* up thinking that you caused your child to have CAS by passing on "bad" genetic material.

Say That Again?! Chapter Summary

It's a tough call when some well-meaning person asks you what causes childhood apraxia of speech. Short of ripping out this chapter and making copies to distribute to everyone you meet, you can sweetly say, "It could be a number of reasons. Too many to count." That's what the Geek Squad told me when I needed a new hard drive for my computer. That's it in a crude kind of nutshell—your little one's hard drive just needs a Geek Squad (enter the SLPs, pediatricians, and other professionals).

Otherwise, you could say, "It's idiopathic" (we don't know what caused it)—which is true for the majority of children with CAS at present.

Keep track of family connections as you learn about them. The more members of your child's family who have a speech-language delay or learning difference, the more likely your child may have CAS or another speech-language difference.

Geneticists and brain researchers are just beginning to find some links between specific genes and CAS. At this point, nothing regarding CAS and genetics is definitive—it's all speculative. The bottom line: we need more research.

Recommended Resources

- Additional information on fragile X syndrome is available from the *National Fragile X Foundation:* www.fragilex.org or 800–688-8765.
- This book by Libby Kumin, PhD, CCC-SLP, is a great resource for learning more about speech and language difficulties in children with Down syndrome: *Early Communication Skills for Children with Down Syndrome: A Guide for Parents and Professionals,* 3rd edition (Woodbine House, 2015).
- I also love this book, *A New Course: A Mother's Journey Navigating Down's Syndrome and Autism* by Teresa Unnerstall (Kat Biggie Press, 2020). Written by a mother, this memoir is sympathetic, engaging, and even humorous at times, plus, Nick was also diagnosed with CAS. You'll find many tips and experiences that will help you on your journey.
- If you want to learn more about genetics, then look to *The Cartoon Guide to Genetics,* by Larry Gonick and Mark Wheelis (HarperCollins, 2014). You just may find yourself laughing as you read it! Another option is *Genetics for Dummies* by Tara Rodden Robinson (For Dummies, 2nd ed. 2010).
- You can download an article from the *Journal of Communication Disorders* entitled "Family Pedigree of Children with Suspected Childhood Apraxia of Speech" by B. A. Lewis, L. A. Freebarin, A. Hansen, and G. Taylor: www.waisman.wisc.edu/phonology/pubs/PUB10.pdf.

- ***Out Came the Sun: One Family's Triumph Over a Rare Genetic Syndrome*** by Judith Scott (Chicago Review Press, 2008) is an uplifting, well-written memoir you may find comfort and hope in.
- In ***What I Thought I Knew*** (Viking, 2009), Alice Eve Cohen writes a candid memoir that reads like a novel about her daughter with a genetic disorder. There are plenty of suggestions on coping intertwined.

Chapter 7

All about Speech Therapy

An Introduction to Ideas & Methods Best Suited for CAS

Imagine you are in grade school and someone asks you what you are going to be when you grow up. You tell her you want to be a doctor. "But, what *kind* of doctor?" she presses. Well, just as with doctors, there are all kinds of speech-language pathologists, therapy styles, and methods out there.

There are lots of types of speech therapy. Your SLP probably has his or her favorite style—which is likely to be a hybrid of standard models. In fact, it has been suggested that kids with CAS benefit best from a multimodal approach; that is—a combination approach.

A SLP ought to be creative and flexible when working with kids. After all, we know kids can be unpredictable, have short attention spans, and tend to be easily frustrated. How an SLP plans treatment sessions is based on your child's age, temperament, and interests, as well as on your SLP's personality and education. Just as a great pediatrician or kindergarten teacher is your new best friend, a skilled pediatric SLP is an invaluable resource. Count yourself lucky if you have found one.

You will likely come across many new terms reflecting strategies commonly used in the world of speech-language pathology. So, let's begin by defining some terms.

The Nuts and Bolts of This Chapter

- What speech therapy consists of, goals of therapy, and how to track progress
- Various types and methods of speech therapy, such as natural (play) therapy, directive approach, individual vs. group therapy, as well as modeling and direct versus indirect instruction
- The top eleven things you and your child's SLP should be doing for success in a motor-programming apraxia approach
- The importance of imitation
- The parent's role in therapy

The Naturalistic Approach

Remember life sciences in biology? Don't worry; I won't make you relive a painfully boring seventh-grade lesson. Humor me for a moment. Where do frogs naturally spend their time? Are you picturing a pond hidden in the woods? What do frogs do? They hop around and eat bugs with their long, sticky tongues. What do frogs sound like? Well, they croak and grunt. This is the natural environment of a frog. If a preschool-aged frog had CAS, he would likely have therapy in the pond on a lily pad with his favorite stuffed fly as a stimulus for croaking.

SLPs often use a naturalistic approach that involves play, particularly with young children. After all, play is the natural medium for kids to learn. A therapy session may last an hour, and in that hour, there are multiple ways your child will be learning. Your SLP will likely use a variety of stimuli—toys, art, books, games, and puzzles, written work, and old-fashioned "drills," possibly in combination with some gross motor/movement time. All of the activities will focus on your child's predetermined therapy goals. Be sure you know your child's therapy goals beforehand.

Think about it: what are you naturally interested in? Let's say it's architecture. You love visiting display homes and you dream of designing your own house some day. You know the difference between a Doric column and a Corinthian column; dentil molding and crown molding. You can *talk* about architecture because you *like* it, because you have an *interest* in it. Your child is no different, although her interests may be.

Parents Ask

What's the deal with movement activities?

You may feel that your child is in therapy to talk, not run around! But according to Diane Bahr, MS, CCC-SLP, and author of *Feed Your Baby* and *Toddler Right*, "Movement activities can encourage vocalizations. Think of how vocal children can become on a playground, even children who are generally quiet. Short movement breaks during therapy can also help a child tolerate relatively long segments of structured speech treatment. Speech work is, after all, a fine motor activity. It can become tedious without breaks for children with speech difficulties."

In figuring out how to work with your child, the SLP usually considers the following:

- your child's age (language is still—and always—developing),
- the severity of the CAS,
- your child's overall knowledge base,
- your child's attitude and temperament, and
- what motivates your child.

You can help with some of these areas. Let your SLP know of any tips and tricks you've used at home, particularly things that motivate your child, even if they're not directly related to speech. For example, you may have found your child is more excited to wash her hands before mealtime when you provide the neat, color-changing soap. She does better staying in bed at night when you offer a reward from the prize box in the morning. You get the idea.

However, if your child needs a lot of motivation to speak, and she is best motivated by food, don't take her to speech with a full tummy; the speech-language pathologist's bargaining power may be lost! (Be sure to tell your child and SLP if snacking during therapy is okay; mention any food allergies).

Your child will also do better at speech-related tasks when she has something to work for. Sorry, but acquiring the ability to communicate thoughts, ideas, and feelings is not the kind of motivation that will get the job done—at least not for your kid.

Another point to keep in mind is that play—and therapy—should always be child-directed but SLP-selected. Once your SLP knows what your little one likes to do and is good at, she will likely present several options for therapy that day. It may be that every option is selected by your child (the game, the kitchen play, and the Play-Doh), or the entire session may be devoted to one activity: Play-Doh.

The important thing is that there are options and your child gets to choose the one(s) that excites her the most. Choice making is an important form of communication. It often pays off when you are attempting to encourage spontaneous speech in "everyday" and new settings. When you think about it, that's what you want for your child—for her to communicate in all settings, not just the SLP's office or the preschool or school program. Your SLP can help you figure out ways to encourage your child's communication at home (see chapter 9).

"This just looks like play," you may say. Well, remember that "play is children's work." It looks unstructured and playful because it is. But, your SLP has a plan. She knows your child's goals and is taking a "backdoor" approach to the anticipated outcome. She is flexible and creative and allowing your child to have some control over the process. This is one key to successful treatment.

Naturalistic Teaching Methods

The idea behind naturalistic teaching methods is that kids are learning language in a meaningful way. Language is usually learned in a social context (play *is* social, and so are daily interactions such as meals, bath time, bedtime, etc.). Remember, speech is not *just* a "task to be learned" or something to be crossed off a to-do list.

Parents, this puts you in the driver's seat as "language educator." You can encourage reciprocity and turn-taking. You can follow your child's lead and expand her utterances, and finally, you can provide positive feedback during your child's interactions. Although speech and language are functional, they should also be "*fun*"ctional! You'll find plenty of ideas in chapter 9.

The Directive Approach

This approach may be a little more drill sergeant–like. It's more structured than the naturalistic approach. The SLP will likely direct the types of activities that take place and when. A large portion of the session may be devoted to drills. For example, the SLP might say a word and then have your child attempt saying it. They may do this several times in a row. It's hard work—for both SLP and child—and it can be a little boring. Drills work best when a child has the maturity to do them. They are used to help a child practice a particular speech skill. Directive therapy is also good for introducing words of increased difficulty, such as words with more than one syllable.

"A child as young as two years of age can participate in drill-like activities when play is incorporated. Speech drill-work provides a child with the practice needed to develop speech-motor plans," says SLP Di Bahr.

Bottom line: Try to find an SLP who uses *both* naturalistic and directive styles.

Tip: Children with CAS want to communicate. They are working so very hard to repeat and mimic language. When you say "ball" and show them a big bouncy ball and then ask, "Can you say *ball*," you mean well. But your child simply cannot repeat the word due to a neurological glitch. Plus, it's not exactly natural; it's not how people communicate or carry on conversations. You can roll the ball, bounce the ball, talk about the ball, but your child will not say "ball" until she has worked out the motor pathways to do so. This takes time and the skill of a SLP. Plus, drills like this may lead your child to shut down and even become resentful. And now everyone's frustrated. Take it slow.

Individual vs. Group Therapy

Speech therapy can be conducted in a couple of different manners. The most frequently used approaches are one-on-one therapy and small or large group therapy. Each of these approaches has its pros and cons, and ideally children would receive therapy in the setting best suited to their needs. But depending on who is paying for your child's therapy (the early intervention program or school vs. you, the parent, vs. your health insurance plan), you may not have a choice as to the setting where therapy is provided.

One-on-One (Individual) Therapy

In this type of therapy, the child and SLP work together closely on the child's specific speech goals. Individual therapy is especially good for beginning therapy with a child and for children with more severe CAS. Children learn comfort and trust. They build a relationship with their SLP. Your child's SLP learns about your child in these sessions, too. He or she can pay close attention to the small utterances your child is making and can closely observe body language.

One-one-one therapy is also good for establishing new skills and learning the rules of grammar, such as usage of pronouns and connectors such as "and" and "or." Think back to when you were learning something new. You may have felt self-conscious at first. Perhaps you didn't want to try playing the piano in a room full of relatives, but you were okay with your piano instructor and your sister in the room. Speech therapy is no different. Kids need privacy to practice something that is new and difficult for them.

One-on-one therapy is best for kids with CAS. The reason is that children and their SLP must focus directly on each other. The child must watch the SLP's mouth and vice versa. It is difficult for an SLP to divide her time and attention between several children while still giving a child with CAS the undivided attention she needs.

Group Therapy

Just as the name implies, this type of therapy involves a group of kids, usually working on common goals. The group could be as large as a preschool classroom of fifteen to twenty kids, or it could be a group of just two children. Group therapy is great for kids working on social interactions related to speech (pragmatics). SLPs can group kids together based on their skill level or based on common goals. Group work can also be used to assess carry-over from private therapy sessions. Problem speech habits that need some extra work in individual therapy may be more apparent in group therapy.

In school settings, group therapy may be the only approach available because SLPs are often stretched to their limits with large caseloads. But group therapy can occur in a private setting as well. The kids with whom SLPs are working are usually at the same developmental level and have similar speech goals. Sometimes, however, kids with widely varied goals are put into a group simply because it's the best fit for their schedules. If this happens to your child, and you feel it's a waste of time, speak up. There is no sense in paying for therapy—in time or money—if it's not working for your family.

On the plus side, group therapy can result in peer bonding! If the other members of the group have similar problems and are at a similar skill level, it can also provide a safe place to practice conversational skills. But it can also be nerve-racking for a child who feels shy about revealing her speech difficulties in front of others.

How Does It Work? A Peek Inside a Group Session

Kelly, my youngest daughter, attended private speech therapy sessions with another little girl of approximately the same age and abilities. While working individually in private therapy, Kelly seemed very comfortable with the SLP and therapy expectations. But when she was with the other little girl and the other SLP—there were actually two SLPs in the one session—she became quiet and less responsive. She was less likely to initiate conversation. While this may seem less than ideal, this experience gave Kelly opportunities to observe turn-taking, play, and the communicative style of a peer. Kelly didn't receive group therapy *every* time she attended private speech therapy, and it didn't last the full session, but it was a good way to get her to open up.

In preschool, my older daughter, Kate, participated in classroom-wide speech games, as well as "pull-out" therapy with another student or two. She had fun with the games and the work she did with her classmates, leading to increased social interactions and peer bonding.

We also used another style of combination therapy with Kate. When Kate was working on pragmatics (such as using a "sweet" voice while orchestrating play with others), we brought little sister Kelly into the hour-long session for about ten to fifteen minutes. It was interesting to see how they played and communicated (and argued!) with each other. This gave the SLP an inside view of what we experienced at home. It also gave the SLP an opportunity to facilitate appropriate interactions between our girls.

What about Online Therapy (Teletherapy)?

During a public health emergency such as the Covid-19 pandemic, your child might be asked to switch to teletherapy, regardless of whether she's been receiving individual or group speech-language therapy.

Teletherapy (or telepractice) refers to speech-language therapy that is delivered via a secure online connection and video conferencing software. If your child is receiving therapy through the public school, and the school as a whole is using online instruction, she and her SLP will have therapy sessions via computer screen rather than in person. Together they will continue to work on your child's speech goals to meet required IEP minutes (unless otherwise notified).

The SLP may use online games and websites to work on speech targets. Vicki, mother of ten-year-old Jack, says, "Our SLP used videos and shared her screen so she and Jack could watch a video together and practice story summarizations, word-finding, and thought-organization."

Allison, a parent in Ohio, says, "Our SLP quickly got Nate on fifteen-minute Zoom calls with us. She used Boom Cards [see box] to interact with Nate. We were able to focus on his specific goals. It wasn't until I was observing the Zoom calls that I fully understood how to work with Nate on his speech."

In fact, "Parent inclusion is vital in teletherapy, as it is essential to the success and continued growth of the child's communication skills," according to Maureen Wilson, MS, CCC-SLP, a school-based SLP in Illinois and founder and author of The Speech Bubble blog. "For example," she says, "a parent may need to facilitate or prompt their child and assist with any technical issues or computer navigation." Jack's mother found this to be true, noting that they needed to first work through technical aspects of Microsoft Teams, and then her son "was able to have engaging sessions with his SLP."

Sometimes attention spans can be an issue. Allison says her five-year old son is only able to tolerate about fifteen-minutes online sessions. Jack, at ten years old, can stay engaged for a little longer. What is considered reasonable may vary depending on your child's age and other factors.

If your child has been receiving private speech-language therapy at a clinic (not school) and that clinic is closed for a public health reason, teletherapy may be a viable option to ensure speech-language skills are maintained.

You can visit the ASHA website to learn more about teletherapy (click on "Telepractice Resources"), although much of this information is geared toward speech-language pathologists and not parents. You can also check the Apraxia Kids website (www.apraxia-kids.org) for pertinent information about speech-language therapy during a public health emergency.

> **Wait! What Are Boom Cards?**
> Boom Cards are digital interactive task cards (something like mini-worksheets) that can provide immediate feedback. They are also self-checking, which is handy when you need to collect data while doing therapy from your living room. They might involve dragging and dropping pieces, typing in the correct answer, clicking on multiple choice answers, etc. They let children play with and manipulate words and pictures while they learn. Giving kids the ability to manipulate something on a screen is a fabulous way to keep them engaged while doing teletherapy. If your SLP uses Boom Cards, he or she will send your child digital links to the cards.

Parent/Family Participation

You and your family must be actively involved in treatment. It is a partnership between you, your child, and your SLP. Generally, you and your child's SLP will discuss options for how therapy will proceed. If you're not given options, speak up and ask. You know your child better than anyone else does and can suggest alternatives and ideas your SLP may not have considered. After all, you (and/or your insurance company) are likely paying big bucks to get these little people talking. (If your child is receiving therapy through an early intervention or public school program, see chapters 3 or 11. You have the right to participate in the development and monitoring of your child's Individualized Family Service Plan or Individualized Education Program.)

Be an active participant in discussing the pros and cons of the various aspects of treatment with your SLP and spouse/significant other so that your child will benefit from everyone's efforts. Also keep in mind that CAS is a dynamic condition—it's always changing—and so should the style of therapy. Maybe you have heard the saying "If you keep doing what you've always done, you're going to keep getting what you've always got"? Don't be afraid to ask questions, make suggestions, and shake it up a bit.

In *Nobody Ever Told Me (or My Mother) That!*, author Diane Bahr talks about the partnership between parents and professionals: "Many parents seem intimidated by professionals. However, professionals are people too. So try to relax when you are working with them. It is best for you and your child if you can work in partnership with any professional your child may need."

Remember, you'll need to be a team player. That means everyone, including your child, is a member of the team. All members have value. *CAS is a complex condition that requires consistent and persistent work to resolve.*

What You Can Do at Home

Before you get to the SLP's office for that first session, make a list of things your child enjoys doing:

- What are her favorite types of books?
- What toys can she play with—independently—for a substantial amount of time?
- What activities can she do for long periods of time (create art, play hide-and-seek, climb, assemble a puzzle)?
- Does she have a favorite character (from TV, movies, books)?
- What does she notice in the "real world?" Babies, trees, dogs? Something else?
- What frightens or intimidates her? (Make note of this so the SLP doesn't suggest barking like a dog if, for example, she's been bitten by one in the past.)
- How does your child learn best? Is she a quiet observer, active go-getter, someone who needs to warm up to a new task first?

A pediatric SLP often has about thirty to sixty children in his or her caseload—most of whom have different interests, learning styles, and speech goals. Your SLP develops a specific lesson plan for each child. Your suggestions for what might work best for *your child* are invaluable.

Therapy Strategies

Before we get into the nitty-gritty details of therapy strategies for CAS in particular, it's good to know that there are two main types of approaches to speech therapy in general:

1) *The Bottom-up Approach.* The SLP introduces easy to hard (simple to more complex) sounds/words such as vowels (V), as in "oh"; consonant-vowel (CV), as in "me"; vowel-consonant (VC), as in "up"; and consonant-vowel-consonant (CVC), as in "mom."
2) *The Hierarchical Approach.* The SLP starts where the child is presently performing; that is, she starts with what the child can say already.

In the table below you will find various traditional, but not necessarily CAS-specific therapy strategies with a brief definition.

Therapy Strategy	Definition
Direct Modeling	Usually in the early stages of therapy, the SLP demonstrates (models) the correct pronunciation of a mispronounced word within a natural conversation. The child looks directly at the SLP's face. There may be immediate or delayed imitation. For example, "Watch me and say it with me. Now, say it as I mouth it. Now, say it as I give you cues. Now, say it alone."
Indirect Modeling	The SLP provides frequent and correct pronunciation of a target letter. Say the target letter is /b/: "I see a *boat*. A *blue boat*. A *big blue boat*. It's *beautiful*." This is a "back-door approach" from the SLP's point of view.
Cues	Can be verbal or nonverbal. SLP might use this strategy to get the child's attention to focus; e.g., "Look at my lips as I say *kitty*." A visual cue may involve showing a picture or a card, or some other visual reminder. The goal here is to shape and stimulate articulators (lips, jaw, tongue), improving functional communication.
Prompts	Can be verbal or nonverbal and may include instructions, gestures, demonstrations, touches, or anything we arrange or do to increase the likelihood that children will make correct responses. Prompts are designed to lead children to the correct answer or response. For example, the SLP may say, "Put the baby in the bed" to demonstrate the concepts of in and out.
Successive Approximation (May also be referred to as "backward chaining") In order to use this approach, your child must be able to imitate words at least 70 percent of the time and be able to produce two syllables in a word.	Breaking a word or phrase down and asking the child to get closer and closer to saying it correctly over time—works **only** with multisyllabic words. For example, Kelly had a hard time saying her name. Our SLP started with "Say *ly [lee]*" and then "Say *Keh*"—before long, she was saying *"Kelly!"*

Expanding	Rephrasing what was said in a more complex thought. "Cookie?" becomes, *"Oh, you want a cookie? Yummy. I love these oatmeal cookies. Here is a cookie for you."*
Fading	Fading means ***progressive elimination*** of a prompt. Once you have mastered a certain skill, you no longer need that "crutch" to keep you going (think training wheels on a two-wheeler). Now your child may only need part of the prompt to respond.
Oral Placement Therapy (OPT) developed by Sara Rosenfeld-Johnson	Oral Placement Therapy uses a combination of: hearing (auditory stimulation), seeing (visual stimulation), and touching (tactile stimulation) the mouth to improve speech clarity. It is a tactile-proprioceptive teaching technique to accompany traditional therapy. Traditional therapy is primarily "hear and see" [me speak], so this approach adds in another layer. OPT can be used with children of many ages and ability levels and incorporated into treatment for CAS but requires facial touch. If this is a concern for your child, it may not be an ideal option. OPT is used *in addition* to other treatments for children who cannot produce or imitate speech sounds using the traditional "hear and see" method. SLPs should spend less than 15 minutes per session on this type of therapy with your child. OPT is also useful for children who may need physical cues for redirection (i.e., focus/attention concerns).
Syllable Flexibility Drills (using **C**onsonant - **V**owel or **V**owel - **C**onsonant words)	Uses what the child can already say. Sequences such as *ba-ba-ba-ba* are repeated 4 to 10 times. Then the vowel is changed: "Now say *bi-bi-bi-bi*." Next, alternate the two sounds: *ba-bi-ba-bi*. Finally, throw in something different: *bi-ba-bo-bu*." The difficulty is gradually increased over time. This approach works on the *movement* of speech.

Awareness through **Auditory Bombardment**	Presents words and phrases with targeted sounds. Similar to indirect modeling, above. Say the targeted sound is /k/. You might read a list of words with the /k/ sound to your child over and over. "I want you to listen as I read these words to you: *key, comb, coat, kitty, candy*. . . ." You spend a minute or so reading, two or three times a day. We made up silly stories about words: "The kitty wore his coat while he ate candy and carried the key." Make it personal to the child if you can. Keep in mind, this is a time for listening. Children may benefit from something to increase attention/focus (e.g., fidget toy). It's often a warm-up before practicing target words or phrases. Cupping your hands over your mouth and moving close to your child's ear, or even using an amplification device on your phone, may help your child hear the subtle changes in speech transitions.
Minimal Pair Therapy	This type of therapy helps kids differentiate between two words that are different in just one way, such as *bay* vs. *boy* and *cop* vs. *cot*. Minimal pairs can also be used in listening activities as well as speech production activities.

When Kate was in speech therapy, our SLP used the ***Touch-Cue Method*** developed by Bahir, Graham-Jones, and Bostwick. This would fit under the category "prompts/ cues" in the chart above. In the most basic sense, it is used for kids who have problems establishing and integrating voluntary oral movements for speech, especially in connected speech. It works like this: The SLP provides touch-cues to the child's face or neck. For example, when Kate was learning to say her own name, her SLP would tap on the front of Kate's neck (above the Adam's apple) for the /k/ sound. When Kate had trouble with the /s/ sound, Ms. Jen slid her finger down Kate's arm from shoulder to wrist, while saying /s/. Ms. Jen taught Kate to make these gestures herself, without watching her SLP for guidance. Eventually, Kate could make these sounds without giving herself the cues. In therapy-speak, phasing out cues is known as "fading."

I had the opportunity to chat with Karen George, MS, CCC-SLP, of Chicago Speech Therapy, who has developed a unique treatment approach in which SLPs perform speech-language therapy in-home. She speaks highly of using integral stimulation in the treatment of CAS. "[Integral stimulation] is also referred to as the 'watch me, listen, do as I do' approach using multimodal cues (gestural modes of body movement, pointing, sign, and conversational gestures) to teach the child new information. What appears to be a natural progression toward more complex speech patterns and movements for a normally developing child is a more effortful, demanding, and slow process for a child affected by CAS. So learning this longer speech routine takes much more practice, just as learning a dance for a recital would take more time for other children."

Ms. George continued on to explain that these important steps should be included for CAS therapy to be effective using integral stimulation:

1. The child watches and listens and then produces the sound or movement simultaneously with the SLP.
2. The SLP demonstrates, and then the child repeats the sound or movement simultaneously while the SLP mouths it.
3. The SLP demonstrates and provides cues and the child repeats.
4. The SLP demonstrates and the child repeats with no cues provided.
5. The SLP elicits the sound or movement without demonstrating (e.g., asking a question with the child responding spontaneously).
6. The child produces the sound or movement in less-directed situations with SLP's encouragement in role-play or games.

Tip: Your child's SLP will determine what type of therapy he or she feels is best suited to your child based on many factors, including age, severity of CAS, your child's interests and abilities, personality, focus, and more. Sometimes a child will "plateau" at a certain level or mode of therapy; progress becomes spotty. Changing it up can work wonders. As one SLP shared, "I had been doing similar things over and over with a child who has severe CAS. When I tried OPT in addition to our other therapies, the results were magical."

Parents Ask

What therapeutic intervention is best for kids with CAS?

I wish I had the answer to this question, because it is frequently asked by parents and discussed among SLPs and researchers. However, the studies that have been completed on the various therapeutic techniques for the treatment of CAS are limited. Therefore, SLPs haven't really identified one therapy that is more effective than others. Most SLPs emphasize a motor-programming approach (see below). Remember, CAS is unique and individual for each child. A combination approach developed by your child's SLP is probably "best."

Motor-Programming Approaches

Of course you are aware now that CAS is a neuro-motor disorder of speech. So wouldn't it make sense to start out with a motor-programming approach to therapy? *The goal here is to voluntarily, accurately, and consistently control speech articulators.* (Remember, articulators are the jaw, lips, and tongue.) Reaching this goal will enable your child to say words and sounds when she *wants* to, or when *asked* to do so.

Before we jump into an explanation of the motor learning approaches to CAS, it is important for you to understand what motor learning is all about. First, a child needs *motivation*. Next, a child needs *focused attention*. She needs to be able to focus on the actual movement of saying the words (e.g., "did you see how that felt when you said _____?") while *also* paying attention to the SLP. Finally, for a motor learning approach to be effective, a child needs to practice. The best example I can give to illustrate this concept is learning to ride a bike. The motivation is "I want to ride a bike just like my big sister." The focused attention is, "I feel wobbly when I look down; maybe if I look straight ahead I will feel more balanced." And the child needs plenty of practice before she is independently riding!

Advanced, Evidence-Based Training Approaches

DTTC and PROMPT (as well as PECS, mentioned earlier) are evidence-based methods for treating children with CAS. They are the only methods *proven* to treat this complex speech disorder.

DTTC and PROMPT require both instructional and independent practice. Speech-language pathologists knowledgeable in DTTC and/or PROMPT have sought additional intensive training and fine-tuned their expertise in treating CAS. Not all SLPs are trained in these methods.

Dynamic Temporal and Tactile Cueing (DTTC)

This research-based treatment approach is a very effective method for children with severe CAS. It's a hybrid approach to motor learning developed by Dr. Edythe Strand and colleagues at the Mayo Clinic. It is based on the 1973 work of John Rosenbek on *adults* with acquired apraxia of speech, *not* CAS. It is used with children who have difficulty with verbal imitation—a common characteristic of CAS. Let's break it down:

1. The child and SLP say the word together very slowly with touch cues and/or gestures.

2. Next, the SLP asks the child to increase her rate so that she is speaking at a more normal rate and there is no groping for words.

3. The SLP begins to fade the cue (saying the word with the child) by first speaking in a quieter voice, then whispering the word with the child, and then just mouthing the word with the child.

4. Then the SLP works directly on imitation and asks the child to wait one or two seconds before the child imitates her.

5. Finally, the SLP asks the child to spontaneously produce the word by saying, "What's this called?" (perhaps pointing to an object, picture, or word).

The key to DTTC is that the SLP works to fine-tune the speaking process so that the child can ultimately respond or speak spontaneously (a process referred to as "task analysis"). DTTC is a good example of a multisensory treatment method, as it involves three of the basic senses: seeing, hearing, and feeling.

PROMPT

PROMPT (not to be confused with prompting) is an acronym that stands for: **P**rompts for **R**estructuring **O**ral **M**uscular **P**honetic **T**argets. It is a sensory-motor-based technique developed by Deborah Hayden, MA, CCC-SLP, in which children develop awareness for verbal communication through multisensory cueing. That is, the SLP acts as an "external programmer" for speech by physically touching—and moving—the child's facial structures (lips, jaw, tongue, and cheeks) in order to "show" the child the correct way to say something. Research shows that one to two sessions weekly of PROMPT therapy can help children with CAS shape muscle movements. See below for more information on PROMPT.

Nanette Cote, MA, CCC-SLP, a pediatric speech-language pathologist in private practice and author of *We Talk on Water: Guide for Developing and Orchestrating Successful Group Social Communication*, indicates the protocol is to begin a speech session with a PROMPT "warm-up," which helps remind the child's motor plan how to move.

Tip: *Only* speech-language pathologists can be trained in PROMPT techniques. Unlike other assignments that may be suggested for home use, PROMPT techniques are reserved for the speech clinic only.

Sounds Like a Plan!

You have heard this notion of a "motor plan/programming" often in your CAS journey. So, just what is a motor plan? In terms of speech, it's the development of timing and coordination strategies necessary to produce a series of speech sounds. For example, without the right timing of sounds, words come out as gibberish. CAS occurs because there is a disruption in a child's ability to learn and control the motor planning aspects of speech, which happens at a neuro-motor level.

There are stages to motor learning. For example, these are the stages described in 1991 by Richard Schmidt:

- **Verbal-cognitive Stage:** The child knows the goals of therapy; makes initial attempts to say target words, but with less attention and effort.
- **Motor Stage:** The child begins to develop motor programs for movement; words become smoother and better timed; more consistent.
- **Autonomous Stage:** Movement gestures are perfectly performed with less effort/attention.

A motor-programming approach has a few rules you should keep in mind for it to work successfully. Here are *the top eleven elements needed for a successful motor-programming "CAS" approach to therapy:*

1. **Intensive Services.** What one defines as "intensive" will vary. Should it be daily? Weekly? Since these kids tend to progress slowly, you will see results faster with intense therapy. Most SLPs suggest twice-weekly appointments. These kids do best with as much therapy as time and money will allow. But beware of burnout. Speech therapy time and money commitments can quickly add up. Remember, you'll need to practice with your child five to seven days a week outside of therapy time. You are helping her develop and change motor habits; doing so requires a lot of practice (and patience)!

2. **Many Repetitions and Drills.** The goal is for your little one to produce words and phrases without really thinking about *how* to make them. She needs to sequence speech movements correctly, and she needs to develop those neuro-pathways. Let your child "rest" her mouth structures after a certain number of repetitions, especially if she is showing any sign of fatigue. You won't necessarily *see* fatigue, but you may *hear* it (your child has problems saying words she could previously say well).

Consider this scenario: You are working with a personal trainer. The next day your muscles are sore, so you take the day off from exercise. The next time you meet with your trainer, you remember some of the exercises because you have done them before—and your body remembers them, too. It's the same idea for your child in therapy. But the "resting portion" may be only a minute or two while the SLP jots down some notes before she asks your child to complete another speech task. If you are working on speech at home, you can have your child take a quick gross motor break: "Okay, now show me five jumping jacks!"

A couple in the Chicago suburbs gleaned this from their child's pediatric neurologist: "Using speech therapy for a child with CAS is comparable to using a personal trainer for an exercise program—[SLPs] can show you what to do and provide a road map, but the real work comes on your own as you incorporate the lessons from speech therapy at home with your child."

3. **A Systematic Approach.** Begin with the most simple task and work up to the most complex task. Find out what your child can do first—in terms of words and sounds—and start building on it. (More on this topic in the "Imitation" section of this chapter.)

4. **Jaw, Tongue, and Lip Strengthening.** Children with CAS or oral apraxia don't need strengthening unless they also have dysarthria. Oral exercise must be applied only *if* a child has dysarthria in addition to CAS. *If your child has "just" CAS, then no strengthening or oral placement exercises are needed.* Instead, what your child needs is automaticity of movement, and possibly increased (or decreased) movement and greater endurance. Please talk with your child's SLP if you think oral exercise and strengthening are concerns.

5. Motor Memory. Back to our earlier analogy of learning to ride a bike. You remember that it was hard and frustrating at times; once you got the hang of it, you never forgot. That's called motor learning. It involves motor programming and muscle memory. Your goal in taking your child to therapy is to help her learn articulator programming and memory so she can communicate.

6. Auditory Discrimination. Many children with CAS have subtle problems with telling the difference between words, or auditory discrimination. Talk to your child's SLP to see if this is the case for your child; he or she will help you determine whether your child needs extra practice in this area. Minimal pair work is often used (see chart on page 109 above).

Parents Ask

What's the difference between positive and negative reinforcement?

Positive reinforcement involves adding something to the environment that increases the chances that the child will repeat a particular action/behavior. So, you give her a reward or praise when she says a word. Hopefully, it increases the likelihood that she'll say it again.

If you are using praise as positive reinforcement, the entirety of your statement is positive. For example: "Yes! That's right. Daddy will be home soon. You got the word *Daddy* right. Hooray for you!" (You ignore the fact that the rest of your child's statement was unintelligible.)

In contrast, suppose you responded to your child like this: "Nope, that's not how you say *Daddy*. Not even close!" That would be negative reinforcement. Negative reinforcement is when you take away something from the child or her surroundings in hopes it will increase the chance that she will respond "correctly" the next time. (It's the punishment approach—which may work in other situations, such as taking away your child's toys if she leaves them scattered around the living room.) There's not really a token you can take away from a child who is learning to talk; but saying something hurtful or degrading would take away her self-esteem or willingness to speak and most likely make her less likely to try the next time around. Always be positive when reinforcing your child's speech attempts.

Tip: In discrimination therapy, SLPs will acknowledge that a child said something different than the target. This might appear negative, but it is crucial in teaching self-monitoring and auditory awareness. It might sound like this: "No, sorry. That's not quite right. I heard _____. What we want to hear is _____. Can you try it again?"

SPEAKING OF APRAXIA

7. Building on Success. Kids with CAS are very aware of what sounds and words they can and cannot say. Has your child ever flat-out refused to say a word when asked? That's because these kids are smart—if they know they won't be successful, why even bother attempting a sound or word? Instead, work in small increments; let your child succeed at an easier task before making it more challenging.

8. Self-Monitoring. This is an important skill that your SLP will teach your child. It will enable her to identify when she is correctly producing verbal sounds and modify those that aren't correct. Your child will learn to monitor her spontaneous speech with the skills of self-monitoring.

9. Rate, Tone, Intonation, and Stress of Speech (Prosody). These are all related to motor planning. Children with CAS have difficulty with prosody (emphasis on words, rising and falling pitch). Poor prosody affects the overall intelligibility (understand-ability) of speech. What helps: practicing rhyming words, tapping out words to a beat, climbing the stairs and saying a word for every step, finger tapping while saying words, and whole body movement while saying/practicing words.

10. Teaching Compensatory Strategies. These are similar to the idea of self-monitoring. Your SLP will teach your child to slow her rate of speech, increase the length of vowel sounds in words, or substitute a developmentally easier sound for one that is harder, such as using a /d/ for the *th* sound rather than omitting the sound (phoneme) completely. (For example, a child may say *dat* instead of *at*, if the word *that* is too hard for her, *eventually* adding the correct *th* sound).

11. Rewarding Success. Even little pieces of success feel good! Give positive reinforcement—all kids need it to stay motivated and cooperative.

A Look Inside a Speech Therapy Session

No doubt you are wondering what therapy will look like. How soon will you begin to see progress? Keep these pointers in mind before we delve into a therapy session:

- *Kids with CAS need frequent, intense 1:1 therapy—at least in the beginning.* Be prepared to be at the speech clinic at least once a week. Most kids with CAS will require some form of speech therapy for at least two to three years.
- *Some SLPs recommend at least two sessions a week.* It depends on the severity of diagnosis, your child's age, attention span, and personality, as well as your time and financial resources. Your child may receive speech in school and privately to meet these criteria. In an ideal world, the SLPs communicate with one another regularly to align treatment plans.
- *Some kids with CAS don't respond as quickly and easily to "traditional" therapy approaches—or at all.* That is, they don't respond to SLPs who say, "Look at me. Do what I say. Do what I do." For this reason, a good SLP should use a combination of creativity, flexibility, drill, and engagement in each session.

- *Your child is learning to recognize different sounds (phonemes) by ear.* It is your SLP's job to assist in that process by providing additional cues—visual, tactile, and proprioceptive (the body's sense of movement in space)—to help your child establish motor plans for speech.

Parents Ask

How often should we practice speech skills/go to speech therapy?

Should you be doing "distributed" practice (spread out across time) or doing it all at once ("mass" or "blocked" practice)? Mass and distributed practice are used in treatment to help the child establish motor plans/programs for words. In mass practice, a word may be practiced as many as 100 times (e.g., 4 sets of 25). In distributed or random practice, the word is practiced among other target words.

In the 1990s, researchers Richard Magill and Jack Fletcher determined that for the development of skills such as speech, distributed practice periods are best for motor learning in CAS. According to a 2010 presentation by Edythe Strand, PhD, CCC-SLP, "Mass practice yields quick development of the skill, but poor generalization for incorporating it into other motor skills. Distributed practice takes longer, but [the child] will get better motor learning in the long run."

So, if your SLP recommends two hours of speech therapy a week, the best scenario would be to break those two hours into four thirty-minute sessions. But with busy lifestyles, that may be near impossible. As far as actual "practice" goes—as often as possible—while still allowing your child to be "just a kid." See chapter 9 for ideas.

Tip: Home practice should only focus on target words and sounds recommended by your child's SLP. This helps with accuracy and is easier to monitor progress.

Welcome to the Two-Way Mirror, Mom and Dad

Let's assume you are sitting in a therapy room with a two-way mirror. You can see your child at work with the SLP, but she can't see you. Ideally, you are alone, your phone is turned off, and you have pen and paper nearby.

Your little one walks into the therapy room with the SLP, and they begin with a brief *warm-up period*. Your SLP may have already selected a few toys, games, and books (stimuli) to work with based on what your child likes to do, and perhaps some target words or phrases that are challenging.

Other SLPs like to have kids pick out their own stimuli by leading them to a toy closet (heaven for any child!). This ensures that the child has chosen something she is really "into," with the hope that it will elicit some spontaneous response.

Assuming everything is in the room, your child may begin with some *exploration of the stimuli*—picking things up, going from toy to toy, and perhaps making some spontaneous utterances.

Our SLP, Ms. Jen, often used "apraxia cards" during sessions. These cards were like large flashcards that showed pictures of common objects or actions. You may know them as Kaufman cards, created by speech-language pathologist and CAS expert, Nancy Kaufman. (From the *Kaufman Speech Praxis Treatment Kit*, these are just one example of "apraxia cards/materials" your SLP may have access to.)

Ms. Jen would select a few of these cards from her stash to drill Kate. The aim of these cards is to help children produce correct articulation. But for children who find correct articulation too challenging, it is often enough to allow them to produce approximations—not the whole word and not even perfectly—of the action or object depicted on the card. Ms. Jen often made two different piles of cards: (1) words that were easy for Kate or "mastered," and (2) words that were a bit more challenging.

My youngest daughter, Kelly, got to where she actually *liked* these cards and would ask, "More cards, please." Needless to say, once she got to this point, we ended therapy!

Parents Ask

What are Kaufman Cards?

SLP Diane Bahr describes the Kaufman Speech Praxis Treatment Kits in her book, *Nobody Ever Told Me (or My Mother!) That* this way: "[These kits] are designed to help children with speech motor-planning problems say word approximations that get closer and closer to the real word. They build speech from the bottom up. The kits help speech-language pathologists to systematically cue speech and fade that cueing over time as the child develops speech." The Kaufman cards are also large and visually appealing to children. For more information on these kits, the Kaufman Children's Center (located in Michigan), and Nancy Kaufman's work please visit www.kidspeech.com.

The Role of Imitation in Therapy

Since a major goal of therapy is to increase your child's voluntary control (automaticity) over the movements for speech, imitation is a huge component to therapy.

You want your child to be intelligible, of course, but don't be surprised if the imitation activities presented in the beginning of treatment have nothing to do with words. Of course the goal is to talk, but sometimes you have to start with something your child will have success with. Here's an example:

Can your child jump? Clap? Touch her toes? Your SLP may have your child watch and learn at first. "I'll jump . . . now you jump."

Your child and the SLP *may* spend a small portion of the session working on imitating nonspeech movements. Look at it as a way of laying the groundwork so that more complex motor tasks—like talking—can be added in subsequent sessions. This builds trust and rapport, and can be fun. It takes the pressure off talking. If you are quiet and patient, you may even hear a spontaneous word or two. The hierarchical approach would then build on these words.

However, an entire session of gross motor imitation is *not* an efficient use of precious speech therapy time. If you notice that this is all your child is doing in therapy, say something to your SLP. It could be that she chose this method of "warm-up" because your child is particularly young (developmentally, gross motor imitation comes before fine motor oral movements), or your child is cognitively delayed.

Imitation tasks evolve from easiest to hardest. For a child who is unable to imitate speech sounds and words, imitation may begin at a gross motor level and progress like this to speech imitation:

1. Gross motor activities: clapping hands or stomping feet
2. Actions with objects/toys: rolling a ball back and forth or banging two blocks together
3. Subtle movements: nodding head or wiggling fingers
4. Oral-facial movements: blowing kisses, sticking out tongue, other facial expressions
5. Vocal play: blowing raspberries

Parents Ask

Does the PROMPT technique use imitation?

Well, no. PROMPT is often used when a child cannot imitate speech. The PROMPT technique uses touch and movement. Deborah Hayden's therapeutic technique was already alluded to on page 112, so let's talk about it.

PROMPT uses "Dynamic Systems Theory" to shape, guide, and educate muscles for speech movements. The SLP will use tactile and kinesthetic prompts such as moving the child's lips or pressing her cheeks in a manner that elicits the correct sound. If you or your child is uncomfortable with the use of touch, then PROMPT may not be the therapy best suited for your family. To use this therapeutic technique, the SLP must be specially trained. SLPs should not train parents or other providers on PROMPT—there's too much room for error. For information on PROMPT techniques, visit www.promptinstitute.com.

In her book *Becoming Verbal with Childhood Apraxia of Speech: New Insights on Piaget for Today's Therapy,* the late Pamela Marshalla, MA, CCC-SLP, devoted an entire chapter to the critical role of imitation in the ability to speak. Most humans can imitate facial expressions, words, sounds, intonation patterns, accents, gestures, actions, and emotions within the first year of life. However, Ms. Marshalla proposed that kids with CAS have a much more difficult time learning how to imitate than typically developing children. According to her book, children with CAS have the following problems with imitation:

- **Late Emergence:** Children with CAS begin the process of imitation development later than "typical" children.

- **Slow Maturation:** Most kids with CAS take longer to move from one stage of imitation to the next.

- **Stagnation:** Most kids with CAS plateau at an early stage of imitation, making it more difficult to advance.

- **Inability:** Some children with severe to profound CAS never do begin the imitation process at all.

- **Scatter:** Sometimes, kids with CAS skip ahead to a more advanced stage of imitation, leaving the earlier stages incomplete.

I remember these stages clearly with Kate—only she *wasn't* a baby when she was in them! Although I knew what was happening—she was experimenting with vocal play as a toddler—I found it exasperating and almost embarrassing. We might be at the grocery store or at a play date and Kate would make "mouth noises" as though she were a six-month-old infant, but she was three and a half or four years old. There were times I just cringed or even told her to be quiet. I look back on those days and wish I had reacted differently.

Kids with CAS *do* have the ability to acquire mature speech-imitation skills; it just may take longer than typical. Keep in mind that imitation is *the* building block to a fully functional communication system.

Tip: You might have heard SLPs use the word *plateau* when describing a child's speech-language progress. But you might want to consider reframing. CAS expert Dave Hammer, MA, CCC-SLP, refers to this stage as the "input phase." This is a period of approximately one month when a child isn't apparently making gains. This period can be misconceived as a plateau, while in fact, the child is absorbing information and creating new pathways just before a burst of improvement surfaces.

More Building Blocks: Approximations and Mean Length of Utterances

Once your child is able to imitate speech sounds, the SLP might begin to have her work on **approximations** of words—for example, "nana" for "banana." Of course, the goal will be for your child to say words with increasing accuracy, but this can be slow. If your child is only saying a couple of sounds, her SLP will choose words to approximate based on those sounds. This is a hierarchical approach.

After approximations comes **increasing the length of utterances**. A common speech pathology term is **mean length of utterance (MLU).** This refers to the number of language units (morphemes), on average, that the child says in one phrase/sentence.

Researchers have documented the average MLU for children of all ages, and these averages are one indicator that is often used to measure your child's progress or the amount of speech delay. The MLU is sometimes used in writing goals for speech therapy provided through early intervention or special education programs in the public schools. For example, you may see a goal like this: "Jack will increase his MLU from 3.5 morphemes to 5.0 morphemes in structured conversation by the end of the school year." If the goal has short-term objectives, the objectives will involve teaching the various age-appropriate language structures that his speech is lacking (e.g., present progressive tense, plurals, possessives, or vocabulary).

Below-average MLUs may be used in justifying a child's need for speech therapy from the school/EI program. For more information on MLU, visit Speech & Language Kids (www.speechandlanguagekids.com/increasing-sentence-length-mlu/), and you will find an MLU/age-equivalent chart and a protocol for calculating MLU.

Once your child is able to say longer words and phrases, your speech pathologist will begin working on:

- **Accuracy:** what percentage of the time your child says a word correctly. Often used in writing goals for speech therapy; e.g., "Jack will produce 20 one-syllable words with 90% accuracy by (date)"
- **Clarity:** meaning how clearly—or intelligibly—your child is speaking those words
- **Increasing vocabulary:** understanding the *meanings* of words is not usually a problem for children with CAS, but getting them to branch out and *use* those words can be
- **Pragmatics:** the "social appropriateness" of conversation

As you see, there are a lot of skills your SLP is working on. That's a big reason why kids with CAS need frequent and intense therapy.

Functional Expressions

A major piece of therapy for CAS is to provide the child with some functional expressions—words, phrases, or gestures that can assist in helping her get what she wants and needs. Examples of functional expressions include the following:

- "More, please"
- "Help (me)"
- "I need . . . "
- "I want . . . "
- "Please"
- "Thank you"

You can work on these phrases in real-life situations where the phrases would come in handy, particularly in motivating situations when your child actually wants a particular item or needs help with something she enjoys doing. For example, I used to have my daughter Kate place her order when we went out to eat. While it may seem like "mean ol' mom" here, I actually viewed our weekly lunch dates as therapeutic. Kate got to the point where she could order without a problem. (Of course, if she stumbled, I was there to help.)

How Can Parents Assist with Speech Therapy?

■ *Ask if you can observe sessions.* This may be the single most important thing you do for your child. It helps you understand what the SLP is doing with your child and gives you some tricks for learning to communicate more effectively with your child. Plus, you will see that the techniques your SLP uses are not "rocket science." Once you see them, you can usually do them at home. This is crucial for home practice. If observing is not routinely done in your clinic, ask if there is a way to videotape a session.

■ *Observe unobtrusively.* You may watch from a two-way mirror so that your child is not distracted by your presence. You could observe for just a brief period, say, ten to twenty minutes of each session. You might just observe by listening—perhaps sitting in the hallway with the therapy door propped open. Listen to the interactions between your child and the SLP. Some parents sit in the room for the entire session. When I did this, however, I became anxious waiting for those words to come. Sometimes it was boring; other times the SLP and I got to talking about something relevant to therapy, but then Kate got less therapy time. When I left those therapy sessions, however, I felt more motivated and eager to model good communication at home.

■ *Know what your child's therapy goals are at all times.* If you don't know, ask. It's best to have them in writing so you can refer back to them. Plus, it makes you feel good when you can cross off an achieved goal. (Note that if your child is receiving speech therapy through an early intervention program or public school, the goals will be written in your child's IFSP or IEP.)

Margaret Fish, MS, CCC-SLP, says this about a child's treatment goals: "In addition to providing a warm and supportive environment for children, one of the best things that families can do for a child with CAS is to locate a therapist [SLP] who understands the unique needs of children with motor speech challenges. Request that your SLP explain the goals and methods, as well as the types of things you can be doing at home to support your child's communication skill development."

■ *Get to know your SLP.* Because of the intensity of CAS therapy, your SLP may become like a member of the family. We even invited ours to a birthday party! If the SLP doesn't mind sharing his or her business email, get it. Send therapy-related emails occasionally. Ask his opinion on something you read; update him on progress at home. But don't bombard him—remember your child is just one of many he treats. Developing a close working relationship with your child's SLP shows that you are interested and engaged and keeps your family on his radar.

Ronda Wojcicki, MS, CCC-SLP, urges parents to get involved: "Get involved with your child's teacher, SLP, local speech and hearing association. Participate with your child in therapy and learn how to take what they are doing in therapy and bring it to the home environment and elsewhere. This is a family journey, so treat it as such. And remember to celebrate each and every small victory along the way—this is how we ultimately get where we are going."

Nanette Cote, MA, CCC-SLP, cautions against getting too close: "Since I practice from a home office, setting and maintaining boundaries is something I work really hard at. It's considered best practice to use every minute [of our sessions] prioritizing the child's needs. Once my clients graduate from services, I offer to connect via social media as a way to keep in touch and hear about continued progress."

- *Ensure that therapy is an active process for you, as well as your child.* Bring reading material that directly relates to the technique your SLP is using. Read it in the waiting room and share it with your SLP. Use the waiting room time to review your child's progress. Create a timeline of improvements for you and your child to review, or make a list of goals you'd like your child to achieve. It can really be motivating!

- *Give your child incentives.* Perhaps you can take your child to the park after her session. Three sessions of speech therapy could result in a trip to the Dollar Store or an ice cream cone. Make it fun (and spontaneous), and you and your child will avoid burnout.

- *Track and celebrate progress.* Celebrate your child's small successes with CAS. Remember, every little word, phrase, or sentence is a result of much effort.

> "The frequent and consistent speech therapy and the actual carry-over into [my son's] classroom created a big difference in his speech, language, articulation, reading, and fluency. Since then, we've seen incremental improvement each year, but not as great as the first year or two he was there: that was his "burst." But then, with our son, we are dealing with a lot more than CAS (ASD, ADHD, anxiety issues, global sensory issues, etc.) so we are constantly changing gears and directions to solve the issue du jour. Progress is progress, and baby steps are big steps in our world. We've climbed a mountain since he was originally diagnosed at 20 months old."—Holly, mother of son with CAS.

"Branded" Therapy Methods

In your CAS journey, you may come across some "branded" therapy styles—that is, methods that were developed by one or more individuals who have published materials or hold training sessions to teach others how to use their methods. I will break them down for you here:

"Branded" Therapy Methods Sometimes Used for CAS

Method/ Program	How It's Used	Where to Learn More
Language Is the Key: A Program for Building Language and Literacy (LIK) Kevin N. Cole, Mary Maddox, and Young Sook Lim (2006) You may come across this program as CLAS (culturally and linguistically appropriate services)	Uses constructive interactions between books and play (see below). The program uses "dialogic reading" and teaches parents to ask open-ended questions (what, why, how) and make comments by responding to and adding more to the child's utterances. Best suited for a child who has delayed language development but normal cognitive function.	Washington Learning Systems, the company that creates and markets LIK, can be found at: http://www.clas.uiuc. edu/fulltext/cl01113/ cl01113.html Parents can view the *Language Is the Key: Video Programs for Building Language & Literacy in Early Childhood*, a video in the program *Talking and Books*, at above website.
It Takes Two to Talk: The Hanen Program for Parents Ayala Hanen Manolson, SLP (1985)	Teaches parents to use methods designed to facilitate speech development. Parents are taught to recognize their child's stage and style of communication, motivation, how to adjust daily routines and follow the child's lead in communication. Best for kids who are late talkers and preschoolers with cognitive and developmental delays.	*It Takes Two to Talk: A Practical Guide for Parents of Children with Language Delays*, 5th edition, by Elaine Weitzman The Hanen Centre website: www.hanen.org

Picture Exchange Communication System (PECS) Lori Frost and Andy Bondy (1994)	An evidence-based visual communication method developed to help children with autism communicate. Children are taught to give pictures to others in order to express their needs, wants, and observations. Children work up from exchanging a single picture (e.g., cookie) to sentence strips expressing a complete thought (e.g., I want a big chocolate chip cookie, please). Does not inhibit children from developing speech. PECS serves as a bridge to speech through supporting expressive language development, providing natural means for modeling target words repeatedly, improving social communication, and developing a picture vocabulary system. It is best suited for children who lack initiation for communication. If your child has this communicative intent, then another low-tech visual picture system or speech generating device may better meet his needs.	*A Picture's Worth: PECS and Other Visual Communication Strategies in Autism*, 2nd edition, by Andy Bondy and Lori Frost (Woodbine House, 2011) Available from: www.woodbinehouse. com *Complete Visual Reinforcement System Set for PECS: Picture Exchange Communication System* PECS materials available from Pyramid Educational Systems: www.pecs.com

Criteria for Choosing Books and Toys in the Language Is Key Program

Children are more stimulated to talk with lively and colorful illustrations. Vary the content of the books. Children are *least likely* to converse with counting books, name-the-color books, or ABC books. Allow children to choose books; read them over and over if they insist (repetition helps them internalize the words). Allow children to flip pages until they come to one they like. Remember, the goal is not to read the book cover to cover, but to facilitate language development. (Teri Peterson, MS, CCC-SLP, has written a book with this strategy in mind. Look for *The Big Book of Exclamations!*) Nanette Cote enthusiastically recommends working with books in therapy, "I love using titles with lift-the-flaps, removable stickers, or textured pages. These lend for opportunities to engage and interact with literacy. Sensory bins with pictures from the book are another great way to engage children in book readings while working on speech."

The key here is to observe your child's interests and follow her lead in the types of toys, books, and activities she gravitates toward. What items get her to vocalize most in free play? As your child plays, talk about what she is doing with the toy. ("Oh, I see you are stacking the blocks.")

Some SLP favorites for working with children include inexpensive wind-up toys, textured puzzles, Pop the Pirate, Elefun, magnetic or stationary marble/ball tracks, Play-Doh-style compounds, and Velcro foods. More on this topic in chapter 9.

I Am Not a Speech Pathologist

I am not a speech pathologist. If you have questions and concerns about the techniques presented in this chapter, I urge you to ask your child's SLP or to do some of your own research.

The strategies presented in this chapter are a general guide to working with kids with CAS. As your child progresses in therapy—age and maturity—other areas of speech will need practice, such as correct sentence structure and grammar, as these are known to be problematic for kids with CAS.

At some point in therapy, your child will need to work on intelligibility and speech precision. Intelligibility is the understandability of her speech, and depends on the correct sound production, including

- stressing certain words within sentences,
- pitch, volume, rate, and rhythm,
- phonological awareness (preliteracy skills), and
- articulation.

Your child will also need to practice these areas related to speech-language:

- spelling, reading, decoding, comprehension (literacy skills);
- listener awareness (repeating herself or making corrections if the listener doesn't understand her; adjusting how she speaks to others depending on their age, status, relationship—e.g., you speak differently to a little child than to a teacher or a friend);
- self-advocacy (learning communicative strengths and weaknesses and how to communicate with teachers, coaches, and friends about these issues).

As I've emphasized in this chapter, experts recommend that therapy for kids with CAS be frequent, intense, and extend over the course of several years. There's a lot of stuff to sort out and a lot of coaching to get these kids with CAS to be effective communicators! Have faith and take it step by step. You and your child will get there.

Bridging Research and Practice

By now, I am sure you've realized that *there is no one method for treating CAS.* Why? Well, for starters there is not enough scientific evidence as to which method works best because researchers are still a little foggy as to what causes CAS, so we have several unanswered questions:

- Do kids with CAS have problems talking because formulating motor routines and patterns is particularly difficult for them?
- Do kids with CAS have problems storing verbal routines in their brain?
- Do kids with CAS have problems adequately retrieving the routines that have been stored?

See chapter 6 for more information on what may cause symptoms of CAS.

Say That Again?! Chapter Summary

This chapter has been all about speech therapy—the types and subtypes that are available to help your child communicate. Your child's SLP will carefully map out a treatment plan designed to assist your son or daughter in producing intelligible speech based on attributes specific to your child (age, attention span, motivation, intelligence, etc.). However, a large piece to the therapeutic approaches used for CAS is *motor learning*, a process of gathering the skills necessary for producing a desired action (in this case—speech). Your child will get better with practice, self-confidence, intrinsic motivation, direct instruction, and modeling. Please discuss the best treatment approach with your child's SLP!

Finally, please remember this: *the key to success with CAS is frequent, intense, long-term therapy, and plenty of practice at home.* Chapter 9 is devoted to explaining how you can help your child at home. Practicing outside of therapy helps make speech skills automatic. Following through at home can keep therapy on track and maybe even speed up the process.

Recommended Resources

Some of these resources might be too costly for many families. That's because many are written as textbooks for speech-language pathology students or for clinicians in practice. They are mentioned only for use as a guide, never as a diagnostic or treatment tool, and should only be referenced if you are seeking additional information. You may want to consider Amazon's or Barnes & Nobles's rental programs, which enable you to borrow textbooks for a designated amount of time for a smaller fee than purchasing outright. You can also borrow books from the library, ask if your SLP is willing to share, search second-hand bookstores, or ask a parent group on social media if anyone has a copy they'd be willing to lend or sell.

- *It Takes Two to Talk: A Practical Guide for Parents of Children with Language Delays*, 5th edition, by Elaine Weitzman and illustrated by Pat Cupples (Hanen Centre, 2017). If you are interested in learning more about this program, this is a must-read. Published by the Hanen Centre: www.hanen.org.

- *Bjorem Speech.* Jennie Bjorem, MA, CCC-SLP, offers a variety of books and products on her website designed for multiple speech disorders. She has special expertise and training in CAS. For more information and a product guide, please visit: https://www.bjoremspeech.com.

- For more information on *Oral Placement Therapy*, please visit *Talk Tools,* developed by Sara Rosenfeld-Johnson, MS, CCC-SLP: https://talktools.com/pages/what-is-opt. Here you can learn about the process, watch videos of it in practice, read success stories, and more.

- *A Picture's Worth: PECS and Other Visual Communication Strategies in Autism* by Andy Bondy and Lori Frost (Woodbine House, 2011). Although this evidence-based communication strategy was originally developed for children on the autism spectrum, it can be used with any children with limited speech skills, such as those with CAS.

- You may also be interested in *learning more about the PECS program*. Go to www.pecs.com and then select your country's flag. Here you'll be directed to a wealth of information, including an overview of the potential benefits of the PECS program as well as brochures, free materials, videos, and research. The website for US-based customers is https://pecsusa.com/.

- For more information about prompts and cues, check out the website of SLP Maureen Wilson, *The Speech Bubble:* http://www.thespeechbubbleslp.com/2017/02/prompts-and-cues-little-words-big-impact.html.

- You may like this set of *free, printable cue cards from Speechy Musings*, developed by a Wisconsin-based pediatric speech-language pathologist with outpatient therapy experience: https://www.teacherspayteachers.com/Product/Speech-Sound-Cue-Cards-Freebie-for-Speech-Therapy-2196455.

- *Kaufman cards.* If your SLP uses these with your child, you may be tempted to purchase and use them at home. *They are not for everyone and should be used only at your SLP's recommendation.* They are also on the pricey side. You may want to see if you can borrow them from your SLP or a local parenting group. For more information, see https://www.northernspeech.com/apraxia-childhood/kaufman-k-slp-treatment-kit-1-basic-level/.

- *Teach Me How to Say It Right: Helping Your Child with Articulation Disorders* by Dorothy P. Dougherty, CCC-SLP (New Harbinger Publications, 2005). While this book is about articulation disorders (CAS is *not* a disorder of articulation), you may still find some helpful information on working with your child at home, as well as on speech sound development.

- ***We Talk on Water: Guide for Developing and Orchestrating Successful Group Social Communication (2019)*** by Nanette Cote, MA, CCC-SLP, may be helpful to you—especially if you are an SLP reading this—and if a child you are working with loves to swim. Being in the water can be relaxing and fun for children and they may forget they are there for speech work. Plus, it helps with SLP burnout. For more information, see https://napervilletherapediatrics.com/.

- ***The Marshalla Guide: A Topical Anthology of Speech Movement Techniques for Motor Speech Disorders and Articulation Deficits*** (Marshalla Speech & Language, 2019) is a book by an SLP for other SLPs and is considered the magnum opus of Pam Marshalla, CCC-SLP. It may be a bit overwhelming for a parent but is immensely valuable. This gorgeous, comprehensive illustrated guide compiles four decades of therapy with modern research, organized by category. For more information, see https://pammarshalla.com/product/the-marshalla-guide/.

- ***The SLP's Guide to Treating Childhood Apraxia of Speech*** by Cari Ebert and David Hammer (Speech Corner, 2018), both nationally recognized speakers, have teamed up in this professional resource. It provides practicing SLPs hands-on information needed to effectively treat toddlers, preschoolers, and early school-aged children who have or are suspected of having CAS. This title is relatively short—and a bit pricey—but parents may still find it worthwhile.

- ***Here's How to Treat Childhood Apraxia of Speech***, 2nd edition, by Margaret (Dee) Fish (Plural Publishing, 2015) may be best suited for students in an SLP program, but it's written in such a way that motivated parents can glean valuable insight into their child's speech-language therapy.

Helping Your Child

Chapter 8

Fish Oil, Diet, Horses, Music, and More

Complementary and Alternative Medical Approaches

"If there is something else out there that will help my son, then I want to know about it!"

—Small Talk: All About Apraxia Participant

When I first learned of Kate's CAS diagnosis, I thought the only thing I could do was to schlep her to and from speech therapy a couple of times a week. Then I found out that we would need to do speech therapy homework, since much of her progress would be made at home.

When I started getting serious about learning about CAS, a whole new world opened up. For better or worse, I was introduced to the idea of complementary and alternative medicine (CAM). Well, maybe "reintroduced" is a better word. I am a nurse, after all, and I had heard patients praise such therapies. Heck, I've even tried some ideas on my own. Visualization, listening to relaxing music, and even yoga can all be classified as CAM. If you've ever lit a delicious-smelling candle and listened to classical music to relax after an exhausting day, then you, too, have experienced some form of CAM.

Just as with most things in life, you often have a choice. This chapter will outline some of the more mainstream alternative approaches to conventional therapy such as B12 vitamins, omega-3 fatty acids, dietary changes, and nutritional supplementation—and some you may not have thought of or heard about before. The goal of this chapter is not to discount or offer substitutes for traditional therapy, but to offer a supplemental approach.

- An overview of complementary and alternative medicine (CAM), including who is qualified to treat individuals with these methods
- Nutritional modifications and how the food we put into our bodies affects the greater whole—including our ability to communicate
- Sensory-based therapies—including hippotherapy (horse riding), vision therapy, and therapeutic listening, among others
- Medically based therapies, including pranic healers, chiropractors, and others
- Finally, a series of questions to get you asking the right questions to determine if a particular therapy is "right" for you and your child

So What *Is* Complementary and Alternative Medicine?

Complementary and alternative medicine (CAM) is a constellation of medical and therapeutic practices and products not currently thought to be part of conventional medicine. Examples of CAM practitioners are chiropractors and acupuncturists; examples of CAM products are dietary supplements.

Integrative medicine (IM) combines mainstream medical therapies with CAM therapies. It treats the whole person, not just the disease. It's the best of both worlds—science and western medicine plus *evidence-based* complementary therapy. Treating the individual through a dynamic team of partners, integrative medicine helps heal the mind, body, and spirit. Biofeedback, yoga instructors, massage therapists, and recreational therapists all fall under that umbrella we call integrative medicine.

Some of the therapies available may just be too "out there" for you to consider. Have an open mind as you read through the next few pages, though. Something just may work for your child. As with anything, do your homework first. These techniques, ideas, and therapies should never replace traditional speech therapy. Also, bear in mind that there is no point in trying to treat symptoms your child does not have. For example, a gluten-free diet will not help your child if he does not have gluten intolerance or celiac disease. If you are concerned, or just curious, you can ask your pediatrician to consider a blood test to indicate whether your child might have an intolerance or allergy.

Nutritional Intervention: Gluten-Free Diets, Fatty Acids, and More

There are books upon books written on the subject of adding ingredients to or eliminating ingredients from one's diet to aid in the body's performance. Most parents either want a general overview or already *know* their child has a food intolerance or allergy and have taken appropriate steps.

Let's assume you fall into the "just the facts, ma'am" category. Here's a quick and easy guide to some of the benefits of diet modification. Please continue to seek out other resources—including your child's pediatrician—should you choose to travel along this nutritional journey.

	Omega Essential Fatty Acids (EFAs)	Gluten-Free/ Casein-Free Diet	B-12 (Cobalamin)
What it is:	Fatty acids that the body doesn't produce naturally but are essential to the development and function of the brain, nerves, muscles, and organs.	A diet that eliminates wheat and dairy products. ***Please have your child tested for gluten and casein sensitivities before assuming there is a problem.*** Going this route takes a lot of time, commitment, and disruption to the child's—and family's—eating routine.	Water-soluble vitamin
Where it's found naturally:	***Omega 3 fatty acids*** (DHA) are found in flaxseed oil, walnuts, dark green leafy veggies (spinach, kale), and cold-water fish like salmon, trout, cod, and sardines (3–4 oz./week). ***Omega 6 fatty acids*** can be found in animal fats and linoleic acid (the primary oil added to processed food), and used in sunflower, safflower, and soybean oils.	***Gluten*** is a protein found in wheat, barley, and rye, as well as in oats that have been contaminated by wheat, barley, or rye. ***Casein*** is a protein in dairy products such as milk, ice cream, cheese, and yogurt.	Often found in red meat, also in dairy and eggs; the body doesn't naturally make B-12.

What's the deal?	Some suggestions are that EFAs *may be able* to offer therapeutic benefits to depression, bipolar, ADHD, autism, heart disease, diabetes, autoimmune disease, and communication. It helps communication in the sense that it may improve attention and focus.	Typically, the body digests these proteins down into peptides. Some kids can't digest them well. They enter the bloodstream and *may* cause problems with brain development, as well as bloating, diarrhea, and other gastrointestinal problems.	B-12 works with folic acid to make DNA and red blood cells. It converts carbohydrates, fats, and proteins from food into energy. Also important in protecting nerve cells.
How it *could* help kids with CAS:	One study from the Univ. of British Columbia found a positive correlation between amount of DHA in breast milk and the language development of children. Some folks feel EFAs help communication by improving focus.	*Nutritional Neuroscience* indicated a reduction in autistic behavior, increase in social and communication skills in kids who went on gluten-free, casein-free diets. These findings were determined after 12 years of studies on kids with autism. The Univ. of Sunderland in the UK found parents reported improvements in communication and concentration in kids with autism after a 3-month casein/gluten-free diet	Scientifically proven to target the communication center of the brain. However, it doesn't necessarily mean that children with CAS need more B-12 in their diets, but perhaps they are not metabolizing it as they should. Please check with your child's doctor to determine if your child has a B-12 deficiency.

Side effects:	Mild tummy ache and fishy taste and/or smell; to avoid, use smaller doses throughout the day, mix with food (some say it's great when added to popcorn or smoothies). Another concern is that it could be contaminated with methyl mercury, especially over the long-term treatment in small kids. According to the CDC, mercury can be passed from mother to her fetus, and can cause brain damage, incoordination, blindness, seizures, and inability to speak.	It's a pain in the you-know-what! Constant monitoring of your food sources and intake can be exhausting. Lots of learning and meal planning involved. You have to stick with it, even bringing your own snacks to a birthday party.	Found to be a safe and nontoxic vitamin. If taken in excess, you're just nourishing your toilet bowl! May have some interactions with antibiotics, so tell your doctor if you are giving your child B-12 supplements.
What you can try at home:	Have your child eat more fish, give her a supplement. Talk with your pediatrician before you do anything.	Read and learn about the diet. Try eliminating some of the above foods, one category at a time, and keep track of effects on your child.	Incorporate more red meat. Find out if your child really has a B-12 deficiency by having a blood test; proceed if your doctor recommends it.

Products to consider:	ProEFA, Nordic Naturals, Carlson Kids, & Dr. Sears Chewies	Nowadays there are a lot of products stocked on grocery store shelves that are labeled gluten-free	Sublingual (under the tongue) B-12 supplements that dissolve in your mouth are best because they go right into the bloodstream, bypassing the digestive system.
Resources	*The Omega-3 Connection* (Stoll), *Children with Starving Brains* (McCandless), *The LCP Solution* (Stordy), and *Cure Your Child with Food: The Hidden Connection Between Nutrition and Childhood Ailments* (Dorfman)	*The Living Gluten Free Answer Book* (Bowland), *Getting Your Kid on a Gluten-Free Casein-Free Diet* (Lord), *Special Diets for Special Kids* (Lewis), *Gluten-Free Kids* (Korn), and *Cure Your Child with Food: The Hidden Connection Between Nutrition and Childhood Ailments* (Dorfman)	*"Could It Be B-12: An Epidemic of Misdiagnosis"* (Pacholock and Stuart)

Some Things to Keep in Mind about Supplements

■ Supplements are *not* monitored by the FDA; prescription medications are.

■ *Never, ever give your child supplements solely on the recommendation of a friend or something you've read!* I cannot stress this enough. This chapter is not intended to replace medical advice.

■ Your child's pediatrician should *always* be consulted before giving your child any type of supplements.

■ When you are selecting vitamins or any other supplements, be sure to look for companies that get their products tested by an outside source/third party. Look for US Pharmacopeia (USP), Consumer Lab, or NSF International on the label.

■ Who will monitor the safety of dosages? A doctor typically does that, but if you are self-medicating your child, you'll need some professional guidance.

- If anyone claims that a particular product helps children with speech and communication concerns, ask for a source or a citation for that claim. If you do this in a tactful, diplomatic manner, they should be happy to oblige.

- If you are concerned that fish oil supplements could contain mercury, make sure the brand you are using has been tested for purity by a third party.

- A registered dietician (RD) may be helpful in making some dietary changes/modifications. Find one at www.eatright.org, website of the American Dietetic Association.

Fishing for an Omega-3 Fatty Acid Product?

Here's a sampling of various omega-3 fatty acids (a.k.a. fish oil, PUFAs) you may want to consider for your child with CAS:

Coromega Kids Omega-3 Squeeze, produced by European Reference Botanical Laboratories located in Carlsbad, CA. Coromega is a form of fish oil in a creamy, orange-flavored, pudding-like substance. Some come in portable, single-dose packets. Parents find it easy to add to juice or yogurt or blend in a smoothie; taking it "straight" is generally not preferred. Kids don't usually mind the taste. You can order directly from the company: www.coromega.com.

Efalex is a fish oil supplement rich in DHA. This is the very product that was used in clinical trials with ADHD, dyslexia, and CAS in the US and UK. It is manufactured by Nutricia USA (Clearwater, FL). Check out their website at www.nutricia.com.

ProEFA (Ultimate Omega, Complete Omega) is the Nordic Naturals version of omega-3 fatty acids found in naturally occurring ratios. You can order directly through the company, www.nordicnaturals.com.

Dr. Sears Go Fish Brainy Kidz Children's Omega-3 DHA Soft Chews is an all-natural fruit-based supplement that supports brain development, no fishy taste or smell. This product is free of wheat, yeast, gluten, milk, and nut derivatives. From a "safe source," meaning that every batch of oil is third-party tested and certified for batch purity and to be free of detectable levels of over 250 environmental contaminants, including mercury, heavy metals, dioxins, PCBs, and pesticides.

Carlson for Kids are vitamins and supplements designed with kids' nutritional needs in mind. All of their products are free of gluten, wheat, milk, casein, nuts, and eggs. They offer liquid fish oil, as well as cod liver oil from fish caught in Norwegian waters and bottled at the site. Kids often prefer it mixed with a favorite food such as chocolate milk. Lemon flavor may be tasty in lemon yogurt. Visit www.carlsonlabs.com for more information.

Sensory-Based Therapies

We all experience the world through our senses—including seeing, hearing, touching, smelling, and tasting (there's also the vestibular and proprioceptive senses, which are very important, but often less talked about). It is through our senses that we make *sense* of the sometimes-overwhelming stimuli coming at us.

Most folks learn how to combine multiple senses in childhood so that they can effectively juggle them at one time. As a child, I used to say something along these lines: "We are always using our brain even when we don't think we are!" I thought I was making an astute observation, but what I was probably trying to explain had something to do with the idea of sensory integration. For example, as you walk outdoors, you *see* the colorful fall foliage, you *feel* the warmth of the sun, you *hear* a school bus coming to a squeaky stop, you *taste* the gum you are chewing, and you *smell* the fire burning off in the distance. You are aware of these things, although you may not consciously be thinking about all of them.

But you *do* consciously think about the bus coming to a squeaky stop. Why? Your sense of hearing is alerting you that there is a possibility of danger. Questions run through your mind: Where is my body in time and space? Could I—or my child(ren)—get hit by that bus?

Some kids (and even adults) have a hard time sorting out sensory stimulation. They may have what is referred to as **sensory processing disorder (SPD)**. The older term for the same phenomenon was sensory integration disorder (SID). You can find more information on SPD/SID in Appendix A.

Sensory Integration Therapy

Sensory integration therapy is used with kids who have a hard time organizing their senses and their world. It's often recommended for children who have autism but can be beneficial to any child who has trouble regulating his senses.

Sensory integration therapy is done by an occupational therapist (OT) and is generally fun, adaptive (working at correcting a deficit or problem), and child directed. You might find kids in an OT session swinging in a hammock or other indoor swing (working on the *vestibular* sensation—movement in space). Or they may be dancing to music (*sound and movement*), playing at a table filled with water or dried beans (*touch*), crawling through tunnels (*touch/space*), doing *balance* beam work, tracking objects or lights with eyes (*vision*), and possibly doing spinning exercises (*balance and vision*). All of these ideas and activities are rooted in various disciplines: neuroscience, developmental psychology, occupational therapy (OT), and education.

Kate participated in OT for help with a mild sensory integration concern, and it worked wonders. She was better able to focus, attend in her classroom, and seek out opportunities to satisfy her need for sensory input. Will it work for your child? Possibly. That is, it wouldn't help with the CAS per se, but might help your child with underlying problems with tolerating sensations or focusing. The effectiveness is a bit controversial.

In *The Out-of-Sync Child* by Carol Stock Kranowitz, we learn that there have been just a few well-designed studies to support sensory integration therapy for kids. About half of the scientific literature suggests it's beneficial; the other half says there's no effect. Perhaps sensory integration therapy may be more useful in younger, versus older kids (again, it's that idea that younger kids benefit from early intervention) Generally, the goal of sensory integration therapy is for kids to be better able to play, learn, and interact with peers—all of which are the *occupation* of a child.

Tip: Movement awakens the sensory system, which can help your child increase attention to tasks. For example, crawling through a tunnel can help provide deep pressure to the joints, making it less taxing to communicate or respond to a question right after the exercise. Your SLP may collaborate with OTs for suggestions about ways to alert your child's sensory system, especially if your child is working with a private OT or one in school.

Hippotherapy

What do *hippos* have to do with *anything*? Actually, *hippos* is a Greek word meaning horse, so hippotherapy is horse-riding therapy.

Kids with abnormal muscle tone (high tone or low tone), poor posture, impaired communication, behavioral and cognitive disabilities, and some medical conditions (Down syndrome and cerebral palsy, especially) may benefit from the therapeutic effects of hippotherapy.

Physical therapists, OTs, and SLPs *may* recommend hippotherapy. The theory is that the rhythmic movement of a horse and the rider's need to constantly adjust to the horse's movements help improve muscle tone, balance, posture, coordination, strength, flexibility, and cognitive skills. Children who are motivated to ride a horse may also be motivated to try to speak to the horse in order to control its movements (e.g., you need to say "Walk on" or "giddy-up" to get it moving, "whoa," to stop, etc.).

Hippotherapy has been shown scientifically to help children with developmental disabilities such as spina bifida, Down syndrome, cerebral palsy, multiple sclerosis, attention deficit, and autism spectrum disorders. Studies have yet to prove its effectiveness with CAS, but one can project similar results.

If you remember back to the discussion about stimulating your child's vestibular system (motor/sensory) to produce more speech, it's the same idea here. Your little one's motor and sensory systems are working hard to ride that horse, so he might as well practice speech sounds too. Keep in mind, just as with traditional speech therapy, children will need repeated exposure to this therapeutic intervention. It is not a "quick fix." For example, if your child is working very hard just to stay on that horse, he may not have the extra reserves to put forth vocalizing. But then again, he might.

Need more to convince you? Think back to chapter 2, in which we talked about the underlying mechanics of speech: postural control, respiration, motor control, timing, and rhythm. Since riding a horse helps in all those areas, it stands to reason that it could also be helpful in speech production.

You may also consider the therapeutic use of an exercise ball in speech therapy. Your SLP may place your child on top of the ball, hold him there, and gently bounce him up and down. The hope here is that your child is better able to make more vocalizations than when he is sitting still.

Sandi Foreman, COTA/L, pediatric occupational therapist, says this about riding horses as a therapeutic intervention: "Hippotherapy is such a great tool for a variety of diagnoses! It provides great sensory input, is good for strength, balance, and motor planning [of limbs and body]. It is so motivational for the kids. The best part is that it is fun and rewarding for both the client and the therapist!"

The American Hippotherapy Association describes physical gains in the form of "balance, posture, mobility, and function; as well as psychological gains in cognitive, behavioral, and communication functions of clients of all ages." The AHS further asserts that people with a variety of diagnoses may benefit from hippotherapy, including language disabilities.

According to Friends for Therapeutic Equine Activities in Winfield, Illinois, the therapeutic results include such things as improved motivation, self-confidence, self-esteem, balance and coordination, cardiorespiratory function, sensory-motor organization, language and cognitive skills, and increased confidence and self-control.

Parents Share

Experiences with Hippotherapy

One mother commented: "My four-year-old daughter [with CAS] went once a week and loved it! She worked with an OT who had her reaching for different objects, throwing balls into hoops as she rode. Since kids with apraxia [CAS] have trouble with planning movements of the muscles of the mouth to make the proper sounds, I thought it helped her with motor planning, as well as coordinating all of the muscles in her entire body. Overall, hippotherapy helped her mouth muscles, overall coordination, and balance."

Another mother thought her child was able to "open up" more with the horse than with people. "[There was] something about not feeling any pressure to talk to people . . . he could just talk to the horse!"

Other parents who have used hippotherapy as part of their child's treatment program have indicated improvements in mood, happiness, exercise, confidence, and animal bonding.

Is Hippotherapy Right for Your Child?

You may be asking yourself, "How do I know if hippotherapy is right for my child?" Here's a list of questions that may help you decide:

1. First and foremost, you will want to **assess whether your child has a fear of large animals.** This sounds relatively easy, but you may be surprised at your child's reaction.

2. Is there a **suitable therapeutic riding facility in your area?** You can start by asking others in your community or at your school, searching online, or posting a question on a Facebook page.

3. **Is therapeutic riding covered by your insurance company?** If so, talk with your child's pediatrician. To receive insurance coverage for hippotherapy, you may need a doctor's prescription.

4. **What are your other time commitments**, and how much time can you commit to hippotherapy? (The drive to and from the facility should factor in to this equation.) Most kids have the best benefits when they have at least one hour a week of therapeutic riding.

5. **What qualifications do staff have?** You'll want involved, educated, specially trained, and professional staff working with your child. In some cases, there are three staff members to one child!

Jill, mom of Finley with CAS and other developmental disabilities, points out one thing to keep in mind if you are hoping for insurance coverage: "Be aware of how you inquire about riding programs. Hippotherapy is not the same as therapeutic riding, according to some facilities. In our experience, 'therapeutic riding' was not covered by insurance, but 'hippotherapy' was." Horse Play Therapy offers a great explanation of what therapeutic riding versus hippotherapy consists of. Check it out here: www.horseplaytherapy.org/hippotherapy-vs-therapeuticadaptive-riding.

Therapeutic riding lessons vary in price, often depending on where you are located (facilities in larger cities tend to charge more, as do those on either coast). In my research, I came across a range of prices, from about $75 to $115 per one-hour class to a low of $35 per half hour. You may also find places that offer package rates or that require an initial evaluation fee. Some insurance companies may cover a portion of the expense. Check to see if yours does.

Therapeutic Listening/Auditory Integration Therapy

Because children are generally not great listeners, I would wager that most parents would gladly enroll their child with CAS in a therapeutic listening course without really knowing what it is!

While therapeutic listening (sometimes called Auditory Integration Therapy) may be able to help regulate a child's listening skills, it's not a cure-all. What therapeutic listening really aims to accomplish is to train a child's ears to attend to and discriminate among sounds.

Children listen—through specially designed, costly earphones—to music that has been carefully engineered so that certain sound frequencies are modulated or distorted. They listen for a prescribed amount of time each day while going about their regular business. The theory behind therapeutic listening programs is that the electronically altered music stimulates neural pathways in the brain. The brain is then supposed to be better able to tune in to higher frequencies that make up human speech.

Does it help? Some folks contend that therapeutic listening *does* help with organizing thoughts, attention, behavior, and speech-language difficulties, while plenty of others suggest it *doesn't*. Many scientists will tell you it is not effective or that it is still experimental. For example, some doctors say that patients responded negatively. And studies completed at MIT and Northeastern University indicate that the frequencies in the music could be harmful to one's ears. The American Speech Language Hearing Association (ASHA) studied the Berard Auditory Integration Therapy (the most commonly used program in the US) and then the ASHA executive board adopted a stance against using the therapy in March 2003. They found that these particular programs did not meet scientific standards for safety and effectiveness.

Vision Therapy

We've got another sense that helps us see the big picture, literally. Our eyes bring a wealth of knowledge and stimulation to our minds. Together, OTs and developmental optometrists have developed vision therapy to home in on visual discrimination and hand-eye coordination. Trained providers use fun, educational activities to strengthen eye musculature. The therapy can help children tune out environmental distractions by integrating various inputs from other senses. Let me explain.

When we began seeing an OT for Kate's attention-control issues, her OT told me that Kate was frequently distracted by visual stimulation. *Everything* was interesting and exciting for Kate to look at. It's like when you are vacationing in a new place—you look around and flashing lights and attractions catch your eye. You can't get enough. Or maybe you do, and you become overwhelmed. That may be how your child feels too.

Our OT said that Kate had difficulty focusing her eyes on something for a significant (or even normal) amount of time. She was darting from activity to activity, losing interest quickly, and getting distracted. Most kids have a tendency to do this anyway—they *are* kids, after all!

But there is a difference between being a "typical kid" and being a child with a visual tracking problem. (**Note: *There is no reason to believe that a child with CAS will have a visual tracking problem.***) A child can have both CAS *and* visual tracking concerns, but they are independent problems.

Kids with tracking problems have weaker musculature around their eyeball(s). Vision therapy presents exercises to do at home to strengthen them. For example, your child may be asked to track a light source with his eyes only (without moving his head or body to follow the light). Or he might look at two objects at the same time, but focus on one first (in the foreground), then the other (in the background), which helps with visual discrimination.

Of course, you want to know if vision therapy will help *your* child with CAS. It *might.* Remember, though: while vision therapy may help improve focus and decrease distractibility, it does not directly improve motor speech issues such as CAS. However, if you suspect the reason your child is not progressing in speech therapy is because of a visual tracking problem, then you may want to mention it to your SLP or OT.

It's also worth noting that there is not much awareness of vision therapy. Therefore, there is not much scientific evidence to prove its effectiveness. It's typically not covered by insurance.

Other suggestions that may help your child if she has a visual tracking problem include the following:

- Declutter work and play spaces your child frequents (more on this in chapter 10).

- Ask your child's teacher to make accommodations in worksheets—for example, removing unnecessary graphics or increasing the text size.

- Talk about a toy, game, or activity to help your child understand what is expected before presenting him with the new (visually stimulating) item. This helped Kate.

For a fuller idea of how vision therapy might help your child, visit the websites listed in the resource section of this chapter.

Talk Yoga

Children love to mimic their parents, and so when a child-parent yoga class became available at our local YMCA, we went. I found that many of the poses were familiar and augmented the work that Kate was doing in OT. And then I stumbled across Talk Yoga, the creation of SLPs Kim Hughes, MA, CCC-SLP, and Amy Roberts, MS, CCC-SLP, who are both certified yoga instructors.

It all started with an after-school program, two fun-loving pediatric speech-language pathologists teaching yoga poses and vocabulary to children. These children had a variety of diagnoses, including autism, attention-deficit disorder, neurological challenges, and learning disabilities. Later the program shifted to a new and improved method called Talk Yoga.

Kim and Amy see this concept as a melding of traditional speech therapy and yoga. It's empowering to children who often feel they cannot do anything quite right. Yoga is individual, go-at-your-own-pace, and offers no competition. Kim and Amy feel strongly that yoga improves learning and communication skills by integrating the mind and body. While children are moving, having fun, and playing, they are learning to express themselves and improve receptive language skills.

Children learn Talk Yoga poses to address articulation, yoga sequences, breathing techniques, and more. For example, children are taught an articulation pose coordinating movements of articulators (lips, tongue, cheeks, breath, jaw, etc.) with movements of the legs, arms, or entire body. Movement, breath, mindfulness, and intention are all emphasized, resulting in a more integrated approach to treatment. As children learn to coordinate their movements with the sound, the neural pathways for that particular motor plan are further developed and strengthened. Amy and Kim have seen children with various speech and language needs grow in their self-confidence as they practice and play with their articulation sound poses and show improvement in their areas of need.

For a fuller understanding of how Talk Yoga may help your child, please refer to the resources section at the end of this chapter.

Medically Based Approaches

Some people you'll encounter on your CAS journey will tell you that there are medically based approaches that may help your child's CAS. For most of these approaches—including cord blood/stem cell transplant and hyperbaric O_2 chamber therapy—there have not been any scientific studies of their effectiveness in treating CAS, so I feel it would be irresponsible to delve into them here. I think it is worth discussing chiropractic treatment, however, because many insurance plans will pay for this, and some case studies published in the literature show that it *may* be effective for children with CAS.

Parents Ask

Can the style/difficulty of birth cause CAS?

I am not aware of any major studies linking communication delays—specifically CAS—and style of birth (C-section versus vaginal) or difficult birth. Many of the birth histories reviewed at speech clinics, however, indicate some concerns perinatally (around the time of birth), such as cords wrapped around the child's neck, loss of oxygen at birth, and emergency C-sections.

There is really no reason to believe that C-sections "cause" CAS. But note that a child born via C-section does not experience that tight "squeeze" through the birth canal that usually activates the lungs and accessory muscles associated with breath control. If the C-section was in response to an emergency situation (e.g., loss of oxygen), that may have affected speech development.

Be honest when your SLP asks you about your child's birth. Don't beat yourself up over the possibility that the style of your child's birth caused CAS. Chances are nothing could have prevented this.

Chiropractors

Some people strongly believe in the healing touch of a chiropractor. If you are interested in having a chiropractor help your child with CAS, make sure he or she is familiar with kids and their issues. Doctors of Chiropractic (DC) medicine do not treat disease but instead remove spinal nerve stress. That is really a fancy term for a "pinched nerve." Spinal nerve stress interferes with the proper function of the nervous system, according to chiropractors.

Dr. Tony Ebel, a chiropractor in Crystal Lake, Illinois, says the reason that chiropractic treatment can help children with CAS is that there are "kinks" in the upper neck and occiput region that prevent messages from flowing normally between the brain, nervous system, and muscular/motor system. Chiropractors are trained to find and detect this misalignment (subluxation) through touch (palpation) and examination. A chiropractic exam looks for the three components of the subluxation—misalignment, fixation, and nerve interference. A chiropractor then uses specific, gentle adjustments to correct and remove the misalignment, allowing proper neurological function to return.

So, is there any research to support using chiropractic adjustments for children with CAS? There are some case studies but no randomized control studies (RCT) that I'm aware of. A 2009 *case study* (Cuthbert and Barras) followed 157 children with developmental delay syndromes, including dyspraxia (CAS), dyslexia, attention-deficit/hyperactivity disorder, and learning disabilities who received chiropractic care. Individual and group data showed that at the end of treatment, the 157 children showed improvements in several areas, including in ability to concentrate, maintain focus and attention, and control impulsivity, as well as in their performance at home and school. However, the researchers did not say specifically whether the children with CAS improved, or if the children with CAS also had other concerns such as ADHD (a comorbid condition).

Please consider talking with your child's pediatrician or others for recommendations of a chiropractor who works well with children. The "best of the best" have received either a certification and/or diplomate in pediatrics through the International Chiropractic Pediatric Association (ICPA). The "Find a Doctor" portion of the website would likely be the best place to start (www.icpa4kids.org). You may want to bear in mind, however, that there are many articles about specific aspects of chiropractic care (as well as other types of complementary and alternative treatments) on the Quackwatch website: www.quackwatch.org.

Music Therapy

Anthropologists may call music the "universal language," and they just may be right. Think of an opera singer singing in Italian. You may not know any Italian, yet you know that the performer is very emotional about something. You can sense her hurt, passion, love, etc. without really understanding the words she is using.

Music therapy is an established healthcare profession that uses music and music experiences to attain *nonmusical goals*—motor, cognitive, social, emotional, and speech communication. Kimberly Sena Moore, PhD, a board-certified neurologic music therapist in private practice, gives several examples of how children with CAS may benefit from music therapy:

"Music therapists (MT) can use rhythm to help organize the oral-motor mechanisms (e.g., speaking in a steady rate where each syllable equals one beat), or they may use singing to help practice speech production. MTs may also select—or compose—specific songs in order to practice specific issues in speech production." For example, the song "The Witch Doctor" by Ross Bagdasarian (a.k.a. David Seville) is especially helpful for practicing vowels, as it repeats "Oo ee oo ah ah ting tang walla walla bing bang" several times throughout the chorus. Finally, a music therapist may use musical improvisation to learn and practice back-and-forth "dialogue" between speaker and listener, which is an important component of communication.

Emily Sevick, assistant professor of music therapy at Western Illinois University, is a strong proponent of singing and its connection to the oral-motor piece of CAS. She explains: "[Singing] is something that can address many important aspects of speaking, such as breath support, tongue movement, and lip movement. Singing can also be used to teach new vocabulary concepts. Songs can range from singing simple nursery rhymes or current songs on the radio to highly structured songs that focus on one particular letter sound or other language concept."

Why Does Music Work as a Therapeutic Intervention?

According to "Music, Rhythm, and Their Potential Benefits for Childhood Apraxia of Speech" by music therapist Kimberly Sena Moore, music therapy works for these reasons:

- *Music is a core function of the brain.* Our brains are wired to respond to music, as proven in various studies on babies as young as one day old.

- *Our bodies naturally move to music.* That is, we move to a rhythm without thinking much about it. Tapping our toes to the beat, for example, is usually an unconscious movement.

- *Children generally respond well to music.*

- *Music shares neural circuits with speech.*

- *Music can make learning easier.* For example, the ABC song helps kids memorize the letters in the alphabet. Try it with other things your kids are expected to know or remember such as their phone number, address, or spelling words!

- *Music is predictable, structured, and organized.* Think of a favorite song. There is a verse with one melody that is followed by a chorus with a different melody, which is usually the same every time it is sung. As we know, kids with CAS need lots of repetition, so go ahead and belt out those tunes!

- *Music can help improve attention skills.* Listening to and reciting music takes concentration, and that, in turn, improves attention.

- *Music is a noninvasive, safe, and motivating intervention—plus, it's FUN!*

Ms. Sena Moore ends with this observation: "Music therapy is a natural fit when targeting speech, language, and communication goals. From using singing to help rewire the brain for speech to using rhythm to coordinate oral motor skills, music therapy works because of the unique way music engages and changes our brains." For more information about Ms. Sena-Moore and how music therapy can help your child, visit her website at www.musictherapymaven.com.

On top of the benefits mentioned above, music therapy can help with managing stress, promoting wellness, and enhancing memory. It can also help children to improve communication and express feelings. Hmm . . . now, that might be something to sing about!

Does Research Support Music Therapy for Kids with CAS?

Perhaps. One clinical case study of a three-year-old girl with CAS found that she was able to produce many syllables, combination sounds, and words by the end of therapy (she was nearly nonverbal when she started therapy). She received twenty-four therapy sessions over a period of nine months.

A critical look at this study makes it difficult to say whether this little girl's improvement had anything to do with her developmental age, or if she was receiving speech therapy in addition to music therapy. More randomized controlled studies need to be done to determine the effectiveness of music therapy on kids with CAS.

What Can You Do to Encourage Speech through Music?

- Encourage your child to dance to the beat and clap his hands when the song mentions a certain word or phrase.
- Try fill-in-the-blank singing: "Old McDonald had a ____." (This fill-in-the-blank style of eliciting a response is called the cloze task in speech-language pathology.)
- You can also practice repeat-after-me style of singing.
- See if your child can match pitches. Go really high and then really low with your voice. Can your child imitate you?
- Have your child imitate musical instrument sounds. You play the kazoo and then have your child play the kazoo in the same manner you did, likewise for other instruments like drums, cymbals, and maracas. (We will talk more about incorporating music at home in the next chapter.)

Ask your SLP about incorporating more music into therapy sessions if you think this is something your child may respond to. To make your case, you may want to refer to these possible benefits of using music in treatment noted in *Here's How to Treat Childhood Apraxia of Speech*, by Margaret (Dee) Fish, MS, CCC-SLP: "Incorporating music into treatment facilitates opportunities to repeat target utterances multiple times, practice producing varied intonation patterns, and model and produce target utterances at a reduced rate by prolonging the vowels."

If you want to pursue formal music therapy, you can ask the American Music Therapy Association for help finding a music therapist at www.musictherapy.org.

Do Nontraditional Therapies Help?

Sometimes you will find scientific research that supports the treatment claims you hear or read about regarding CAM products, but sometimes you won't. Many folks will ask, "So, if it's not scientific, why bother?"

It's been my experience that parents want to know what else may help their child. Since we live in a society in which "more" sometimes equates to "better," why stop at "just" speech therapy?

Knowing about—even trying—additional therapies or remedies gives hope to parents whose kids are struggling. *For children with CAS alone, it is just as beneficial to work with them on a frequent, intense basis to remediate symptoms associated with CAS.* If your child has additional concerns, complementary and alternative medicine (CAM) provides options to augment more traditional therapy. For instance, one parent in my Small Talk: All About Apraxia group noted:

"We had really hit a plateau in speech therapy. Once we started occupational therapy [OT], my daughter really took off in terms of speech and language. We still continued with speech therapy, but I firmly believe it was the addition of OT that did the trick."

While many "claims to cure" are anecdotal success stories, it never hurts to be a smart consumer. Ask questions, be critical, and then go with your gut, as discussed in the next section.

Assessing Alternative Treatments

When you go online, it's likely you will find hundreds of websites, Facebook pages, Twitter feeds, blogs, and message boards that will tell you that "ABC Wonder Remedy" will cure, or dramatically improve, CAS. That's why you need to get really good at *assessing* alternative treatments. Here are a few tips to keep in mind:

- *Consider the source.* You don't believe just anything you see, hear, or read, right? Sites you can generally trust include websites of a government agency, national organization for a specific disorder, nonprofit organizations, a medical school, or a speech pathology department page within a university website.

- *Buyer Beware:* if you're on a website with success articles and products for sale, be extra cautious before whipping out that credit card.

- *Sounds like an empirical question.* Want to know if a study is valid? Find out if any scientific studies have been done using the scientific procedure you learned about in school. Think hypothesis, data collection, results, conclusions . . . then go beyond that and think "controlled studies," "peer review," "reputable journal," and "randomized control trial." A good study needs all of those elements. Sometimes you will run across studies that *sound* good, but they are limited by sample size (too small to make generalizations) or are testimonials—sometimes called anecdotal—from just one doctor, one SLP, or one patient. A treatment could very well still "work," but for the results to really be valid and conclusive, it should be tested using the scientific method, which involves having a control group as well as an experimental group, and sometimes a "blind" study in which researchers are not told which group has had which treatment, so as not influence their conclusions.

- **Really? Or are you just saying that?** Fads come and go. The media will report something is a "breakthrough," and it's not yet ready for the public market. You need confirmation and not just speculation on a new claim. Always go to the primary source—a journal article in an academic publication or the reputable website associated with the claim.

- **Says who? Is there an expert in the house?** Expert opinion should be objective, meaning the expert has nothing to gain personally or professionally from the product or claim. What does your SLP have to say about something you are willing to try? What does ASHA have to say about it? Check it out at www.ASHA.org.

- **Go with your gut.** You know when something feels "off." Listen to that little voice and then sleep on it, ask around, make a pro and con list, whatever you need to do to feel better about things. If the treatment could cause a problem, especially for your kid—but even to your bank account—be conservative. Quackwatch.org is a good place to check out dubious-sounding therapies or even therapies that just sound "too good to be true."

Say That Again?! Chapter Summary

I don't mean to suggest that any of the approaches covered above are cures. They may not even help. But then again, you may have just found *your* magic bullet. Kids are individuals, and just as they do not all like the same toys or colors, they also don't respond to the same CAM approach in the same way.

Whatever approach you decide to try, do your homework. Take a close look at the resources in the following section to further your knowledge on the subject. Make certain there is no risk to your child. It's best to try one approach at a time. Take careful notes and be systematic about it. Trying several at a time to increase the likelihood of progress can be confusing, and you may have a hard time determining just what was helpful—was it the gluten-free diet or the fish oil that helped your little pumpkin talk? Pick and choose a few approaches, but don't knock yourself out, or you could be trying them until your kid is thirty!

Recommended Resources

- If you want to know more about hippotherapy (therapeutic horseback riding), look into **Special Needs, Special Horses: A Guide to the Benefits of Therapeutic Horseback Riding** by Naomi Scott and J. Warren Evans. In addition, you may want to visit the website of Horsefeathers Center in Lake Forest, IL, at www.horse-featherscenter.org for additional information on benefits of hippotherapy.

- *The Out-of-Sync Child: Recognizing and Coping with Sensory Processing Disorder* by Carol Stock Kranowitz and Lucy Jane Miller is a great resource for parents who are looking for ways to understand a child who has different modes of interpreting vision, hearing, motor skills, and nutrition, among others.

- If you liked *The Out-of-Sync Child* (above), then try this one next: *Growing an In-Sync Child: Simple, Fun Activities to Help Every Child Develop* by perceptual-motor therapist Joye Newman.

- *Raising a Sensory Smart Child: The Definitive Handbook* by parent Lindsey Biel and pediatric occupational therapist Nancy Peske will give you some hints, tips, and understanding of sensory issues from a practical view.

- Two additional resources for information on sensory processing difficulties: *Sensational Kids: Hope and Help for Kids with Sensory Processing Disorder* by Lucy Jane Miller and *The Sensory Processing Disorder Answer Book: Practical Answers to the Top 25 Questions Parents Ask* by Tara Delaney, MS, OTR/L.

- For information on **chiropractic treatment**, try the websites of Anthony J. Ebel, DC, CACCP (www.PremierWellnessChiro.com) or Katie Stull, DC (www.stull-chiropractic.com), both of whom provided me with information helpful in writing this chapter.

- *The International Chiropractic Pediatric Association* is a helpful online resource if you are interested in looking at chiropractic care for your child: www.icpa4kids.com. You may also appreciate the *Intersect4Kids program*, a very advanced certification for chiropractors in the area of neurodevelopmental disorders, spectrum/sensory challenges. Their website is www.intersect4kids.com.

- *Cure Your Child with Food: The Hidden Connection between Nutrition and Childhood Ailments* by Kelly Dorfman (Workman Publishing Company, 2013) presents a parent-friendly explanation of theories about possible connections between nutrition and chronic childhood ailments such as ear infections, allergies, and ADHD. You may also gain valuable information from Ms. Dorfman's website: www.kellydorfman.com.

- *Healing the New Childhood Epidemics: Groundbreaking Program for the 4-A Disorders: Autism, ADHD, Asthma & Allergies,* by Kenneth Bock and Cameron Stauth (Ballantine Books, 2008).

- The **American Hippotherapy Association** can provide you with guidance and information on hippotherapy/therapeutic riding: 970–818-1322; info@theahainc.org; www.americanhippotherapyassociation.org.

- The Listening Program (TLP) is one of the main companies that specialize in *auditory integration therapy.* Their website provides an overview of the program and help finding a provider: www.thelisteningprogram.com. You can also check out Vital Links (www.vitallinks.com), which has a similar product.

■ For more information on *vision therapy*, refer to the Optometrists Network: www.visiontherapy.org.

■ Learn more about *Talk Yoga* here: https://www.talkyogaslp.com/.

■ *Seeing through New Eyes: Changing the Lives of Children with Autism, Asperger's Syndrome, and Other Developmental Disabilities through Vision Therapy* by Melvin Kaplan (Jessica Kingsley Publishers, 2008).

■ *The Holistic Pediatric Association* at www.hpakids.org is a good source for information on treating kids in a holistic manner.

■ Timothy Culbert and Karen Olness have written a book called *Integrative Pediatrics* (Oxford University Press, 2009) with guidelines on Complementary Medicine in an easy-to-read, evidence-based manner.

■ Hilary McClafferty, MD, FAAP, a pediatrician and associate professor in the Department of Medicine at the University of Arizona College of Medicine in Tucson, Arizona, has a text that may inform and educate on matters of integrative medicine when it comes to your child, *Integrative Pediatrics* (Routledge, February 2017).

■ For more information on music therapy, check out the *American Music Therapy Association:* www.musictherapy.org; 301–589-3300.

■ *Music, Language, and the Brain* by Aniruddah D. Patel (Oxford University Press, 2010) is a comprehensive volume about the neuroscience behind language and music.

■ You may find these various *music therapy websites* helpful to you and your children:

- Milestone Music Therapy: www.milestone-musictherapy.com
- Listen and Learn Music: www.listenlearnmusic.com
- Kimberly Sena Moore's website: www.musictherapymaven.com

■ The article "Music, Rhythm, and Their Potential Benefits for Childhood Apraxia of Speech" by music therapist Kimberly Sena Moore is available here: www.pediastaff.com/blog/music-rhythm-and-their-potential-benefits-for-childhood-apraxia-of-speech-647 (originally published online, May 28, 2010).

Chapter 9

What You Can Do at Home

Tapping into Your Inner Speech-Language Pathologist

"I learned the most from the sessions on what I can do at home to help my son. I didn't know there was so much I could actually do. I had thought only the SLP could do some of this stuff. Don't get me wrong; they do a lot. But I can do some pretty cool things to help my son too."
—Small Talk: All About Apraxia parent participant

This might be the chapter we have all been waiting for. It's the one I am the most eager to write. You may have turned to this chapter first, for it is the one thing you can actually feel good about doing—making a difference in your child's struggles with childhood apraxia of speech.

Here you will find tips and ideas for helping your child make progress in a fun and nurturing speech-rich environment at home and on the go. Simple toys and books can become therapeutic; music and games can promote speech development. This chapter will enable you to combine all aspects of your parenting brain: teaching, nurturing, creating, role-playing, and limit-setting. So get ready!

Even adults remember new information best when they are having fun. If you had a traditional education, you grew up with desks, blackboards, and the teacher at the front of the class. You were taught that this is how people learned. It might be time to shift your view and throw out the flashcards! This chapter does not take place in a classroom. It does not even suggest you turn your dining room into a speech clinic (although that's not necessarily a bad idea). But it *is* about learning how to help your child overcome CAS in a natural environment: your home and community.

Here are a few ideas to get you started:

- *Have a family game night.* Traditional favorites will do the trick. The speech pay-offs here: turn-taking, counting, requesting, being a good sport, and other communication opportunities.

- *Visit your public library.* Let your child find some books of interest and then read them to her. Speech payoff: child-directed learning, introduction to new vocabulary, one-on-one time with you in which you are modeling pronunciation and articulation. You might even hear some sounds or word approximations from your child!

- *Experience and connect with nature.* Speech payoff: identify and describe what you see, hear, and smell. Think holistically—this is more than *just* a walk in the park.

- *Exercise* by biking or sledding, walking, or swinging. Speech payoff: movement can help trigger vocalizations and words. Exercise also increases self-confidence, which these kiddos need more than anything. Children with CAS often crave movement.

- *Do some art.* Speech payoff: unleashing creative potential and giving you something to talk about (e.g., "What color should we make the banana?".) Practice saying "banana" or "yellow" while you're at it.

- *Listen to music.* Speech payoff: kids need physical movement, and what better way to get them moving than with some rockin' tunes? Even if they can't get the lyrics out, they can hum along. Plus, music has a positive effect on mood—even yours!

- *Bake cookies or cupcakes.* Speech payoff: identifying ingredients as you toss them into the bowl, having your child repeat the words (flour, sugar, butter, etc.) if she is able, talking about shapes as you roll out sugar cookies. Share your cookies with friends and neighbors and let your child do *some* of the talking—if possible—when the two of you deliver the goodies. It can be as simple as saying "hi" or "cookie" or "bake" (an approximation will do).

The Nuts and Bolts of This Chapter

- Your "toolbox" with a host of fun ideas to get your child talking, playing, and learning
- How to have fun with speech and language each day in a variety of settings, as you move through your family's daily routines
- Gross motor, musical, and multimedia avenues to get your child's speech system warmed up and ready to go, and to actually facilitate speech
- How to identify your child's learning style and preferences and how to best tap into these

Learning Styles

Before we have a deeper discussion about what you can do at home, it's important to talk about different styles of learning. Each of us learns best in different and unique ways. Sure, we can learn in a classroom by reading books and sitting at desks in neat, straight lines. But is this the *best* way for everyone to learn? How do you learn best? How does your child learn best? Don't be discouraged if the two of you learn in different ways. We'll touch on melding those differences later in this chapter.

When I sat down to write this chapter (at a coffee shop, where I tend to do my best writing and learning), it came as no surprise that I had several piles of information corresponding to different learning styles. The biggest pile was about gross motor/sensory/whole-body/kinesthetic learning. By now, you know why: *CAS is a disorder of the motor-speech system.* Many children with CAS may also have other motor programming problems such as oral and/or limb apraxia. Adequate sensory processing is necessary for good motor programming.

But there are lots of other learning styles and preferences. Without getting into too much of the psychology of learning and different educational theories, let's review them in brief. Be sure to note the traits that sound most like your child.

Howard Gardner, a developmental psychologist and professor of education, suggests that humans have multiple intelligences. Most individuals are more skilled in some areas than others, which leads to a preferred or certain style of learning. Gardner has identified eight different types of intelligences, all of which work together to create a whole. Here they are:

Multiple Intelligences

Area	Description	Strengths
LINGUISTIC	**Strong awareness of:** ■ Sounds ■ Rhythms ■ Words	**May be adept at:** ■ Organizational abilities ■ Logical deduction ■ Good memory of spoken words & written language ■ Structured & sequenced instruction
LOGICAL-MATHEMATICAL	**Proficient in:** ■ Logic ■ Patterning ■ Conceptualization ■ Abstraction	**Likely enjoys:** ■ Problem-solving ■ Patterns ■ How and why things work

MUSICAL- RHYTHMIC	**Easily discriminates:** ■ Auditory tone ■ Pitch ■ Rhythm	**Generally good at:** ■ Auditory patterning ■ Remembering things that he or she hears
VISUAL-SPATIAL	**Naturally:** ■ Understands the relation-ships between objects, concepts, or images ■ Looks at events from different viewpoints.	**These learners:** ■ Can mentally create and visualize very well ■ Good at drawing maps and diagrams ■ Look at the big picture first, then fill in details
BODILY- KINESTHETIC	**Loves to:** ■ Move body through time and space ■ Perform sequential move-ments	**Generally:** ■ Has a good sense of time ■ Understands proportion ■ Predicts sequences well ■ Can visualize move-ments before they occur
INTERPERSONAL	**Highly proficient at:** ■ Perceiving moods ■ Empathizes well with others' feelings	**Typically:** ■ Interacts well with others ■ Natural leader ■ Can do the above well because they can sense emotions, needs, desires, and intentions of others
INTRAPERSONAL	**Confident in:** ■ Knowing self well ■ Believing strongly in one's values and goals	**These individuals:** ■ Can reflect well on their own thoughts and feel-ings ■ Are introspective ■ Analyze their own be-havior through reflection.
NATURALISTIC	**Highly perceptive of:** ■ Things in the natural world ■ Plants ■ Animals	**Generally, it is easy to:** ■ Organize things into categories ■ Make detailed observa-tions ■ Recognize patterns

Did you see yourself in any of these categories? Your child? Perhaps you saw attributes in more than one category that describe you and/or your child.

Despite the many strengths identified by Gardner, schools, teachers, and even parents tend to expect children to have just one of three learning styles: auditory, visual, and/or kinesthetic.

How do you prefer to learn new material? By **seeing** it done (demonstration), **reading** about new information, **hearing** someone else describe what to do, or **doing** the new task until you feel you've got it?

Of course, your little one with CAS likely can't tell which learning style she prefers. It takes time and introspection to figure out one's best learning style, and most children have no idea what theirs is. It's up to you to observe and see how your child responds to different approaches. Particularly good teaching instruction will employ *seeing, doing, hearing*, and *reading*.

Before we can help our children at home with speech and language, it is helpful to have some idea of how they best learn, so we can best help. The bottom line with this information on learning styles and intelligences is this:

- Your child will not fall neatly into one camp.
- You will see bits and pieces of your child's traits in each category, but there will be one category that seems to be the "best fit."
- Kids with CAS are individuals, just like other children. It is your job to find out how you can best help *your child with CAS.*
- Hopefully this information will help you hone your skills so you can best help your child.

Parenting Primer

There are a few things you need to keep in mind as your "golden rules" in working with your child with CAS:

- **Have your child repeat, repeat, repeat!** Movement repetitions build strong motor planning/programming/gestures. *Can you say that again?*
- **Provide lots of opportunities throughout the day to get your child to talk or vocalize—about** **anything.** Your child will begin to see that communication is indeed a fun part of life.
- **Be goofy and funny.** If you are relaxed and your kiddo is relaxed, words will come easier.
- **Make talking and speech practice more about your lifestyle and less about "sit and speak" time.**
- **Team up with your SLP.** Have him or her give you ideas for homework and report back to him or her. Let the SLP know what your kid does well at home and see if it works as well in the clinic. Think of your SLP-parent-child connection as a

circle with no beginning and no end; make it appear as if you are driving a fancy automatic car—smooth and effortless, even if it's really a jumpy five-speed jeep.

- **The more talking feels like work, the less willing your kid will be to do it.**

- **Imitation is huge too.** "Can you say what I say?" Try it. If imitation is too hard, try doing it in unison. Even singing the ABC song is a type of imitation in the form of chanting memorization.

- **You are a parent or caregiver first.** You do not need to become your child's SLP. Kids are smart. They will know what you're up to and won't participate if you act too much like their SLP.

- **Your goal is to complement your SLP's efforts in your own home.** Talk to your SLP about a reasonable amount of home practice. This will also depend on your child's age. As one CAS parent named Mike says, "An SLP is like a personal trainer at the gym. You go, your trainer works with you for an hour and teaches you things to do on your own, but it's up to you to do the rest."

Homemade Speech and Language Lessons

Feeling ready to kick it up to high gear? Grab a notebook or a highlighter. You'll want to make a list of favorite activities—ones you think your child will respond to best, based on personality, interests, personal motivators, and age. Your willingness and ability are other factors to contribute—time, effort, support, and sometimes money. Remember, your goal here is not to get your child to say things perfectly, but to encourage speech communication.

Gross Motor and Whole Body Activities

1: Bounce Your Way to Words!

What you need: A trampoline appropriate for your space and budget. You can find small basic trampolines in the sporting goods department of your favorite retailer for about $30. You might even be able to find one second-hand through a friend or other reputable source. Bigger (outdoor) ones come with a higher price tag and other concerns like space, insurance, possible injuries, and neighbor kids. Look for one made just for one child; a stabilizer bar is helpful. Keep it in a place in your home where your child will see it and use it.

What you do: Let your child bounce on it for at least fifteen minutes a day over a period of several months; you're bound to see a jump in words. You can also have your child jump and practice saying target sounds and words.

Speech payoff: It's fun! The underlying issue in CAS is neurological motor planning. Jumping requires motor programming. Movement helps your child's mind and body work together more effectively.

2: Box It Up, Please

What you need: Boxes—big, little, and in-between sizes—plus imagination. Make sure there are no sharp brads or corners and then let the kids have at it!

What you do: Create toys, forts, stages, and playhouses. Probe your child to describe—using words—what she is doing. Is she making a robot? Ask her to identify and describe body parts. "Building" a dollhouse or castle can focus on words like *window*, *door*, *inside*, *outside*, and the many other descriptions that can go with building.

Speech payoff: Kids use their imaginations and creativity to paint, cut, tape, fold, and construct. It builds problem-solving skills and a larger vocabulary.

3: Freeze Frame

What you need: Music (CD player, radio, iTunes, etc.) and kids. You might even want to try JustDance, technically a party game featuring top 40 hits that can be accessed via a gaming platform like Xbox, Nintendo Switch, PlayStation, Wii; you can also use your smartphone to connect. Designed in conjunction with child development experts to encourage healthy movement, you can read more about it at www.ubisoft.com.

What you do: Put on some tunes and have the kids dance, wiggle, jump, and move to the music. When the music stops, everyone freezes and says a word, phrase, or approximation of a word, either related to how they're posing, or some other target word or phrase you determine ahead of time. The key is they have to say *something*!

Speech payoff: Besides providing fun and exercise, it works the vestibular system and helps those words come out.

4: Rollin', Rollin'— Keep Those Kids Rollin'

What you need: Kid(s), adult(s), and a flat, open, safe place to roll around.

What you do: Lie down, grab your child, and gather her to your chest with your arms. Roll back and forth saying, "I've got . . . mommy/daddy/baby brother/teacher/friend/neighbor/grandparent." You and your child take turns saying who they've "got." If your child can't say the entire phrase, "I've got Papa," just have her say "Papa." You can even use fill-in-the-blank to help your child: "I've got _____."

Speech payoff: You can practice names of family members in a nonthreatening, on-the-spot manner. Aunt Lauren isn't really there when you are practicing this activity, but the next time you see her, your child will be more comfortable with saying her name. It also encourages parent-child bonding and stimulates the all-important vestibular system.

5: Get in the Swing of It!

What you need: Swings at the park, in your backyard, or even hanging from the rafters in your basement.

What you do: Push your child as long as she will allow, and you have energy for. As you push, think of target sounds, words, or phrases to work on with your child. Practice the ABCs, work on perfecting her name, count to ten, etc. Do this at least once a day for fifteen to twenty minutes over the course of a few months, and you just may see a surge in talking.

Speech payoff: Can you say *vestibular system*?

> **Parents Ask**
>
> ***What's the big deal about motion, again?***
> The first couple of chapters explain that CAS is a disorder of the neuromotor system. In fact, physical and occupational therapists who have worked with children with speech disorders have commented that children become much more vocal when engaged in movement such as rocking, swinging, bouncing, sliding, or even rock climbing. These activities are often referred to as *vestibular stimulation* activities.
>
> We found that Kate did much better in her speech therapy sessions when we complemented them with occupational therapy. I would go as far as to say that it was the combination of speech and occupational therapies that was the "key" that unlocked Kate's voice.

6: Do a Little Dance, Make a Little Word

What you need: Adult and child.

What you do: The adult calls out different kinds of movements: "Touch the sky way up high—touch your toes way down low—wiggle your hips—rub your tummy." The child plays along and can repeat words as she feels ready. Add in other body parts like nose, ears, hair, mouth, tongue, knees, etc.

Speech payoff: Whole body movements can help get your little pumpkin talking; they also encourage listening to directions and enhance receptive language and identification of body parts.

7: If We Could Talk Like the Animals

What you need: Nothing but you and a child with CAS.

What you do: Can you make a great pig noise? Do it—but really act like a pig by rolling around (as if in the mud). After you are done oinking, say the name of the animal. Bark like a dog, jump like one, pant and lick like one. Meow like a cat, rub your head on a loved one, purr, and curl up like a cat.

Variation: As your child gets better at this, she has to identify the animal by name ("dog") before moving on to the next one.

Speech payoff: Besides the fun and giggles you're sure to get, it helps your child learn about different animals and their sounds. Plus, making animal sounds may be less intimidating than saying actual words. In fact, the Kaufman Speech Praxis Treatment Kit: Basic level begins with animal sounds. These are often some of the first words children say.

8: Roll to Me, Baby

What you need: Kid(s) and a ball.

What you do: Sit on the floor, legs apart, and take turns rolling the ball back and forth (or tossing the ball in the air as your child's skills improve). Practice saying target words or telling about a favorite something (food, color, season, friend, etc.) while you roll/toss the ball. Do this until you (or she) tires of it, but aim for at least six passes. If your child is nonverbal, you roll the ball and say "Mommy's turn." When it is your child's turn, say "Kate's turn" for her.

Speech payoff: This is a wonderful way to encourage conversational turn-taking: speaker + listener = conversation. Teach this concept early.

9: Take a Hike

What you need: Yourself and a fun/interesting place to walk.

What you do: Walk around your park, neighborhood, or local arboretum with your family. Using the letters of the alphabet as a guide, find items along your path that begin with the letter, sound, or word your child is working on in therapy. First choose words and sounds your child already knows and build upon that base.

Variation: Label every tree (or other item) you see as you pass by (a form of concentrated practice; auditory bombardment).

Speech payoff: Repetition, whole-body learning, develops a love of nature, plus it's a fun way to sneak in speech drills.

10: Stage a Scavenger Hunt

What you need: Four or five items that interest your child and that target a sound, word, or phrase you are working on.

What you do: Show the items to your child and then hide them around your house. Set a timer for an appropriate amount of time and have her look for the items. When she finds the item, have her identify what it is, three times. After three attempts at saying the target sound, reward her with something of value (a sticker, a food treat, more play, a video game, movie, or something else).

Variation: Make it a mobile scavenger hunt by doing it in the car. First, list items you might spot on the route you choose. Sneaky parents will think of the target sounds that are challenging (e.g., the *st* sound in the words *stop sign, store, stone,* for the child who has advanced to this level). You could even draw pictures of a stop sign, store, stone, etc. or cut them out of magazines. When you drive by that spot, your child shouts out what she found.

Speech payoff: Kids, like adults, get bored with the same ol' routine. This activity shakes it up a bit, plus it encourages memory and works on repetition.

11: Create an Obstacle Course

What you need: Whatever you have on hand and don't mind your kids crawling through, jumping in, bouncing on, or climbing on top of—chairs, blankets, trampolines, etc. Throw in some directives, too. "Do two somersaults and now three jumping jacks!"

What you do: Design the course and then have your child complete the activities. You can make it more challenging by having your child say key words/phrases/sounds at each station. Encourage verbalization at the end ("I'm a winner," "Hooray," or another similar phrase). Afterward, you can pull out the speech flashcards. You may be amazed at how much faster and easier your child responds once the body (and brain) have been "warmed up" with a vestibular/movement activity.

Speech payoff: Fun, silly play beats boredom any day, and it just might be what your rough-and-tumble kid needs to stimulate the verbal part of her brain.

12: Switch It Up

What you need: Flashcards (make your own or buy some); speech exercises or worksheets from your SLP; objects from around the house that correspond to sounds, words, or phrases you are currently targeting; coloring books. You'll need access to music and your child(ren).

What you do: Arrange the items you gathered on the floor. Then start the music and the dancing. When the music stops, have your child pick an item from the floor to talk about, or practice. Do several rounds.

Speech payoff: Again, it's work disguised as fun involving movement, rhythm, and vestibular activation.

13: Target Toss

What you need: Hula hoop and bean bags, foam balls, or other soft toys.

What you do: Set the hula hoop on the floor (or grass). Invite your child to stand a certain distance away from the hula hoop and toss or drop beanbags, foam balls, or other soft toys into it. Each time she tosses something into the target, have your child say "toss/throw in" or a target sound, word, or phrase.

Speech payoff: Fun for little ones, especially when targets are large and accuracy is not important. Plus, it's active fun for little minds.

14: Fall Fun

What you need: Rake (child-sized is best), kid, and lots of fall leaves.

What you do: Help your child rake leaves in the yard. Talk about the sounds the leaves make as you rake them. You can stress the words "in" and "out" as you put leaves into bags.

Speech payoff: Working together promotes bonding and teamwork, respect for nature, and, again, it's a whole-body movement that not only exercises the body, but the mind as well.

15: Touch & Talk

What you need: Container, rice or beans, and various small objects.

What you do: Fill the container with uncooked rice or beans, add small objects, shake it up, and then have your child reach in and find an object (look for objects that contain target sounds or words). Talk about what the object does, looks like, and what other things can go with it. Description is a powerful language development activity.

Speech payoff: This activity is great for touchy-feely kids who learn best by doing. It encourages problem-solving, language development, and critical thinking skills (what can we do with it? what else goes with that?).

16: Be a Superhero

What you need: Something your child can use as a cape or crown.

What you do: Pretend your little one is a superhero—"Super Word Boy/Girl" or the like. Let her run—but not aggressively—in a safe place, with her cape or crown. Encourage neat words that superheroes often use: "Kaboom, bam, boink, and pow," and let your child have fun saving the day with verbal power!

Speech payoff: This activity is a great outlet for kids' supercharged energy. Those silly action words are a lot of fun to say. Plus, when speech drills and therapy wear them down, this feels like play, yet you know it's secretly work.

17: Block Head

What you need: Table blocks, colored stacking blocks, cardboard brick blocks, even empty food boxes.

What you do: Have your child build with blocks. Encourage her to talk about what she is building. For example, "I see you are building a tall tower . . . how do you get to the top?" Or, "Who lives in the house?" If your child is reluctant to answer questions, make statements and give her time to respond. Some children with speech concerns are sensitive to too many questions.

Speech payoff: Again, it's active play that ties together gross and fine motor work (speech is fine motor work). Your child is actively playing with something that already interests her and may not notice that you are getting her to talk about what she is doing. Words just might "pop" out.

Books/Words

We all know that books can open a whole new world of imagination, but they can also help open a whole new world of speech. Here are some ideas for using books, magazines, and catalogs to get some word practice in for your child.

1: Vacation Time

What you need: Nothing!

What you do: Pretend you are going on a trip to the beach. Ask your child to help you "pack." Have her make suggestions by giving prompts: "We wear this when we go swimming" or "So we don't get sunburned, we will need to bring ____." Fill-in-the-blank is a *great* way to encourage speech production. Suggest a couple of silly items that your child knows won't be going in your suitcase to the beach. Try a pretend vacation to the mountains next.

Speech payoff: It's a fun way to pass the time if you are waiting. It also develops vocabulary, word associations, and critical thinking skills. You can focus on target sounds/words/phrases.

2: Art Appreciation

What you need: Picture books or real artwork at home or around town. Try these books: *Can You Find It Inside?* and *Can You Find It Outside?* by Jessica Schulte. They're great hardcover art appreciation books for kids in which you search and discover famous pieces of art based on rhyme-style clues.

What you do: Study the pictures/illustrations/art. Ask your child questions about what's happening. Together, you can create a story. "Who lives here?" "Why do you think he's sad?" For less verbal kids, just identifying what you—the adult—see in the picture can encourage your child to vocalize. The more you talk, the more she learns. Just be sure to give your child time to respond. Some adults are uncomfortable with silence, especially when their communication partner is struggling. You will get better at this!

Speech payoff: Exposure to new media and styles of art increases observational skills and attention to detail and encourages storytelling.

3: A Picture Is Worth 1000 Words

What you need: Magazine, scissors, and glue.

What you do: Cut out magazine pictures of things that interest your child—people, places, and things like toys and food. Look for pictures of a single object, say pizza, Grandma, etc. Then glue the images to a note card or construction paper. When you have a sizeable collection of photos (it will vary based on your child's age, attention span, and verbal ability), arrange the cards on the floor and use the pictures to create a story. You can target specific speech sounds, words, or phrases.

Variation: Rip an action picture/photo from the magazine. Ask your child to tell you about it. Where are the people going, what are they eating, are they happy or sad? Can your child ask *you* about the picture? This can help your child develop question-asking skills.

Speech payoff: This can target sequencing (see below) and stirs the creative juices to develop storytelling. It can get your child talking about things that interest her.

4: Folding Fun

What you need: Kumon *Let's Fold!* and *Let's Cut!* workbooks for preschool (ages 2–5 years), available from most places that carry books.

What you do: Pick a few activities from the book and do them together with your child. Ask her about what you are doing. For example, one activity is a picture of a little boy smiling. When you open the folded part, he's crying. You could ask your child to say "smile" (working on an *s* blend or ask her to say "cry"). Ask other questions such as "Why is she happy?" Even if your child answers with "I don't know" (or some variation of it—as long as it's verbal), it still counts!

Variation: If your child is reluctant to answer questions, try comments or fill-in-the-blank.

Speech payoff: Fun, engaging, and one-on-one time with a parent. The activities are varied and can be used just about anywhere. Keep a Kumon workbook in your car or bag and see where it takes you.

5: The Big Book of Exclamations

What you need: *The Big Book of Exclamations 2* (Chatterbox Books, 2017), written by SLP Teri K. Peterson, MS, CCC-SLP. There's a board-style book, too—thicker pages, rounded edges, not available on Amazon. Look for it at www.thebigbookofexclamations.com or www.chatterboxbooks.com.

What you do: *Look* at it with your child. This book is not a traditional storybook. The captivating illustrations give your child lots of opportunity to practice speech words and sounds in a fun, nonthreatening way. It helps parents learn to talk about the illustrations in books. Teri's technique is useful for other illustrated books as well. (See "Literacy Is Key" in chapter 7 and dialogic reading later in this chapter as well as in chapter 12 for more tips on this style of looking at books with your child).

Speech payoff: If you're a bookworm, you'll find this is a fun way to bond with your child while sneaking in speech practice. Check out Ms. Peterson's website for more information: www.thebigbookofexclamations.com.

6: Auditory Bombardment

What you need: List of words beginning with the same sound (a target sound for your child). For example, sixteen words beginning with a *k* or hard *c* such as *coat, cane, cage, kick, camp, kite, court, cup, cut, cab, card, cone, king, kid, kiss,* and *key.*

What you do: While your kiddo is sitting at the table, playing quietly in the sandbox, or any another quiet moment, read the list aloud several times slowly and clearly. Read the list a couple of times a day. It will only take you a minute or two to get through the words. This is more of a listening exercise and not exactly one your child will repeat.

Variation: Have your child search through magazines and catalogs looking for items on the list. Make a collage. I used to make up silly stories like this about the words on the page: The kid kicked the cat's cage and then kissed the king.

Speech payoff: Your child will hear that beginning letter sound over and over and begin to internalize it. Speech requires auditory recognition and discrimination of sounds.

7: Magic Words

What you need: Good manners.

What you do: Model those "magic words" (*thank you, please,* etc.) wherever you go. The more often you do this in the presence of your children, the more likely they will do the same. Thank your kids for small things too: "*Thank* you for playing so nicely with your sister. *Thank* you for taking your plate to the sink. *Thank* you for getting buckled up so quickly in the car." After you have modeled polite words for a while, see if your child can imitate you or say the words in unison with you. Unison can be easier than imitation. This is sort of like the auditory bombardment idea above. Your child hears it so many times he'll eventually get it. You'll need to exaggerate the words and get your child to look in the person's eyes and say it (even an approximation) with you or right after you say it.

Speech payoff: Children with CAS may not be able to say much, but it's no excuse for not being polite. Explain that a "thank you" or "please" makes people feel good, and when people feel good, they may help you again in the future. Watch folks smile when your child uses manners, even if it is just an approximation.

8: Act It Out

What you need: Nothing.

What you do: Think charades with a therapy twist. Bring therapy ideas home and get creative. For instance, the *j* sound is typically very tricky. You can turn that into a jump-a-thon at home in a sort of "say it, do it" fashion. Act out the word *push*; exaggerate the *p* sound as you push open doors, or push a toy ride-on around the room. Have your child bring in a grocery bag. Say, "It's *heavy*. So *heavy*. Can you say *heavy*?" Exaggerate the *h* sound. (Keep in mind, some SLPs may not want you to work with hard/tricky words at home with your child at first. They want to see you and your child be successful at home with easier sounds and words before making homework more challenging. Check with your SLP first.)

Speech payoff: It's a fun way to entertain and engage (whole-body) kids with their speech practice. It shows them you are serious about their interests/activities and that you have found a way to incorporate them at home. Plus, it might help you get some household chores done!

9: Book Talk (Dialogic Reading)

What you need: Picture books your child likes.

What you do: Read with your child and *let* him interrupt. Allow lots of time for a reading session. Remember, you don't have to read everything on the page. Study the pictures together and ask "wh-" questions (who-what-when-where-why), and see what your child can come up with. You might start just by pointing out the items in the picture. Give choices if your child has a hard time spontaneously identifying objects: "Is this an umbrella or a boot?" When you ask *what* a character is doing in the book, you'll get an answer that works on action words and the "–ing" word ending (running, walking, jumping, washing). You can expand on this and say, "Show me *running*," and allow your child to run around the room once or twice and finish the exercise by saying, "Run!"

Speech payoff: Besides facilitating language development and introducing new vocabulary words, you are engaging in what experts call *dialogic reading*. It's reading as though you were having a conversation—stopping to discuss pictures and new words, and identifying feelings and emotions of the characters. The key with dialogic reading is to read with expression and enthusiasm.

10: Show and Tell for Mom and Dad

What you need: A nifty little item you want to talk to your kids about (e.g., your new iPhone/iPad, a cool new cooking gadget), perhaps at the dinner table.

What you do: Instead of your child and a favorite item being the center of attention, it's *your turn* to "show and tell." You can expose your child to new words like "[app]lication," "download," "garlic press," "nutcracker."

Speech payoff: Your child is likely familiar with the game from school, so you are expanding on that experience by introducing her to new vocabulary. This helps our see-it-touch-it-learn-it learners.

Rhythm/Music

The jury's still out on the role music plays in the learning process. Scientists are continuing to look at whether music supports verbal and math skills. In the meantime, it is fun, and what could it hurt? Music can help kids express themselves, relax, and release tension, and it may even help with attention, focus, and creativity. Here are some products designed with speech improvement in mind, some specifically for CAS:

SPEECHercise CDs

These CDs were created by SLPs to help kids ages three to six with speech disabilities at home, at school, and in the car. They combine silly songs, mouth activities, and speech drills. Plus, there's a parent guide, worksheets, and lyrics if you order the "enhanced music CD." Available at www.twinsisters.com.

Marvelous Mouth Music: Songames for Speech Development

Created by Suzanne Evans Morris, PhD, this product consists of a book and CD and gets kids working on speech breathing and voicing in fun ways. You can find it on Amazon and other sites online.

Therapro

This company helps kids with speech and language difficulties sing simple songs through fun, themed albums such as *Drills for Sounds* and *Rock and Roll with a Language Goal*. Check them out at www.therapro.com/Browse-Category/Talk-It-Rock-It-formerly-Kids-Express-Train.

Make a Sound and Move Around

An SLP and musician created this program consisting of a CD and booklet. The program works on basic communication, socialization, and movement skills. It is best suited for kids aged eighteen months to three years. Available at www.pediatrictherapynetwork.org.

Dr. Jean Feldman's Albums

Dr. Feldman has lots of albums under her belt—all with fun titles sure to get a giggle (*Kiss Your Brain, Going Green,* and *Totally Math*). An educator for over forty years, Dr. Feldman has a way with kids from preschool through the elementary years. Look for her website at www.drjean.org, under "Song Store Lyrics."

Silly Mom Jingles

Even though I can't carry a tune in a bucket, I still sing songs to my kids. After a few poor attempts at singing lullabies, I quickly learned that the better form of song for me is the jingle. I challenge you to think of ways to turn everyday comments or directives into a song. Before you know it, your little ones may just join in on the chorus. Here are a few examples of things I sang/chanted around the house during our daily routines:

- "Yummy to my tummy, yummy to my tummy, yum, yum yum!"
- "Pee pee in the potty, pee pee in the potty, pee pee pee!" (Or substitute "poo poo.") This jingle worked wonders when we were potty-training.
- "This is the way we dry your hair, dry your hair, dry your hair. This is the way we dry your hair so early in the evening."
- "Go with the green light; go with the green light; go with the green light. Go!" or "Stop with the red light, stop with the red light; stop."

Traditional Songs and Rhymes to Teach Your Kids

- ABC song
- "I'm a Little Teapot"
- "Rain, Rain Go Away"
- "Head, Shoulders, Knees and Toes"
- "Twinkle, Twinkle Little Star"
- "Pat a Cake"
- "This Little Piggy"
- "Wheels on the Bus"
- "Pop Goes the Weasel"
- "Itsy Bitsy Spider"
- "Five Little Monkeys Jumping on the Bed"

I like these songs and rhymes because many of them have an action component. Since we know that CAS is a motor-based disorder, these motions go hand-in-hand with the lyrics.

You may also want to try the "call and response" style of singing with your child(ren) in which you say something and they repeat or answer your "call"—as in "Who Stole the Cookies from the Cookie Jar?"

Props

Consider investing in some of these to have on hand for a music experience:

- kazoos to encourage vocal intonation used in signing and speech,
- harmonicas to encourage breath control and direction of air through the mouth,
- a toy microphone that amplifies the voice and increases auditory feedback,
- an echo microphone (Echo Mic) to provide auditory feedback via reverberation (you might find a similar experience with Pop Toobs)

Look for these items at party supply stores and dollar stores.

Sequencing

Sometimes kids with CAS have difficulty following directions or following an orderly sequence of events. They may need extra time to absorb what is being said or asked of them, and they may need directions repeated during the middle of a task. Help them out by offering to strengthen those skills through some fun games. Just remember to vary the activities to keep your child interested and engaged.

1: Follow the Leader and Simon Says

What you need: Child(ren) and a little bit of time (five to twenty minutes).

What you do: You're probably already familiar with these classic childhood games, so start small—simple actions and concepts go a long way in these "do as I do" games. Make them more challenging by giving two or three commands at each turn as your child's skills increase: "Stomp your feet, turn around, touch the ground." It is important that your child have successful listening experiences.

Speech payoff: Attention to detail and memory are stressed, as well as receptive language and sequencing skills.

2: Memory Take-Away

What you need: A commercial memory game, or objects from around the house.

What you do: Instead of playing Memory in the traditional sense, pull out just a few cards with target speech sounds, words, or phrases (from two to five, depending on your child's ability, tolerance, and attention span). Talk about what's on the cards. Place them faceup on the table or floor. Take away one of the cards while your child covers her eyes. Her job is to tell you which card you took away.

Variation: Let you child be the teacher and quiz *you*. Many kids are much more engaged when they're in charge. Switch it around so you're the teacher again. As your child gets better at this, try taking two cards away and then three from a set of five or six. Some children do better with objects than with pictures. Try it both ways and see what works for your child. My daughter did so much better at this activity when we used actual objects that she could touch and relate to.

Speech payoff: Develops memory skills, attention, and focus—which may be a struggle for kids with CAS. It also helps with vocabulary and targeted speech sounds, words, and phrases.

3: Photographic Memory

What you need: Camera and child.

What you do: Take pictures of your child completing activities around the house: washing hands, setting the table, getting ready for bed, heading out the door. Keep the steps in the routine manageable—say, no more than five photographs (steps) of the same routine. Print them out and laminate, or stick them to note cards. Have your child arrange them in order from start to finish. Have her tell you her own story about these sequences to the best of her ability. If she struggles with this, you can tell *her* the story. For a challenge, have her arrange them in *reverse* order!

Variation: Take photos of an item that changes over time—seeds to sprouts to flower (or trees in and out of bloom), seasons, or baby to child to mom to grandmother. If your child is really interested in cameras, consider giving her one of her own. You may appreciate this book: *Picture This: Photography Activities for Early Childhood Learning* by Susan G. Entz (Corwin Press, 2009).

Speech payoff: Kids respond best when they are center stage. So, taking actual photographs of your child doing everyday things will be a motivator to remember steps in an important household routine. Talking about these routines can make your child "the star of the show."

4: First . . . Then

What you need: Not much of anything, unless you'd like to create a picture board, in which case you'll need an 8½ x 11 piece of construction paper, two half-sheets of construction paper, a marker, and a laminator (if you want to get fancy).

What you do: Give your kid simple two-step directions. For example, "*First* wash your hands. *Then* we'll eat." Don't overtalk a request: "I need you to go to the bathroom and wash your hands—they're really dirty and we're eating soon. Gosh, you look like you've been playing in mud all day." See how confusing this could be to your child when all you really want her to do is wash her hands?

Variation: Make a picture board that shows activities of "first" and "then." You can use clip art to show pictures of things your child does around the house—handwashing, toothbrushing, TV watching. Tape a picture of "clean your room" in the "first" category and a picture of a TV in the "then" category. Visually it gets your kid thinking and remembering what to do.

Speech payoff: If your child is a visual learner, she'll love the picture board. You'll find that life is easier and you are less frustrated when your child cooperates with your requests. Think of how you use visual reminders like Post-It notes to remind yourself of something you need to do—it's the same idea for your child.

Household and Family Routines

Kids thrive on routine. One of the best things you can do as a parent is to establish your own daily routine. Remember, there is a difference between a routine and a schedule. A *routine* is a typical pattern of events that happen roughly about the same time each day. For example, after we eat lunch (between 11:30 and 12:30), we have quiet time (for about two hours), followed by some activity or outing (usually around 3:00). A *schedule* is precise, as in every day at 9:30 we have to be at preschool.

1: Visual Routine Sequences

What you need: Pictures (photographs, clip art, or picture software) of daily activities.

What you do: Choose the daily routine you would like to visually depict (getting dressed, eating a meal, getting out the door, packing a backpack). Draw, print, or find clear, simple pictures showing the specific steps involved. Aim for about four steps in each routine; more could be too complex. Post it in an area where you and your child will see it. Point to the steps and repeat them aloud together.

Speech payoff: Not only does this exercise help with sequencing, it also helps with time management and vocabulary development.

2: Speech and Language Star Charts

What you need: A simple chart that shows the days of the week. You can make your own on the computer or with old-fashioned poster board and a marker. Add in some gold stars or other small stickers.

What you do: Tell your child that for every day of the week she completes a speech/language activity (see end of chapter, further reading/resources for hints), she gets a star. She can receive a small prize at the end of the day as a reward for her hard work or she can "bank" the stars for a bigger prize at the end of the week: "If you earn five stars by the end of the week, you can earn a _____." Make sure the prize is something your child is invested in. Keep in mind that rewards don't have to be monetary. Most kids love earning special one-on-one time with Mom or Dad or a trip to the park.

Speech payoff: You can get your child to do just about anything for the right motivator. Just make sure you are targeting a *positive* behavior—one you want her to do most of the time. Some parents may target negative behaviors. For example, when a parent says, "No booger picking," the child may just hear, "Pick my boogers—okay!" and the "no" is ignored. Bringing attention to negative behaviors often reinforces them. If you want a bad habit to end, mention an appropriate alternative.

3: Create a Speech Star Chart

What you need: Poster board, computer printout on which you have created a daily or weekly grid, or a store-bought chart designed for good behavior or chores (Board Dudes Magnetic Dry Erase Rewards Chore Chart, for example). You can even make a list of speech exercises (suggestions below) and use stickers or tally marks to mark off those your child completes.

What you do: Come up with lots of questions that will get your child to answer with words. For example, "name a color in the rainbow"; "tell me two things you wear in the winter (summer, fall, spring)"; "a glove goes on your hand, and a shoe goes on your_____"; "name five animals that belong in the zoo"; "tell me the name of our neighbor's dog"; "ice is cold, and fire is _____"; "tell me what you know about a cat (other animals)." Once you think of a few, you'll be amazed how many more you can come up with! You'll likely just do one or two of these star speech tasks a day; too many may overwhelm your child. When your child completes one, give her a sticker or other incentive. Remember, these are only suggestions. If these examples seem too difficult, tailor them for your child.

Speech payoff: It's a fun way to practice words, sounds, and phrases with your child. It's also another opportunity to engage your child in conversation and work on critical thinking and memory skills.

4: Schedule Playdates with Peers.

What you need: A child and parent you and your little one enjoy spending time with.

What you do: Find a time each week or month you all can get together to talk and play. Playdates don't have to be confined to your family room. Branch out and have them at the park, a bounce place, or a fast food restaurant with kiddie play area.

Speech payoff: It's amazing how peer interactions can work in a positive way. Repeated interactions with kids who speak at developmentally appropriate levels may encourage your child's communication as well. Plus, it gives *you* a chance to catch up with other parents. Try not to make your child's speech issue the main topic of your adult conversation, though.

More information: Here are a couple of resources you may find helpful when planning a playdate:

- *What to Expect at a Play Date* (a children's book) by Heidi Murkoff (Harper Festival, 2001)
- *How to Be a Friend* by Laurie Krasny Brown and Marc Brown, the husband-wife team of the "Arthur" series (Little, Brown & Co, 1998)
- *Let's Talk about Playing with Others* by Joy Berry (available on Kindle from Inspired Studios, 2019)

5: Remember Me Always

What you need: Photos of loved ones, neighbors, friends, babysitters, and pets. Cut and laminate into smaller (e.g., 2 x 2 inch) cards. You'll also need a key ring or binder ring.

What you do: Place the cards on a key ring and toss them in your bag for use in waiting rooms, in the car, or at home. Have your child flip through them while you tell her who's in the picture. Next quiz your child; approximations will do just fine. Then get silly and point to the dog and ask, "Is that Grandpa?" You can also use fill-in-the-blank sentences such as "This is _____." Wait for your child to respond with a word, sound, approximation, or phrase.

Variation: Take photos of your child *doing* things she enjoys—playing at the park, digging in the sand, jumping through the sprinkler. This activity focuses on action words and the suffix "–ing." Ask, "What are you doing here?" to which your child might answer, "Riding [my bike]." Work on expanding those responses as your child's skills grow.

Speech payoff: This is a fun way of encouraging language development and getting your kiddo to say the names of key people in her life. Repetition and repeated exposure don't hurt either.

6: D is for Describe

What you need: An object to talk about.

What you do: Talk about an object—how it looks, sounds, feels, tastes, smells, or makes you feel. Name its parts or talk about what it's made from. For example, talk about an orange: it's heavy, it's orange, it smells sweet, and it feels a little bumpy, maybe even cold. After your child touches and hears you talk about the orange, ask your child to say "orange." She just might surprise you. Again, try the fill-in-the-blank approach here. For example, "The orange feels _____.

Speech payoff: Quite possibly one of the most powerful speech development activities we can do for our kids is to describe things. Touchy-feely learning in a real-life environment is much more effective for kids with CAS than the sit-and-speak approach.

7: Stretch It Out

What you need: A child who can follow simple directions and say about fifty words.

What you do: Help your child put her words into two-word phrases like "more juice" and "go bye-bye." For example, if your child says "Go," stretch it out by saying, "Yes, Mommy go."

Speech payoff: Kids hear appropriate language models. Show delight, pay attention, and respond when she tries to put words together. This way she knows you're listening and understanding her.

Multimedia

In today's technology-saturated world, there's got to be an app for CAS, right? Well, yes and no. If you're looking for useful apps, fast-forward to the end of the chapter to determine if there is some bit of technology that might apply to your family. More old-school forms of technology, including software and TV, are discussed below.

1: Tune In!

What you need: Television, DVD player, and access to programs such as those listed below. Check local listings on www.pbskids.org. Ask your librarian for DVDs, or consider purchasing them.

What you do: Find time to watch the shows or videos with your child. Talk about what you see and learn during commercial breaks, or when you pause or hit "stop."

Speech payoff: Watching TV is a time to rest. Your child isn't likely to become any smarter or overcome CAS by sitting in front of the TV. However, it *will* provide some reinforcement of the ideas and activities you have provided for your child in a more active, hands-on setting.

- *Word World* (PBS Kids): Everyday words are spelled out in the shape of the actual item, helping your visual learner see the words she hears all day.

- *WordGirl* (PBS Kids): She might be small and she might be a cartoon, but this girl knows her words!

- *Emma's Extravagant Expedition* (Amazon Prime Video): An elephant dresses up and introduces your child to advanced vocabulary such as embellish and magnificent.

- *Signing Times* (DVD): These videos teach beginning American Sign Language (ASL) through the help of Leah, a deaf four-year-old, and lots of catchy songs. It's geared for kids between the ages of one and eight, and teaches many first words. Don't be deterred by sign language. It can encourage more verbalization and help you understand those sounds your child is using to communicate.

- *Baby Bumblebee* (DVD). According to the website and many parents, these products—with their real-world images—have helped many kids with autism spectrum disorders, speech and language delays, and general developmental delays. Check it out at www.babybumblebee.com.

- *Preschool Prep Series* (DVD). Geared toward kids aged fifteen months to six years, this DVD series has won many national awards. It teaches shapes, numbers, letters, colors, and words. Look for the DVDs at www.preschoolprepco.com.

Parents Ask

How much TV is OK for my child to watch?

Not much, according to the American Academy of Pediatrics (www.aap. org). Television may provide some supplement to hands-on teaching with your child, but it is not a substitute for education or speech-language therapy.

In 2016, the AAP released new guidelines for media consumption for children, including television. If your child is less than eighteen months, the AAP recommends avoiding all screen media other than video chatting. For children eighteen to twenty-four months of age, an introduction to digital media in the form of high-quality programming is appropriate with a caregiver watching to ensure children understand what they are viewing. For children two to five years old, the AAP recommends limiting television to one hour of high-quality programming and watching together with an adult who can help the child apply the programming to the "real world." For children over six, the AAP stresses setting consistent limits on media consumption, with a note to ensure media and television do not replace adequate sleep, physical activity, and other habits associated with good health.

Finally, the AAP highly suggests that families settle on some media-free times for everyone, such as when driving or at mealtimes, and limit where in the home media can be consumed, such as bedrooms. Having ongoing discussions about media, citizenship, and safety, including respect, is vital. Hands-on exploration, face-to-face communication, and interaction far exceed the benefits of screen time, and also enhance critical thinking. See also the section in chapter 14 on "Exercise and Extracurricular Activities to Help Your Child Thrive."

- *The Kid Should See This* (TKSST) is a carefully curated and constantly growing online library of exciting and educational videos that can easily be watched alongside your youngster. The creator of TKSST describes the videos as "not-made-for-kids, but perfect for them." Each week, about eight to twelve new videos are added to the already massive collection of over 4,000. Explore TKSST at: https://thekidshouldseethis.com/.

Erik Raj, PhD, CCC-SLP, an Assistant Professor and Clinical Supervisor in the Department of Speech-Language Pathology at Monmouth University in New Jersey, says this about TKSST, "I love this website to bits. I talk about it during many of my speaking engagements and I utilize it often. It's a free website and so clutch. I highly recommend it."

2: Computer Fun

What you need: Access to a laptop or tablet computer, and in some cases, child-safe internet access. Your local library may have these resources, including software, to check out. They may even have a computer lab you can use.

What you do: Go online or download software to use with your child and then see those brain connections grow, and the words a-coming. Look into these websites and reasonably priced software programs:

- *Little Bird Tales* (www.littlebirdtales.com/): A darling program for children and their caregivers incorporating storytelling and e-learning in hundreds of ways for all ages, even children who haven't learned to read or write yet. Children enjoy taking their own art, ideas, and even voices to create their own stories. Voices can be recorded online or via an iPad. For children with CAS, hearing their voices repeated back helps with self-correction. There is a free three-week trial.

- *Starfall* (www.starfall.com): This website is a great resource for kids in preschool through early elementary years, including those with special needs. The goal of the website is to make learning to read with phonics fun.

- *School Zone Preschool-Kindergarten Super Scholar* (www.schoolzone.com): This software is designed for kids aged three to six years old. It builds language skills through word searches, crosswords, mazes, pictures, and imaginative puzzles, and builds early math skills. You may also appreciate **On Track: Beginning Sounds** software, which helps children work at recognizing sounds and associating them with words and objects.

- *Boardmaker* (https://goboardmaker.com): Boardmaker is a software program that allows SLPs, teachers, and other adults to make materials using the Picture Communication Symbols (PCS) —line drawings widely used by SLPs. You may be surprised at all of the uses for this program, including making printed materials, communication boards, homemade sequencing games, schedules, and flashcards. Many schools and speech clinics have access to Boardmaker, so purchasing it yourself makes a nice extension for home use.

- **LessonPix** (https://lessonpix.com): This is an easy-to-use and affordable online resource that allows users to create various customized learning materials such as

Bingo boards, picture cards, coloring sheets, etc. LessonPix users have access to thousands of pictures that can be infused into their customized learning materials, and if you need a certain picture that isn't within their library, just click "Request a Picture" on the Menu Bar, and they will create it! For further customization, LessonPix users are able to upload their own photos.

- *Speaking of Speech* (www.speakingofspeech.com): This interactive website is really intended for parents, teachers, and SLPs and provides a host of advice, information on products, resources, and web/internet links.

Tip: When weighing the pros and cons of various online resources for creating customized learning materials (e.g., Boardmaker, SymbolStix, and LessonPix), consider how often you might be using the program and for what purpose. Some have monthly fees, yearly fees, professional/school district, and personal fees. There's no reason to throw good money at a program or website just to use it once.

Toys & Games

Kids play. It's their job and they see it as serious business, just as you see your job as a parent. What are they really getting out of play, you ask? It's an opportunity to learn about the world and how they fit in it. Through play, kids can rehearse scary or worrisome situations (like going to the doctor or dentist), experiment with a new object or idea, and learn what they are good at doing—and not so good at doing. Here are some ideas to slip in speech practice while your little one is hard at play.

Choosing Toys for Your Child

I could give you lots of suggestions for types of toys to purchase or how to play with the ones you already have cluttering your living room. Instead, I'd like to emphasize that *anything and everything can become a therapy tool/prop!* Please, don't rush out and purchase expensive "therapy" toys, unless you just want to (and have an abundant supply of "toy cash").

I highly recommend that you check out the podcast (and website) called Learn With Less, the brainchild of Ayelet Marinovich, MA, CCC-SLP, an amazing SLP in the San Francisco Bay Area. I adore the concept and website so much. Marinovich's message is key: The days are long and we just want the best for our children, so we go out searching for the best and newest toys and gadgets. But really, we should be maximizing what we already have; everyday, mundane items can be just as entertaining and educational. Think: Tupperware and cardboard boxes, sticks and tubes.

The next time you decide it's time for a new toy, keep these tips in mind (they were compiled by the National Lekotek Center, a now-inactive nonprofit organization that was dedicated to making play and learning accessible to children with disabilities):

1. **Multisensory Appeal.** Does the toy respond with lights, sounds, movement to engage the child? Does it have scent, texture, or contrasting colors? Will these aspects of the toy irritate or intrigue your child (or you)?

2. **Method of Activation.** Will the toy provide a challenge, but not to the point of frustration? What is the force required to activate? What are the number and complexity of steps required to activate the toy? Some children with CAS also have limb apraxia and may find some toys too complicated to activate.

3. **Places the Toy will Be Used.** Will the toy be easy to store? Is there a special place in the home for playing and storing the toy? Can the toy be used in a variety of ways?

4. **Opportunities for Success.** Can play be open-ended with no definite right or wrong way of using the toy?

5. **Current Popularity.** Is this a toy that will make your child feel like *any other kid*? That is, she will like it because it's considered a cool toy, and not another "tool" to help with her speech.

6. **Self-Expression.** Does the toy allow for creativity, uniqueness, and making choices? Does it provide experiences with a variety of media?

7. **Adjustability.** Does it have adjustable height, sound volume, speed, and level of difficulty?

8. **Child's Individual Abilities.** Does the toy provide activities that reflect both developmental and chronological ages? Does it reflect *your* child's interest?

9. **Safety and Durability.** Is the toy appropriate for kids of your child's strength and size? Is it moisture resistant? Are the toy and its parts sized appropriately (i.e., not a choking hazard)? Can it be washed and cleaned?

10. **Potential for Interaction.** Will the child be an active participant during use? Will the toy encourage social interaction and engagement with others?

If you are just an ordinary parent like me, you might have fewer criteria than what's on this big, official list. Choose the most important points to you.

Managing Toy Chaos

At our house, we manage toy chaos with "Toy Trade Tuesday." It may well be the very best thing we've done as parents—in terms of managing all of the "kid clutter." Here's how it works: First I organized our toys by "family"—farm, zoo, dress-up/role-play, cars and trucks, building and constructing things, baby dolls, cooking and baking items, and pets and vets.

Then, everything that somehow related to a particular group of toys—puzzles, books, art supplies, stickers, and placemats—went into a large plastic storage bin. I slapped a label on each box and stored eight of them in the basement, leaving one out in the family room where the children spent most of their time playing. The girls were able to keep several special toys out at all times: their favorite stuffed dog, for example, never got packed away, nor did the miniature dollhouses. When Tuesday rolled around each week, it was time to trade the toys the girls had been playing with for one of the bins downstairs. I'd ask the girls, "What should we do for Toy Trade Tuesday?" They almost always had a request. Sometimes I'd try to tie the week at home in with a unit of study at school. (If you decide to try this with your kids, you can have them help you with categorizing your toys—it's a great language categorization activity.)

When we went to the library on Wednesdays, I'd look for books that connected with our theme. On Friday, we had "field trips" and headed to the zoo, visited a working farm, set up the tent in the backyard, or popped into the pet store for a visit. We could almost always relate these activities to the toy theme we chose on Tuesday. The field trips were a fun way to end the week.

Managing your toys like this helps with clutter control. It also helps you concentrate on specific vocabulary and target speech sounds, words, and phrases. It gives you and your kids something to look forward to. Plus, it's exciting to see how much your children have grown and progressed when you pull out a group of toys they haven't seen in a while.

You will also want to regularly add to and update the boxes so that the toys offer a bit of a challenge and change.

Since "Toy Trade Tuesday" has made its way into our life, I have several questions I ask myself before allowing a new toy into our home:

- Does it match with one of our existing toy themes? Which one?
- Is this something the girls will get some challenge and pleasure out of for a while (a year or more)?
- In what ways can I make it educational?
- Will it fit—physically—into my box?

Try "Toy Trade Tuesday" or "Swap-It-Out-Saturday" or "Mix-It-Up-Monday" today! You'll be amazed how your child(ren) respond to this. See the resources section at the end of this chapter for a list of other Toy Trade Tuesday ideas.

If Toy Trade Tuesday sounds too organized for your style, then try this variation: get a tote, basket, or box that you can call your Speech Box. Fill it with special toys, treats, and crafts that only make an appearance at home speech time. Periodically update the box (as a surprise, perhaps, or as a "job well done," with things you know will excite your child.)

Toy Trade Tuesday Themes

Think you may want to adapt Toy Trade Tuesday at your house? You can create as many themed weeks as you have space and toys for. Generally, you'll need about five to ten objects per theme. Look at what you already have and build on it, based on your child's interests. Here's a list to get you started:

- Zoo/Safari/Wild Animals
- Food/Baking/Nutrition
- Seasons/Weather
- Dinosaurs
- Tools, Machines & Measurement
- Family and Homes
- Cultures of the World
- Ocean and Beach
- Shapes/Alphabet/Colors/School
- Transportation
- Community and Careers + Role-Play
- Farm (we combined Farm with Weather)
- Pets
- Earth/Environment/Camping (we added Space Exploration to this one)
- Exercise
- Folk Tales and Nursery Rhymes + Dress-Up

Toys to Encourage Communication

Here are some more qualities you can look for in toys that encourage speech/vocal communication:

- **Amplification and Reverberation.** These toys have the ability to change or make your child's voice louder. Think megaphones, microphones, and echo-phones. Why? They motivate your child to use her voice in a fun and sometimes goofy way. Plus, they provide the auditory feedback some children need to hear the details of targeted speech.

- **Speech.** These toys encourage the development of spoken words. Look for toys or dolls that speak, flashcards that use phonics, etc.

- **Verbal Talk-Back Response.** These toys respond to speech and help develop receptive and expressive language. Be sure to look for toys that have clear, simple voices.

- **Words and Pictures.** These toys use words and pictures that can be pointed to and talked about. Look for: books, puzzles, games, and electronic toys that use the alphabet (e.g., Leap Frog products have a lot of options).

- **Communication.** Remember walkie-talkies from your childhood? It may be fun to introduce them to your child. Old telephones work well too.

- **Pretend Play.** Dressing up and pretending to be someone or something you dream about may help with communication. Hand puppets work in this way, too. Kids can talk "through" the puppet so they tend to feel less self-conscious. Children can use different voices and play with speech sounds. You might be surprised at the speech you hear from your child when she pretends to be someone else.

Parents Share

Puppets are a handful—and may help with speech!

My daughter must have been about twenty months old. She wasn't diagnosed with CAS yet, but we were concerned about her lack of speech. I remember telling my husband that I thought a puppet would help her use her words. While she didn't love the puppet like I thought she would, she did enjoy watching me have conversations with her and the puppet and even made some new sounds during puppet play.

—mother of a girl with CAS

A Few Personal Favorites

I know I said I wouldn't tell you what to run out and buy, but I just have to share the merits of a few playthings:

LEGOs. Whether you have a son or a daughter, you most certainly have a set of LEGOs. They have the utmost power to bring to life a child's imagination, and perhaps her verbal skills as well.

Deb Tomarakos, CCC-SLP, elaborates on the uses of plastic building blocks: "LEGOs or Duplos can be used to work on: receptive and expressive vocabulary skills related to people, places, and animals; following directions; articulation of target sounds that are pictured in the scene; identifying and producing animal and environmental sounds; direction/location concepts (up/down, left/right, beside/front/behind); community workers (policeman, pilot); categories (farm animals, zoo animals, vehicles); color labels and identification."

"For the older crowd," she shares, "I love the **LEGO City Comic Builder.** [It's] a great way to work on story narratives; story sequencing; story elements including setting and characters; main idea formulation; problems and resolutions; sentence formulation; humor; social skills stories." Visit the LEGO website (www.lego.com) to find other ways to target speech/language practice.

Zingo! It's like bingo with a zing—think word lessons and picture matching instead of letters on the bingo card. Each player gets a Zingo board; all of the chips are stored in a kid-friendly slider case. Each player takes a turn sliding the device to reveal what chips are doled out. The chips have both a picture *and* spelling of a common object (house, shoe, bird, sun). We started using this with our daughter when she was about three and a half. We'd have her practice saying the words as they appeared on the chips. As she got older, we'd have her string together more words, "I have a ___(sun)," or "Here's a sun!" "Does anyone have a ____ (house, bird, sun, etc.)?" The game teaches turn-taking, patience, listening, sight words, and target word practice.

What's in Ned's Head. This toy from Fat Brain Toys may appease your sensory-seeker or the child who enjoys "gross stuff." Basically, Ned's head is a large plush "head," with an assortment of gross stuff inside (a large tooth, a frog, a lab rat, Ned's lost lunch—rubber vomit, an alien, a worm, moldy cheese, among others). The players are dealt one card each with a picture of an item in the head. They all then reach into Ned's head through his mouth or ear holes—to try to find their item. You can practice having your child say these "gross things"; they may be icky enough to illicit some chatter.

Play with Your Food

1: Table Talk and Toss

What you need: Just you and your family members at the dinner table, plus any school papers and artwork your child created that day.

What you do: Whatever kid-created pieces of paper come out of your child's backpack go directly on the table as though they were placemats. At dinner, ask your child to tell you about what she created. Ask open-ended questions, such as "How did you come up with this idea?" or "Tell me about this" (and point to what you want more information on). Be sure to show positive interest.

Speech payoff: It gives your child a chance to share something meaningful about her day and offers yet another opportunity to practice new words. Plus, when dinner's over, you either save the paper or toss it in the recycling bin, reducing the mounds of paper that are sure to make their home on your kitchen counter.

2: Favorite Part of the Day

What you need: Family members talking.

What you do: My family found that this activity was best done at our dinner table. Bedtime also works. Go from person to person and ask about their favorite part of the day. You may need to give choices—even silly ones—to prompt your child, depending on her verbal skills. "Was your favorite part of the day getting in trouble for coloring on the wall?" "Was your favorite part of the day going to the doughnut shop? What color donut did you get?"

Speech payoff: It's a great way to hear the highlights of everyone's day, and it encourages communication.

3: This or That

What you need: A couple of food or beverage options at meal or snack time (this also works with just about anything at just about any time).

What you do: Offer your child a choice between two items: "Would you like milk or juice?" As you say "milk," hold the milk jug up and clearly enunciate. Do the same for juice. "Would you like hot dogs or chicken nuggets?" Then wait for a response from your child. Any response besides a grunt or a point will do (unless that is all your child can do at the time). After a speech attempt, clearly say, "Okay! Chicken nuggets it is! Can you say 'chicken'?"

Speech payoff: It can be grueling to wait for a response when it would be easier to fill the glass with chocolate milk and present it to your kid, but giving her some say in the matter will make her feel empowered. Choice-making is a basic part of communication; young children are eager to make their own choices.

4: Mealtime Prayers

What you need: Mealtime prayer and child(ren).

What you do: If your family says a mealtime prayer, see if you can modify your traditional prayer to make it more fun and kid-friendly. Can you add gestures? (We give everyone a high five at the end of ours.) Ask your child to lead the prayer and coach her along, or use fill-in-the-blank if you say a routine prayer.

Speech payoff: Having a family tradition at the table can be a fun way to bond and connect. Saying words in unison (almost like a chant) can be easier than having your child say it on her own.

5: Handful of Goodies

What you need: M&Ms, Skittles, or another small candy; a small bowl; and a child who likes candy. Make sure you and your child are comfortable with the size of candy, as they may pose a choking hazard.

What you do: Have the bowl of candy on the dinner table. When everyone is finished with the meal, have them reach in and grab a few. Each family member is to say something for *each* M&M they grabbed. It can be as simple as a sound your child is learning in therapy (like the "st" blend), a target word (*me*), first name, etc. Eat the M&Ms one at a time as a special treat.

Speech payoff: The candy serves as an incentive. "If you can say ___, then you can eat the M&M." The whole family is doing it, too—safety in numbers and good role modeling, right?

> **Dinner Games & Activity Cards**
> You may want to invest in this deck of *51 Family Time Fun Dinner Games* cards designed for dinnertime conversations. It comes in a handy container with a lid so you can take it with you on the go (restaurants, camping, picnics). The cards provide great prompts for conversations, thought-provoking questions, memory games, and more. This product even comes in a beginner series (ages 3 and up). The regular series is best for kids five to twelve years. Look for them in various catalogs, bookstores, and online.

Arts & Crafts

Art is not just about the outcome—the final masterpiece. The process is equally important. Kids can express their originality and feelings through art, while improving their coordination (fine motor), learning colors and textures, and developing pride in their artistic accomplishments. Take time to talk with your child about the art she is creating. Encourage confidence and satisfaction in creativity by asking questions like these:

- "Tell me about your picture!"
- "How did you decide what to draw?"
- "I like the colors you used. How did you decide which ones you wanted in your picture?"
- "Where would you like us to hang it?"
- "Should we send it to Grandma?"

If your child does not respond well to questions, comment about her work and wait for her response. For example, "Oh, I see you drew a big bright sun." Stop and wait. It may take a moment for your kid to come up with a response.

1: Draw & Label

What you need: A child at the table with markers, crayons, a blank sheet of paper, and imagination.

What you do: Let her work for as long as she wants. Listen and make observations. When she's finished, say, "I like your picture. Tell me about it." Point to items on the page. Ask her to describe it for you. Any little word will do. Write down what she says in quotations right next to the image. Put her name on it and date it. You can save these in a binder so that you can go back and look at her progress—not just artistically—but verbally too.

Speech payoff: It's fun and interesting to see what our kids are drawing; consider it a little window to their world. Plus, it helps catalog where she's been—in terms of ability.

2: Sketchbook

What you need: Find a notebook with plain paper—one that's spiral-bound works best. Add crayons, markers, colored pencils—whatever media you feel most comfortable with.

What you do: Allow your child to make several entries daily (maybe during quiet time)—label and date them. What's really fun is to make the sketchbook into a sort of scrapbook. Collect pictures, articles, ticket stubs, leaves, feathers—whatever fascinates your child. Have her describe the item, the scents, colors, and textures and capture that in the book.

Speech payoff: In many ways, this activity combines the elements of learning—collecting, identifying, researching, and talking. It introduces new experiences and vocabulary. Again, it's a good way to measure progress.

3: Pen Pals

What you need: A friend or family member (cousin or grandparent) who lives in another zip code.

What you do: Provide your child with envelopes, stamps, pens, paper, stickers. Your child can draw or write a biography of herself and include artwork and other tidbits about her life. The pen pal will hopefully respond with similar items. When letters arrive in the mail, talk about what you've received. This activity is probably best suited to older kids.

Speech payoff: It gives kids the message that communication—even if written—is very important.

Parents as Partners in CAS Treatment

No pressure here, but you are very much a partner in your child's speech-language treatment. Don't let her know that, though, or she'll be less likely to go along with your ideas! You need to be clever. Here are some suggestions for tapping into your inner speech-language pathologist.

1: Car Schooling

What you need: A vehicle and an adult willing to go for a drive.

What you do: While you are running errands with the kids, quiz them on some of the words and sounds you know they know. For example, "Where do Nana and Papa live?" Or, "Who lives in St. Louis?" Other ideas: "What does a dog say? Who's at work? Who's driving the van?" etc. Then throw in a new word your child is working on, or one you'd like her to say. Practice it.

Speech payoff: The back seat is a safe place for your little ones to practice those new words and sounds. There's less performance anxiety. Plus, they are a captive audience. One time when I was doing this activity, Kate said, "No more talking!" I considered that a success—her first three-word phrase!

Please keep safety in mind. I found this type of activity was best done as we were traveling roads I was familiar with. Speech work shouldn't cause you to become a distracted driver!

2: Teach and Drive

What you need: Vehicle and parent running errands.

What you do: Tape a kid-friendly lesson to the back of the headrest in your vehicle—right in front of your child's eyes. These lessons could be as simple as a worksheet from your SLP's office on a target sound or a picture of a family pet. Make sure your lesson includes pictures/drawings if your child isn't reading yet. Your child will see the "lesson" each time she's in the car and eventually will learn things such as her ABCs, phone number, and what sound the letter *l* makes.

Speech payoff: Repeated exposure, repetition, and something on which to focus on while you are driving.

Keep safety in mind. Speech work shouldn't cause you to become a distracted driver!

3: From Sounds to Words

What you need: A little person who has a few sounds such as "da" and "ba" in her repertoire.

What you do: Encourage your child to build on sounds she already has by introducing words that begin with that same sound. For example, if she can say "ba," build on that by encouraging her to imitate you when you say, "bottle," "ball," "book," "baby," and "bath." Emphasize and exaggerate these words throughout the day whenever you get the chance. For example say, "*ba-ba*—bottle."

Speech payoff: It exposes kiddos to new words containing sounds they can already say.

4: Expand-o-matic

What you need: A child who can say about ten or fifteen words spontaneously.

What you do: When your child says a one-word sentence with clear intent she wants you to *do* something, expand on what she said. For example, she's at the kitchen table and offers you her cup, saying "more?" You can expand by saying, "Oh, you want more milk? Okay! More milk coming right up. More milk."

Speech payoff: In a brief interaction, you have repeated the request three times and have modeled more words while completing a simple task for your child. She will surprise you in the future by saying more than "more!"

5: Parallel Talk

What you need: A happy child engaged in play.

What you do: Describe what your child is doing with her play. "I see you are playing with your cars. It looks like they are driving really fast. Vroom, vroom. Beep, beep. I like the blue car best. Do you like the blue car too?"

Speech payoff: This sort of parallel talk (talking about what your child is doing in short phrases and sentences) helps your child attach words to the actions and objects she is experiencing. It really takes the pressure off speech production and can give your child the freedom to comment.

6: Make a Speech Sounds Practice Book

What you need: All of those worksheets your SLP hands you after a session with your child, plus a small three-ring binder or folder with brads and some sheet protectors.

What you do: Let your child decorate and color the "pages" so she feels a bit of ownership. Give her free rein on the cover too. Review the items in the book several times a day at your convenience with your child. We often looked over ours at breakfast and lunch and as a part of our regular reading routine.

Speech payoff: Putting worksheets from your child's speech sessions into a binder is a great way to make an individualized study guide. It directly strengthens the skills that your SLP is working on with your child. You can look back and see the progress your child has made. Date the pages and put the new ones on top. This helps manage the paper clutter you are sure to accumulate from weekly worksheets!

7: Who's in Your Family?

What you need: Various objects from around the house that represent a hobby or interest of each family member.

What you do: It's fun if you can make this a family activity. Gather at least one object per family member (e.g., Mom's favorite magazine or book, Dad's remote control or newspaper, baby brother's rattle, big sister's video game). Put the items in a pile in the middle of the room. Ask your child to match the item with the "right" person. Practice saying that person's name and the name of the object. Combine them into two-word phrases such as "Daddy's remote."

Variation: Hide the objects (tell or show your child what they are first); take turns having different family members select objects for the game. Name the objects as they are found, as in "Mom's book."

Speech payoff: An exercise like this involves the whole family, can be fun, and helps your child make connections, develop critical thinking skills, and improve vocabulary.

8: "Play" Speech Therapy

What you need: You, your child, and a pile of stuffed animals or dolls.

What you do: Set up a pretend speech therapy session with your child's favorite little critters. Let your child be the SLP, or you can pretend to be the SLP. Teach the toys while your child watches.

Speech payoff: If your child loves her animals or dolls and likes playing teacher, this type of activity will be right up her alley. Your child is doing a couple of important things—role-playing, processing what she's learned in therapy, and spending time with a caring adult. You just may be surprised to hear what your child can say when she takes on the teaching role. It's sort of like a tea party with a twist!

OK—that's a big list of things to try. Don't feel as if you have to try them all. None of them are designed to be *the* magic bullet either. The ideas presented are just a fun way to get that much-needed speech practice in.

Encourage, Encourage, Encourage!

Once your child starts talking more, you'll need to give her lots of praise and encouragement. Here are some tips to keep in mind as you work with your child:

■ *Your child will do her best communicating when she's not under pressure.* How well do you communicate when you are in that important meeting or on a stage? For this reason, don't insist that your child demonstrate her speech skills in front of an audience (even if it's just Grandma and Grandpa). Instead, let your child's speech come out more naturally, particularly with folks she is unfamiliar with.

- *Allow (and encourage) your child to use whatever props she needs to communicate to her very best ability.* That means letting her use gestures, sign, show you pictures, or act it out.

- *Validate your child's desire to communicate with you.* When I couldn't understand what our daughter was trying to tell us, I would say, "Kate, I know you are trying to tell us something really important, but we're having a hard time understanding." Depending on the situation, I might add, "Show us [what you are trying to explain, do, want]." It worked 99 percent of the time.

- *If you can understand some of what your child is trying to say, let her know.* "I see . . . you are talking about George and the Man with the Yellow Hat, but I didn't understand what you said after that. Tell me again." She's going to feel a lot better knowing that something got through and will do her best to revise what she just said so you can "get" the rest.

- *Our SLP often said to give choices with small parts of the day.* It's all about having some control in the choices they make. For example, you might say something like, "Do you want milk or juice?" An approximation of the word such as "ju" is good enough, but a grunt is not. Finish the word yourself by saying, "*Juice*! OK, you want *juice*. I'll get you some *juice*." Then, if you're as goofy as I am, you might break into a song about juice. "Juicy, juicy juice. . . . yum, I love juice. Juice helps me grow strong and gives me important vitamins. I love juice, don't you?"

- *Do not demand that your child use speech to make requests.* For example, "Tell me what you want to drink. You won't get anything unless you can tell me what you want." Yikes! Your child may never feel ready to talk if she's under that kind of pressure.

Parents Ask

What is an approximation?

When you are working hard to help your child talk, you just might accept anything as an attempt to say the word correctly. That's an "approximation." But you must not respond to grunts, squeals, crying, and fussing as an appropriate approximation. Set the record straight beforehand by saying something like, "I need you to try and use your words. It's OK if it's not perfect. Just try to say ____." When your child feels confident and not so pressured, she'll try it. It might take a minute; be patient.

At first, it's OK to accept practically anything that pops out of her mouth that sounds like speech. Give her lots of praise when that happens—a smile, a hug, and a victory jump have worked wonders with us! Your child will quickly learn that in order to get what she wants, she is going to have to try to say something. One day, a true breakthrough will happen, and she will attempt to talk with you without your prompting!

Where's the Research?

Many of the suggestions in this book are rooted in the research world. An October 2008 article in the *American Journal of Speech and Language Pathology*, "When 'Simon Says' Doesn't Work: Alternatives to Imitation for Facilitating Early Speech Development," discusses ways SLPs can provide evidence-based strategies to facilitate speech in kids who are not readily imitating sounds. The suggestions in the article include the following:

- *Provide access to AAC.* There is evidence to suggest an augmentative and alternative communication (AAC) device *does* facilitate speech development.

- *Minimize the pressure to speak.* High pressure requests are direct requests to speak, whereas a low pressure technique would be modeling what you want to hear.

- *Imitate the child.* You've likely heard certain sounds from this child before. Remember what they are and pick targets that get the child to produce words based on those sounds.

- *Use exaggerated intonation and a slowed tempo.* This helps with intelligibility.

- *Augment auditory, visual, tactile, and proprioceptive feedback.* Children with CAS need appropriate sensory input to progress. This is a different approach than traditional articulation treatment.

- *Avoid emphasis on nonspeech-like articulation movements.* We learn to talk better when we practice talking! Work on tasks in context so children are better able to generalize in different environments.

What's AAC? Does My Child Need It?

The American Speech-Language-Hearing Association (ASHA) defines augmentative and alternative communication (AAC) as the means to "temporarily or permanently compensate for the impairments, activity limitations, and participation restrictions of individuals with severe disorders of speech-language production and/or comprehension."

ASHA proposes a continuum of AAC. That is, there are multiple ways in which communication can be assisted. For example, *unaided communication* involves using one's body to convey a message—through gestures, showing, even word approximations. *Aided communication* requires the use of an *external tool* to communicate a thought, feeling, message, need, or want. For example, a child may find it easier to communicate using a picture/symbol such as one produced with SymbolStix or Boardmaker, or writing down a request in a notebook. Higher-tech ideas may include using an iPhone or iPad, a voice output communication aid (VOCA) such as a Tobii Dynavox device, or something similar.

Not all children with CAS need AAC. But if a child has very limited expressive speech or reduced intelligibility, AAC can be very helpful. Talk to your child's SLP to determine if this would be appropriate for your child.

Tip: If you and your child's SLP determine AAC is the right choice for your son or daughter, you may appreciate this book, designed and written by Eden Molineux, MS, CCC-SLP: *Something to Say about My Communication Device.* Illustrations are vivid and eye-catching. Learn more here: https://somethingtosay.net/.

Parents Ask

Should I teach my child with CAS sign language?

Would it do more harm than good? I am afraid he'll then be more comfortable never talking. I know he is capable of making all the sounds, but I get the sense he doesn't want to say anything for fear of making a mistake. He does use picture boards to get his point across. Should I do more? Should I teach him American Sign Language (ASL), or not?

Teaching signs (ASL) might appear at first to be more work and maybe a crutch. But it's not. We used several signs with Kate, and it worked wonders. She would sign "more," and "all done," and even "I love you," which melted our hearts.

One mother I spoke with said this: "I love sign language, love, love, love it! It made life so much better. My children were happier because they could communicate. As soon as they developed the word for the sign, they phased the sign out."

Alexa, mother of a three-year-old son said: "Since it's hard for Mason to get the words out, it helps give him time to get the word together in his head. It also seems to help him remember how to say the word."

Finally, Randy, a father of two said: "Signing was life changing for my son. It does not inhibit the desire to speak. Studies have shown that learning signs helps create new language pathways in the brain. It can only help."

According to Nanette Cote, MA, CCC-SLP, "Anything you can do to enhance communication will allow for more opportunities to model sounds, words, and phrases. As an SLP for over twenty-five years, I can assuredly tell you that nothing prohibits speech. No program, tactic, picture, communication book, speech-generating device, sibling, or family member prevents another from progressing with speech. So many make this assumption based on their own subjective opinion. There is much evidence out there that contradicts this mind-set."

If you're interested in exploring this further, check out these sites:
Signing Time at https://www.signingtime.com/
Baby Signs at https://pathways.org/

Benefits of AAC

According to Margaret (Dee) Fish, MS, CCC-SLP, kids with CAS can benefit from AAC in the following ways:

■ Increased efficiency and effectiveness of communication	■ Decreased reliance on familiar adults to serve as interpreters
■ Increased *quality* and *quantity* of the child's language	■ Reduced challenging behaviors caused by limited ability to express ideas
■ Increased opportunities for social interaction across a wider variety of setting, with a wider variety of individuals, and for a wider range of communication functions	■ Decreased communicative passivity

From Margaret Fish, *Here's How to Treat Childhood Apraxia of Speech*, 2nd ed. (p. 279) (San Diego: Plural Publishing, Inc., 2015). All rights reserved. Used with permission.

Let's Get Tech-y

There is no doubt our children will be exposed to technology from a young age. You may find that introducing your child with CAS to mobile devices, such as an iPad or iPhone, early on actually helps her communication skills. In fact, many organizations these days are advocating that children with special needs have access to an iPad or similar tablet. For example, eLearning Industry lists a plethora of free (iPad) apps for children with special needs (https://elearningindustry.com/free-special-needs-ipad-apps-part-1). They include apps geared toward children with special needs in general, as well as autism, behavioral needs, speech, and vision concerns.

Not only are iPads and other tablets less expensive than most electronic devices used in speech-language therapy (which can run well over $1,000), but they are sleek and trendy. Children with an iPad at their fingertips are less likely to be stigmatized for being "different." Plus, it's lightweight and can be customized for each child's communication needs. Still, the expense of an iPad may simply be out of reach for some families.

If you decide that you'd like an iPad for your child with CAS, don't give up hope because it is too expensive. Many companies and foundations are developing programs that award iPads to deserving families. You can start by asking your school, your speech clinic, or your early intervention coordinator if they know of anything along those lines.

According to Mirla G. Raz, MEd, CCC-SLP, a pediatric speech-language pathologist in Arizona and author of the *Help Me Talk Books*, the iPad is "an extremely motivating device [for children] . . . a wonderful gadget with a multitude of uses." But she points out that parents must weigh whether the initial cost of the iPad plus the sometimes steep prices of apps is worth it.

Erik X. Raj, PhD, CCC-SLP, gives smartphones and tablets high marks for their ability to motivate children with speech delay. "As an SLP, I am simply in love with what we can do with mobile technology—more specifically, how it can be used to excite our children and motivate them to use their voice to the best of their abilities. Something as simple as a photo manipulating app that can add silly sunglasses and a wig can trigger so much communication when used in a shared manner. When a caring adult sits side by side with a child with these types of apps, and when they treat the app like a shared book reading, wow, that's what I love."

App development for both Android and iOS-based devices has exploded in recent years. And they can be a great resource if you know where to look and how to use them. For starters, remember that apps cannot replace the dedicated, in-person practice of having your child work with an SLP. Apps also cannot be your child's only source of "home practice" either. As with everything, moderation and balance are key.

That said, there are some really great apps that target articulation, expressive and receptive language, fluency, voice, swallowing, preliteracy skills, and even training for AAC. There's been a recent push for evidence-based and peer-reviewed apps, so be sure you and your SLP are working with those terms. Here are a couple apps you might want to consider:

Your Face Is Learning, an award-winning app created by Erik X. Raj, is super cute and a great blend of traditional therapy-meets-technology. Users can personalize early learning worksheets in ways that have never been done before. With just a few taps on your device, you can snap a photo of your child's face, and it automatically gets added to a massive amount of category-specific early learning worksheets. Categories include letters, sounds, numbers, colors, shapes, and more. You can print or email your worksheets or save them to your device. Thanks to this app, children now have access to spectacular worksheets that make their educational experiences more memorable, amusing, and effective. For a child, the personalized touch of seeing your own face on your worksheet is second to none. Available for Apple devices from the App Store.

Smarty Ears is a company that focuses on speech-language pathology-focused software. It has developed numerous apps for the assessment and treatment of children with various communication difficulties. Their website is packed with loads of great information that can help you explore their apps to see if any of them might benefit your child's speech-language needs. For example, *Apraxia Farm* (formerly called *Apraxia Ville*) was designed by certified SLPs and created specifically to help children with CAS and severe speech-sound disorders. You'll find multiple levels, vowel and consonant targets, and the ability to create custom words geared to your child. You can find more apps like *Apraxia Farm* by visiting https://www.smartyearsapps.com/.

Articulation Station by Little Bee Speech is a fabulous app for iPhones featuring flashcard-style "cards" that are bright, colorful, and engaging for young children. You may appreciate the ability to customize your own word sets and also record your child's voice with a playback mode. One mother said, "This [feature] actually encouraged my son to speak more and to try out new sounds." Another parent said, "This is the best I found for my son. It's intuitive, colorful, and keeps his attention." For more information about Articulation Station or other speech-language-therapy-related apps by Little Bee Speech, visit http://littlebeespeech.com/.

Parents Share

"We Love Our iPad!"

In a Small Talk: All About Apraxia meeting, a parent participant pulled out a shiny new iPad purchased for a three-and-a-half-year-old boy with CAS. "We love this thing," he crooned. This dad couldn't be happier with the results and functionality the iPad brought for his son's speech. "It's cool, it's portable, and it's fun. He will ask for his iPad so he can communicate something more complex. It's great!" Yet there is a cost to all of this.

Courtney, the mother of a child with CAS in Coloma, Michigan, offers advice on affordable apps: "I won't spend huge amounts of money on an app when there are so many good low-cost or free ones available. We really like Phonics Word Family, Word Wagon, *Parents Magazine* apps, and Tic-Tac-Talk. "We didn't particularly like Speech Tutor. While the idea behind it is good, it just doesn't seem to connect with kids; plus, it's pricey." However, many seem to like this one. You can look into this husband-wife SLP team, the app, and their consultation process here: https://www.speechtutor.org/app. Courtney did positively endorse the more pricey Artik Pix: "It's probably the most functional app we've purchased." She also points out that many book apps are free—such as the popular BOB series for learning to read and Sandra Boynton books for children.

An iPad may be useful for your child at school as well. The mother of a six-year-old who has CAS and cri du chat syndrome says that her daughter "uses her iPad at school daily to help with her communication. She can press a button and the iPad will talk for her. Not only can Finley participate, but it helps cut down on behavior problems due to being nonverbal. It's empowering."

Sound Touch by SoundTouch Interactive LDT is another great app that works with your iPhone. Children can tap on an image of an animal to hear its sound. The mother of a nonverbal son with autism had this to say: "We've had these apps on [my son's] iPad for years. He's eight and still plays with them regularly. The repetition of words paired with photos is great vocabulary practice for receptive language. Also, having five different pictures for the same thing helps generalize within a category. For example, dogs can be different sizes, shapes, and colors and still be dogs. The app also helped desensitize my son to sounds that were once upsetting like police sirens, rooster crowing, elephant trumpeting." Sound Touch is available in over thirty-five languages, but there is a fee associated with use. For more information, visit the Apple App Store.

There are plenty of other apps available, some at low cost or no cost (and some upward of hundreds of dollars). It's best to check with your SLP for his or her recommendations based on your child's particular therapy goals. Keep in mind that some of these apps may be fun for your child but might not actually be doing anything therapeutically. Nothing replaces face-to-face skills and practice.

Say That Again?! Chapter Summary

Holy cow! That was quite a list. Did you take note of the activities you want to try with your child? The key to success with kids with CAS is to give them plenty of opportunities during the day to practice their speech and language skills. Better yet, disguise this "work" as fun. Keep your environment and approach healthy and supportive by remembering to be goofy and funny and not always a serious teach-and-talk type of parent. Be sure to keep your SLP in the loop, and let him or her keep you in the loop too. You are partners in this process, after all!

Finally, I want to reiterate that *kids with CAS are unique individuals. It is your job to find out how you can best help your child with CAS!*

- *PlanToys* markets toys created with the help of developmental specialists and design experts. They are also the world's first and foremost manufacturer of wooden toys—very sustainable and eco-friendly. Visit their website at www.plantoys.com.

- *Mindfull Games* is a company founded by Kristin Edmonds, a former SLP. The company focuses on improving literacy and standardized scores, along with speech development: www.mindfullgames.com.

- For more *educationally based toys,* as well as *balance boards, exercise balls, foam mats and blocks, and trampolines,* check out these catalog/internet companies:

  - Beyond Play: www.beyondplay.com
  - Discovery Toys: www.discoverytoys.com
  - Great Ideas for Teaching: www.greatideasforteaching.com
  - Learning Resources: www.learningresources.com
  - Pocket Full of Therapy: www.shoponline.pfot.com
  - Therapy Shoppe: www.therapyshoppe.com
  - Toys to Grow On: www.toystogrow.co.uk/
  - Super Duper, Inc.: www.superduperinc.com

- Titles of interest to stock your *recreation resource* shelf: *The Secret of Play* (DK Publishers, 2008) by Ann Pleshette Murphy, former editor-in-chief of *Parents* magazine, as well as *Unplugged Play* by Bobbi Conner—700 kid-tested activities to keep your 1–10 year old active and engaged (Workman Publishing Group, 2007), *Get Out!: 150 Easy Ways for Kids & Grown-Ups to Get Into Nature and Build a Greener Future* (Free Spirit Press, 2009) by Judy Molland, and *Last Child in the Woods: Saving our Children from Nature Deficit Disorder,* Richard Louv (Algonquin Books, 2008) are great books for parents concerned about too much screen time (TV, computers, etc.).

■ *Let's Talk Together: 55 Home Activities for Early Speech Language Development* by Cory Poland and Amy Chouinard (Talking Child Press, 2008) offers many ideas for stimulating speech and language in every room of the house.

■ *The Kaufman Speech Praxis Treatment Approach* by Nancy Kaufman, MA, CCC-SLP. Many parents find the *Kaufman Speech Praxis Workout Book* colorful, engaging, and reproducible. It's designed to help kids develop expressive language after mastering some basic sounds. See www.northernspeech.com or www.kidspeech.com.

■ *Closing the Gap* is a comprehensive special-needs website providing information and reviews of assistive technology (AT) products. Some resources can only be accessed by members only, but some archives are accessible to all. Go to www.closingthegap.com and click on "Resource Directory." Across the gray banner near the top of the page, you will see "Magazine Archives." Click on that and then scroll down to the left-hand side, where you can search by keyword or topic. You may find articles by Joan Tanenhaus helpful.

■ Eager for super-fresh, digital technology–focused approaches to speech-language therapy? Erik X. Raj, PhD, CCC-SLP, has you covered. His website is hip, up-to-date, and offers many resources, including awesome apps (designed by him) and other products like worksheets and posters for your speech space/home/clinic. He also offers workshops (for SLPs working with children ages five and up) which will quench your thirst in the best possible way. Check it out at https://erikxraj.com/.

■ Websites you may want to look into:

  ● The Discovery Center in the UK: www.boxofideas.org

  ● Kiz Club: www.kizclub.com (free printables for kids)

  ● Teachers with Apps: www.teacherswithapps.com (a good website for evaluating apps and technology for your child—not exactly speech-specific, but it's education-driven and you might stumble upon some great apps for your child)

  ● CommonSense Media: www.commonsensemedia.org (does an excellent job of curating apps, books, movies, and television with parent grades, reviews, and more)

Chapter 10

An Eye for Design

Creating a Language-Rich Environment & Encouraging Sound Sleep

Do you pore over the kids' decorating catalogs that clog your mailbox? Are you envious of the designs on HGTV, Pinterest, and the like? Do you wish to create a "learning lab" in your basement that the preschool envies? What if you just want to get organized? Then this is the chapter for you! I'll help you discover the joy of designing a special niche where your child with CAS can flourish. This chapter will focus on becoming very familiar with your child's interests, passions, and strengths and making them become a reality in your own home—all with a financially friendly approach.

For some of you, decorating and organizing is a no-brainer. You love it and are good at it. Your kids benefit by having age-appropriate toys at their fingertips and you love the clutter-free lifestyle. Plus, you relish the fact that your living environment reflects what is most near and dear to you.

But not everyone has a knack or even an interest in interior design. *You don't have to!* Many of the ideas presented here don't require much decorating talent, just a little know-how and some awareness. You may be surprised by the hints and tips within this chapter that just may help your child with speech and language.

- You are probably wondering why this is important: "Decorating is so not my thing!" you say, "and how does this relate to CAS anyway?" In a nutshell: *You have better access to materials.* Having to spend less time looking for items means you are more efficient and relaxed and inspired.

- *When kids (and parents) work and live in a well-planned environment, it helps keep the focus on learning and living.* The focus is *less* on cleaning up, locating, and managing chaos.

- *You'll feel empowered to do your work as a "speech assistant."* Parents have lots to worry about; why not make this aspect of your job a little easier?

- *Your child benefits from a sense of welcome and belonging.* Enhancing your child's emotional and communicative security is a wonderful result you'll be proud to claim.

Before you get started, you must remember two things:

- No environment is perfect.
- You'll probably never be able to create the most perfect room or house, but you can *enhance* what you already have.

The Nuts and Bolts of This Chapter

- How to turn your home into a speech-rich environment, even if you don't care about decorating
- The indirect relationship between one's environment and the individual benefits gained from a well-planned space
- Transforming rooms in your home into more kid-friendly areas
- Research to back this all up, as well as thoughts from parents who have been there
- Hints and tips for working with your child as you decorate and design
- A discussion on sleep and the connection to CAS

Thinking about a Space

What's in a room? How is the space arranged? How do you use the room? How does the room use you?

That last question is a bit of a trick question. When a space is well planned, it should be serving you, *not you serving the room*. So, if something just isn't working, make it work. That might mean being a bit unconventional.

For example, my kitchen pantry was not conveniently located near the place where I stored the kids' plastic snack cups. I kept going back and forth from cabinet to pantry filling snack cups. Not only was it annoying, but it was inefficient. Then it dawned on me: *Why not just keep these two items together?* So, I purchased an inexpensive plastic tote to store snack cups *in the pantry*. Genius? No, but now my kitchen was serving me, not me serving my kitchen.

Your Five-Mile Radius

Your home and your child's space(s) should be powerful, inviting places to grow and learn. Think about the world of a child—it's pretty small when you get right down to it! Now, think of your world as an adult. You have a home where you sleep, eat, bathe, rest, work (this is a loaded task—could mean chasing after kids, home office, cleaning, maintenance), and entertain. In addition, you may be employed outside the home, and probably have a handful of places you go to regularly: the grocery store, child's school, health club, place of worship, favorite eateries, and the local park.

Chances are you don't venture too far out of your "comfort zone." In fact, most everything you do regularly (other than work) is probably within a five- to ten-mile radius of your home. Using this example of "the world ain't so big," I will show just how important your home is to your child's growth.

Really? Yes. Behavior, thoughts, and feelings are shaped by lots of things, including genes, neurochemistry, history, and relationships, but also surroundings.

Think of a cluttered kitchen counter. Dishes to be done, mail to sort, bills to pay, bulging backpacks, a flashing light indicating new voice mail, a lost sock, a novel to finish. Agh! Your *behavior* may be to ignore or tackle the mess, your *thoughts* may be, "Who cares?" or "Yikes, I've got to do something about this!" Your *feelings* may be, "I'm such a slob," or "I love the abstract pattern of clutter on my counter. I feel so artistic."

Now those genes and the way your neurochemistry handles it are a little more complex. Let's just say that it's because of your genes that shape your personality and thus your immediate reaction to a cluttered kitchen counter.

History and relationships come into the picture in two ways. For example, maybe your mom always kept a spotless kitchen, so you do too. See how history (past kitchen neatness) and relationships (your mom) come together? History could also mean "personal history," as well: "Before I had kids, my house was a wreck; what's the point now that these little tornados have arrived?"

Your cluttered kitchen counter is screaming, "Do something with me—take care of this, take care of that!" If your home is cluttered, your children's thoughts, behaviors, and feelings might be too.

Creating a Great Space

The very best spaces are a result of thought, inspiration, knowledge, and information. When approaching a room to be decorated, it helps to keep these things in mind:

- overall vision for the space
- how the space will be used and by whom
- the room's inspiration piece (often becomes the theme)
- your "splurge" item
- what you can create yourself
- showcasing a collection of your child's interests, passions, and personality
- matching sets aren't always a "good thing"
- combining and blending accessories, colors, and pieces often creates the best look
- decorating is a process that takes time, planning, coordination, and an eye to tie it all together—and it should be fun!

With those ideas in mind, let's get started with your child's bedroom.

Your Child's Bedroom

Many parents might assume that their kids don't really care about how their room looks or the stuff they keep in it. That's actually a poor assumption—many kids *do* have a clear preference for how their space looks. Please ask your child if it's okay to decorate or redecorate before you dive in. Young kids become quite attached to belongings and personal spaces, even if you think less of them.

A child's bedroom is more than just a place to sleep. It's a little sanctuary from the world—a place to escape from the stresses of everyday life, to relax, to read, to daydream, and to just be.

A child's room should be filled with things that matter and interest him. Make a list of those things now. Be honest. It doesn't matter if *you* like Thomas the Train or Tinker Bell, just get the ideas down; you can always pare it down later. Here are some ideas to get you started:

- (your child's) favorite colors (see below)
- favorite TV shows
- favorite type of music
- favorite books
- collections
- sports (spectator or participant)
- Fascinations (bugs, space, nature, princesses)

> ### Does Your Child Have a Favorite Color?
>
> If your child has a favorite color, help him understand how the color can be used in the room. As a parent, you may not want bright orange paint splashed on the walls, but perhaps you could deal with a warm terra cotta?
>
> If your child isn't sure what his favorite color is, make a game out of it to determine if there is a clear theme to color preference. Sort objects and toys around the house together. Crayons, markers, blocks, Play-Doh that he gravitates toward could indicate a preference for a color. What colors are in some of his favorite clothes? What colors does he regularly use in his artwork?

Do Colors Influence Mood?

Yes! Warmer colors (orange, brown, red) tend to stimulate activity, whereas cooler colors (blues, greens) can produce feelings of calm.

RED	Increases restlessness and attention. Use sparingly.
ORANGE	Similar to red, but friendly. Use to increase feelings of friendship.

YELLOW	Sharp focus, cheerful, use to draw attention to achievement and/or themes in the room.
GREEN	Decreases muscular tension; good for concentration.
BLUE	Does not attract attention; can be too calming (decreases focus).
PURPLE	Combination of active red and passive blue; neutral and pleasing.
BLACK, WHITE, GRAY	Emotionally neutral, unless used in large areas.

Plan Before You Decorate

Decorating your child's room should be fun! As parents, it gives us an opportunity to recreate some of our own childhood dreams. Think back to what you were passionate about as a child. Chances are, you and your child have similar ideas.

Your goal at this stage should be to design a room that matches your child's individuality and grows with him. He won't love SpongeBob forever, so avoid a costly under-the-sea mural or pineapple wallpaper!

Start by evaluating the space. Walk around the room at various times of day. Make notes. Too big, too small? Too hot, too cold? Too dark, too bright? What storage/closets already exist? Sketch out a floor plan of the room, including doors, windows, built-ins, and closets. Rough-in furnishings and rugs. Involve your child by showing him a more detailed plan with colors and specific objects.

Next, think about what your child needs. It's easy to get caught up in "wants," but try to be as objective about this part of the exercise as possible. Think about how your child uses (or will use) his bedroom. Will homework be done in the room? Arts and crafts projects? Reading together or alone? Getting dressed? Listening to music? Playing with friends or siblings? Speech practice?

A child's room is his sanctuary. A child's room ought to reflect nearly every aspect of his life. Consider having these elements in the room:

- **Sanctuary:** Make it a place to get away from the stress of everyday life. Develop a place to read, relax, daydream, and feel an overall sense of welcome.
- **Knowledge:** Include items such as a desk, books, computer, puzzle, globe, or maps.
- **Family:** Casual photos of your child with beloved family members work especially well. Consider enlarging and framing favorite candid shots for wall decor. Use matching frames, or matching mats, or make all photos black and white, sepia, or color for a cohesive look. You can have different frames if you keep some other element (such as the mat color) the same.
- **Possessions:** Display collections of any kind neatly and artistically.
- **Recognition:** Highlight awards, trophies, and other accomplishments.
- **Friendship:** Photos with friends, games, and a table with two to four chairs encourage friendship.

- **Creativity:** Blocks, creative playthings, art supplies, computer, materials, and items that are shiny or catch your eye work well.
- **Diversity:** Include music, posters, books that depict various cultures.
- **Careers:** Capitalize on any possible vocational interests with books about careers or items such as mobiles or an aquarium.
- **Pride and Ownership:** Add something that is uniquely your child's. Consider special artwork (frame some he has created), a growth chart, his name spelled out in wooden letters, or a favorite item from babyhood (birth certificate, blankie, or booties).

Bedroom Considerations Specific to CAS

Aside from not being able to communicate as effectively as typically developing kiddos, your child with CAS presents his own unique challenges. Think of *your* child in this exercise and jot down your answers as you go along. This will help you plan a speech-rich environment for him.

- What motivates him? Excites him?
- How does he respond to external stimuli?
- How does he respond to internal stimuli?
- Is he active?
- Is he quiet and reserved?
- Is music calming or distracting?
- Are too many objects, toys, or decorations overwhelming?
- Does your child have difficulty settling down after a long day?
- How does your child self-soothe?

With those ideas in mind, consider these decorating and design tips:

If your child needs a calming influence, consider

- soft lighting such as table lamps,
- painting the room in muted colors,
- wall-to-wall carpeting,
- soft, smooth textures, and
- rounded corners on furniture.

If your child could benefit from gentle stimulation, consider

- overhead and table lighting, or a task lamp over a desk,
- brighter colors,
- hardwood flooring with area rugs to determine "stations" for certain tasks,
- glossy finishes on furniture,

- square corners on furniture,
- interesting textures such as corduroy or ruffles.

Just because your child has some communication (and possibly sensory) issues doesn't mean his room should be devoid of "fun stuff." Get creative, use your parenting intuition, and let him know that his room is a safe, fun, and inviting place.

At four years old, Kate was a friendly, outgoing girl with high energy needs. She loved gross motor activity, art, the color purple, flowers, dogs, and books. She had a difficult time unwinding at the end of the day and needed much sensory stimulation.

Quick Plan: Initially, we thought the theme for the room could be a garden/flower or dog theme. Keeping in mind that we wanted the room to grow with her, we involved her in the decision. We actually went for a "doggies and daisies" theme for Kate. It reflected her interest in gardening and her love for animals. Together, we selected items that we could agree on that went along with the overall theme. We chose items that could easily be replaced, should she grow bored with them. For example, the peel-and-stick wildflowers on her wall are not permanent and the stuffed dogs can easily be relocated.

- Kate's **high energy** meant she needed a wide-open space to play, jump, twirl, and stretch out without feeling restricted. I scooted furniture to the edges of the room in hopes it would prevent bumps and bruises (it did, mostly).
- Since Kate loved (and still loves) **art**, I involved her in selecting pieces of wall art. I also had her create her own with finger paint on a blank canvas and framed some of her favorite artwork from preschool that coordinated with her room.
- **Books** are a big deal to Kate (and her family), so I made sure they were prominently displayed. You might consider turning books into art by installing a book ledge along the wall and purchasing beautifully illustrated hardcover children's books that coordinate with the room's overall theme.
- Achieving Kate's high need for **sensory stimulation** was done by incorporating various textures and surfaces. Beanbag chairs provided the cocoon-like feel she desired (consider also floppy pillows or floor cushions). We even kept fidget toys and oral stimulation pieces in her room for times she needed extra input.
- Kate's day concluded with a **bath, calming lotion** (lavender, vanilla, chamomile scents work well), relaxing music, and quiet reflection time.

I am not suggesting that your child with CAS is just like Kate. The key with CAS is it is as unique as your child. CAS does not present itself the same way every time.

Your Child with CAS Doesn't Talk Much . . . Yet

In reading through this chapter, you no doubt noticed me suggesting you get your child's input. Don't despair if your child isn't saying, "Well, Mom, what I'd really like is a sanctuary I can call my own. I'd like the walls painted quaking grass and the bedspread to be handcrafted by the best quilter in town with all of my favorite colors and coordinating artwork." *No* kid will ever say that unless he is destined to be an interior designer!

What's a Parent to Do?

- Clip photos or pages from a catalog or magazine for your child to cull through with you.
- Take him with you to look at paint chips. "Which color would you like to paint your room?"
- Ask if he'd like to go along to shop for accessories for his train-themed bedroom. You can even "shop" from toys/items in his toy chest, selecting models or toys that fit into whatever his theme might be.
- Try asking questions like, "Where do you like to play/have a playroom? Can you show me?"

Get creative and find ways you can ask for your child's input. Most kids can indicate yes or no. And finally, don't just assume that because your little one can't articulate much doesn't mean he doesn't care.

Designing a Play Space for Your Child

Sure, we spend about a third of our lives sleeping, but that means that two-thirds of our lives is spent awake, doing things, learning things, and enjoying things. Children may spend some of that awake time in their own room, but chances are, they are going to be playing near their parents. This section will focus on developing a playroom just right for *your* child.

Again, you'll have to assess your space. Where do you tend to spend most of your day when you're at home? Are you in the kitchen, a home office, the family room, a basement rec room? Young kids will want Mom and Dad in eyesight, and you might require it too. An ideal play space will be devoted to your child(ren) and will make learning fun and safe.

- *Determine where you will set up shop.* Think of your basement, a loft, the corner of a family room; maybe you can convert a rarely used dining room, living room, or guest bedroom into "kid central"?
- *Try to keep all toys in a designated space.* That way your entire home won't feel like the dumping ground for the local toy store.
- *What kinds of toys do you already have?* Make a list.
- *Which toys do your child(ren) play with the most?*
- *What kinds of playroom furnishings do you own?* Toy box, bookshelves, kiddie table and chairs, easel, storage containers, etc.
- *What are the major traffic ways in and out of the room?*

- *Draw a floor plan.* Include windows, doors, closets, and any built-ins (bookshelves, fireplaces, window seats).

Think of your newly minted play space as a rival to your child's classroom. In classroom speak, the usefulness of a classroom is referred to as "vitality." It's all influenced by the amount of stuff—furniture, decorations, and materials. You may think that more is better. You may feel your kid(s) will be smarter if he has more. Actually, the opposite is true. Clutter depletes energy.

An ideal play space incorporates areas for play and work. And remember, in your child's world, it really *is* work to color in the lines or learn to use scissors. It requires skill and concentration to assemble a puzzle, even if it only has five pieces.

Playroom Considerations Specific to CAS

When you think of a child's preschool classroom, you may envision workstations or "centers"—a kitchen area, a craft and color table, building and constructing, pretend play, and so forth. For your home play space, consider replicating that preschool vibe.

Preschools are also cognizant of allowing the environment to "grow with the child." Teachers are constantly assessing their students to see what they can do, what they are about to do, and what challenges them. You'll want your child's play area at home to grow with him too. For example, once he masters the alphabet, you might replace the ABC wall strip with sight words he is learning to read, such as "and," "the," and "see."

Other things you can do at home:

- Periodically *review* the toys/items in your child's play space for skill level, ease of use, child's interest, etc.
- *Remove* items that seem too "babyish."
- *Replenish* the room with items your child may see as a "reach," or challenge. (We found that introducing items that were slightly beyond Kate's current level gave her renewed interest and motivation to communicate).

Please, don't take this advice as "you need to go out and purchase new toys for your child." You can very well store items your child receives as gifts in a closet and pull them out when he is ready for them. You can arrange a toy-swap in your neighborhood in which you trade toys on a rotating basis. Some communities even have a toy lending program. Garage sales are often good places to get "new" things that may interest your child.

Here are some more ideas for creating a playroom that grows with your child:

- *Have a special section on phonological awareness.* Stock it with magnetic letters, alphabet stamps, letter flashcards, books on letters, workbooks, letter manipulatives (foam-shaped letters, blocks), etc.
- *Label everything.* Use big bold letters and put signs on furnishings: "chair," "table," "easel." Lisa Circelli, an early childhood teacher at the Brokaw Early Learning

Center in Oswego, Illinois, recommends using upper- and lowercase letters in your signage. "Kids need to see the correct way of writing words so they can begin to internalize it."

- *Prominently display alphabet cards at eye level.* Many folks place them at the top of the wall around the perimeter of the room, but children won't see them there.

- *Have a "letter of the day."* Work on that sound for the entire day (even if it is *just* you saying it), point out objects that begin with that sound, look for the letter when you are out and about in the community.

- *Encourage gross motor work.* Engage the vestibular system with a swing or trampoline. Quiz and drill your child on speech homework from the SLP while he moves his body.

- *Create a safe and easily accessible art center.* Stock it with child-safe scissors, glue, construction paper, coloring books, markers, crayons, etc.

Parents Share

Mirror, Mirror, on the Wall

Rita in Ohio shares this experience: "Our six-year-old daughter loves to have mirrors around wherever she is. It's a place where she can go touch base with where her mouth is (proprioception). She spends almost an hour sometimes looking at her mouth, inside [her mouth], sticking out her tongue, and touching her teeth. When she was younger, she did this even more. Eye-level mirrors have been key for us in all living areas."

In fact, speech clinics often use mirrors as a therapy tool—there just may be something to it!

I love this idea from Joy, the mother of twins with global apraxia and fine motor delays:

> One whole end of our family room has a padded floor with table and chairs and our old toy bin, which we stock with all kinds of supplies (including recyclable items like tissue rolls and egg cartons). Both my kids love doing art, but my ulterior motive is to give them as many opportunities as possible to manipulate materials (from tape to a stapler to scissors) and also hold a writing utensil so they can sign all their work and/or write about it. Nobody wants to work on writing letters, since it is so frustrating, but [they] will do artistic challenges that include the basic elements. I am even thinking of doing art challenges and tying it with verbal cues from Handwriting without Tears *and then moving to working on letters if I can sneak it in.*

Robbin, mom of Kennedy (3.6 years with CAS) and Jack (2 years), says her art room has become the therapy room at their house:

> My kids love [our art room]. They have no idea we are working on speech. My daughter's SLP comes to the house and works with her with all the things I have in there. It's great!

Sensory Stimulation and CAS

By now, you should be aware that motion affects the speech and language center nestled deep within your child's brain. But did you know you can create cool features at home that foster good times and social development while allowing your child with CAS to feel comfortable and increase his vestibular stimulation?

- *Got an exposed beam in your basement or attic?* Hang a swing from it, or a hammock (some even come with stands, so no need for an exposed beam).
- *Develop an indoor sports spot.* What you need: space (unfinished basement?), small trampoline, child-sized basketball goal, exercise balls, jump ropes, maybe even a slide, tunnel system, or climbing wall. Add some music and you've got the recipe for burning energy. Kids into gymnastics? Get some mats, make or buy a beam, and voilà—a gymnastics studio.
- *Some kids love to perform.* Consider developing a stage for theatrical productions and allowing him to sing his heart out. It doesn't have to be elaborate—just a slightly raised platform and a toy microphone will do. Who knows—it may even get him to try new words!
- *Some kids with CAS crave sensory stimulation.* Consider converting an old sandbox or under-bed storage box into a messy table. Fill it with popcorn kernels, dried beans (if your child is over three and won't swallow small items), feathers, or ribbon, or make your own slime. Add old measuring devices, bowls and spoons, a kid or two, and bake for hours of play.

Keep in mind: *any* individual learns best when actively engaged in the learning process. And please, don't feel you have to do all—or any—of these suggestions. Pick and choose what works for your family, your space, and your budget.

> Thinking back, if we had the means, we could have put a swing in our basement and a trampoline out back: two very sensory-friendly things for Jack that stimulated his speech. We compromised on two large yoga kind of balls, jumping on the bed, and a Jim Gill CD featuring the "Washing Machine Song," where he'd run himself in circles each night before bed (seriously). Those less-expensive, unobtrusive, yet very kid-friendly items still stimulated the speech and sounds we were looking for, plus fed the vestibular and proprioceptive systems[stimulation]. Sometimes it isn't about what, but more about how.
>
> —Holly, mother of a son with CAS

Creating a Book Nook

In our busy lives, it's hard to find the time and place to practice speech homework assigned by the SLP. One thing that can help: a book nook at home with comfy furnishings (beanbags or floor pillows) where you and your child can snuggle down and look at books together. Pull in a crate or bookshelf to store your materials, and you've got a wonderful area to practice speech in an inviting environment.

If you're short on space, there is no reason not to have your art center in the corner of the family room or kitchen, just as you can also have a quiet reading area in the dining room. It may work well to have "reservations" to use the space: "Dining room closed for speech practice from 2:00 to 2:30 pm," or something along those lines.

■ *Consider making a "book" from the handouts and flashcards your speech pathologist gives you.* Use a folder with brads, or a half-inch or one-inch binder and slip the worksheets into sheet protectors. We kept our notebook in Kate's room and reviewed that week's lesson every night and at naptime. I mixed it in with the other reading we did, so it didn't seem like such a chore.

■ *Practice speech with your child by pointing out pictures in children's books.* This worked wonderfully with Kate when she had difficulties with /s/ blends. "What's this?" I'd say as I pointed to a snail, a snake, a smokestack. I'd look for an /s/ blend on every page. A sigh and a few attempts later, Kate would produce the right blend. This worked because she loves books. If your child isn't the bookish type, don't despair.

Creating a Study Center

By the time your child is in kindergarten, you'll likely see some kind of homework every night. It might just be a worksheet or two, but start looking for small assignments as early as pre-K.

Please have a regular place for your child(ren) to study. Even if you're just working on the ABCs and 123s, practicing handwriting, or drawing shapes, establish a consistent place and keep it sacred. It can be a part of the playroom, in the bedroom, or elsewhere in the home (like the kitchen, a loft, even a wide hallway). The key is that homework is done in this area.

Stock your child's study center with school supplies. Hit the before-school sales and buy double of what your school wants your child to bring. Keep an extra set of supplies at home. Consider purchasing other items like poster board and display boards, binders, report covers, markers, and highlighters. You never know when that last-minute project may crop up.

Make it comfortable with well-appointed child-size desks and chairs. Add a cushion to the seat if sitting for prolonged time. Hang a bulletin board or dry-erase board to post assignments, ideas, task lists, and notes.

Keep some reference materials handy. Consider dictionaries, thesauruses, atlases, and encyclopedias; nowadays, you can find it all on the computer.

Assess when and if you want your child using a computer. At what age do you think having a computer is reasonable? Expected? How will you monitor your child's activity on the computer?

Keep your child's personality and work style in mind when setting up the study area. Ask for his input. If it's an area that's naturally pleasing to your child, he's more likely to use it and succeed there. Let the area grow with your child. Homework is going to be a big part of his life for many years to come. *Last but not least, let it reflect his fun and unique style.*

A filing cabinet or three-ring binder for each child is handy too. It teaches filing and organizational skills and develops a sense of accountability. Parents, you might spend more time managing and looking at this than your child. We kept progress reports, IEP information, and report cards, along with special projects and interests specific to Kate and Kelly.

Music Influences the Environment Too

Music and moods go together like milk and cookies. Songs can make us feel good, evoke happy memories, or help us focus. Kids like music and having some playing in the background adds to the space. You know your child best, so think about how he responds to music. Would classical music help him focus? Would some funky kid music get him up and moving?

Use different types of music at different times of the day and you may be surprised how it affects your child (and your parenting). You can use different music to signal transitions between activities—between playtime and clean-up, for example. Or between awake time and calm-down-and-get-ready-for-bed time. Gross motor time on the indoor trampoline makes for some great speech practice. Put on some tunes, get him jumping, and pull out the flashcards—he may forget he's even "working!"

Why Sleep May Be a Challenge

I have heard from many parents of kids with CAS that sleep can be a problem. Before we jump to conclusions, it's not always CAS that is *the* cause for sleep issues. Just be aware that there is a *correlation* between CAS and poor sleep. Your child, however, may be a terrific sleeper and still have CAS. Again, not all children with CAS are the same.

You'll want to be aware of any potential sensory or medical issues your child may have. See Appendix A for more information on sensory processing.

My four-year-old [with CAS] usually wakes during the night for three or four hours. We've tried melatonin, dietary changes, probiotics, sensory input before bed, strict schedule, white noise machine, blackout curtains, weighted blanket, homeopathy, Epsom salt baths. Short of prescription drugs—you name it, we've tried it. Not one thing has helped. The pediatrician and neurologist shrug their shoulders with a "yep, nature of the beast with these disorders" attitude.

—Amanda, mom to twins with CAS, ADHD, SPD

Sensory Concerns Affecting Your Child's Ability to Relax

While it's easy, in some regards, to call CAS "the bad guy," it isn't *the* source of all concerns for your child. However, if you are truly concerned about the possibility of sensory issues with your child, please seek the services of a pediatric occupational therapist (OT) or consider getting a comprehensive neuropsychological evaluation.

Here are a few ideas you can try if you suspect sensory issues *along with* CAS (but really, these ideas would work with just about any child, regardless of CAS):

Try Kid Yoga. Your child may be very receptive to this idea, especially if he can "share" it with a parent or teenaged sibling as special bonding time. Yoga has powerful, yet soothing effects on the body and mind. For more information, look to *Go Go Yoga for Kids: A Complete Guide to Yoga with Kids* by Sara Weis, the *YogaKids* DVD series, and *Yoga for Families: Connect with Your Kids*. You may also like the book *The ABCs of Yoga for Kids* by Theresa Anne Power, which shows how to teach the formations of letters (and their sounds) through yoga poses.

Explore Visualization or Meditation. Along with, or in lieu of yoga, you and your child may appreciate a little guided visualization just before going to bed. Sit with him in a comfortable spot awhile, taking deep refreshing breaths. Using words, you can create a visual escape to your "destination" of choice: an ocean, wooded forest, mountaintop. Use vibrant descriptions and encourage him to use all his senses as you describe this location—smell the salty sea air, feel the warm breezes. I love these books: *Angel Bear Yoga: Adventure Stories* or *Yoga,* by Christi Eley and *Mindfulness for Kids: 30 Fun Activities to Stay Calm, Happy, and In Control,* by Carole Roman and J. Robin Albertson-Wren.

Relax with a Stress-Relieving Neck Wrap. They come filled with rice or beans, sometimes flaxseed or buckwheat; some may be scented. You can warm them in the microwave. The weight (just a couple of pounds) can be very soothing for kids who have difficulty slowing down. Beanbags can produce a similar result. If you're crafty, you might be able to make your own.

Make a Pig-in-a-Blanket. Try wrapping your child tightly in a heavy quilt, with his head poking out during bedtime stories. The tight feeling can be quite soothing and comforting to some kids (think of swaddling a baby). Unwrap him before tucking him in bed.

Try a Bedtime Snack. Some folks swear that certain foods have magical powers that lull one to sleep (turkey, anyone?). Consider these wonder foods:

- *Cherries* (fresh and dried) are one of the only natural sources of melatonin, the chemical that controls the body's internal clock. Researchers recommend eating them about an hour before you want to fall asleep. Keep in mind, fresh cherries contain pits and could be a choking hazard, especially for kids under three. Even dried cherries should be given with caution.

- *Bananas* are chock-full of potassium and magnesium, which are natural muscle relaxants. Also, bananas contain L-tryptophan (an amino acid), which is converted by the body to serotonin (5-HTP, a neurotransmitter that is a natural relaxant) and melatonin.

- *Toast* is one of those carbohydrate-dense foods triggering insulin production, making one drowsy by releasing tryptophan and serotonin. That's why you often feel tired after eating a muffin for breakfast without a source of protein.

- *Oatmeal* also triggers a rise in blood sugar, just like toast will. Oats also have melatonin.

- *Warm milk* may sound a bit old-fashioned, but there's science behind the magic. Again, the amino acid L-tryptophan is at work here, converting to 5-HTP, releasing serotonin. Milk is high in calcium, too, which promotes that drowsy feeling. (Add a teaspoon of vanilla extract for a little added flavor.)

Consider Heavy Blankets and Quilts. You may want to turn down the thermostat at night (best sleeping temperatures range from 65 to 72 degrees Fahrenheit). The cooler temperatures are actually more conducive to sleep, and heavy blankets often produce a soothing effect for the sleeper.

Getting Back to Sleep

If you're pretty certain that your child doesn't have any additional sensory or medical concerns related to sleep, and you just want some old-fashioned advice on getting him off to dreamland each night, read on.

Although I don't have any specific data proving that sleep difficulties are directly related to CAS, there's no denying that sleep and circadian rhythms are all derived from the nervous system. Since we know CAS is a motor-neurological disorder, then it can be assumed that these two systems are in tandem.

Restless sleep, difficulty falling asleep and staying asleep, being a "light sleeper," and early awakening all qualify as "sleep disturbances."

Here are some simple steps you can do to make sure your child's room is conducive to sleep:

- *Make it dark.* I know this seems obvious, but some kids are bothered by the slightest amount of light creeping under the door or peeking through blinds. You may want to consider a room-darkening shade.

- *Consider painting the walls tranquil and soothing colors.* There is evidence that certain colors may be more relaxing than others. For instance, blue is often used in doctors' offices and prisons because it is known to decrease one's heart rate and blood pressure. Refer to the chart on page 198.

- *Reduce distractions.* Carefully assess your child's room and determine what items may be more distracting to him. Generally speaking, the more stuff that's in his room, the more distracting it's going to be.

- *Keep toys, activities, and playthings in another room.* While this may not always be possible, it's worth considering. A basement, guest room, loft, attic, or sunroom may make a great place to play. You could also repurpose your dining room as a playroom, but you'd have to do without the formal dinner parties—at least for a while.

- *Keep your child's most prized possessions in his room—just limit them.* Please don't read the above advice as "Take everything out of your child's room and paint it blue." As we discussed before, children love the idea of a place they can call their own, with their own belongings and sense of personality.

Say That Again?! Chapter Summary

I hope I have shown you that the environment really *does* shape how we feel about surroundings and influences behavior—good or bad. Perhaps I have given you some ideas of ways you can improve your home, as well as your children's sleep, play, and work areas. If you decide to redecorate or repurpose any rooms in your house, keep these tips in mind:

Have fun and be sure you ask for your child's input. Even though he has CAS, he can still share his preferences. Integrate items that are important and valuable to your child. Think of a theme, but do your best to be subtle about it, because "more" is not always "better." Take your time. Decorating is a process, not just an outcome. Shop around. Talk with other parents. Look at books and magazines and catalogs for inspiration. In fact, look at *anything* and *everything* for inspiration, even the decor of your favorite eatery. Allow your child to have some ownership of the area/room. Consider displaying his name or dedicate a spot for showcasing trophies or artwork.

Remember: clutter depletes energy. Plus, it can be downright overwhelming for kids with CAS whose nervous and motor systems are already overtaxed. Less is more. Consider relaxing music and tranquil wall colors, if your child needs a little extra relief from stimulation. If your child has sensory issues in addition to verbal apraxia, incorporate features that let you sneak in sensory work as well. Finally, I leave you with this thought from "CAS mom" Holly:

In my opinion, every place is a speech-rich environment, whether you are at the grocery store, on the playground, in your own basement, or in your own bathroom. There is always something to point out, talk about, describe, sing about, look at, touch, feel, smell, etc. For us, those were richer experiences than anything I purchased with therapy on my mind.

Recommended Resources

- Looking for some activity-driven pieces to complete your child's playroom? Check out Weplay for items such as **balance boards**, **exercise balls**, **foam mats and blocks**, and **trampolines**: www.weplay.com.tw.

- I love the work of **Ayelet Marinovich**, MA, CCC-SLP, and her Learn with Less concept. Repurposed household items can often be used as toys or props to enhance language and communication. She offers an informative and empowering Podcast too: https://learnwithless.com/.

- You don't have to shop in expensive therapy supply stores or catalogs to outfit your child's physical activity area. You can find many wonderful products made for kids of all abilities through **HearthSong:** www.hearthsong.com. And if you—or someone you know—are handy, maybe you can make your own.

- For **weighted wraps**, you may want to consider these products: North American Healthcare Hot/Cold Comfort Wrap, which can be purchased on www.Amazon.com or the Carex Bed Buddy, www.carex.com/products.

- ***Take Charge of Your Child's Sleep: The All-in-One Resource for Solving Sleep Problems in Kids and Teens*** by Judith A. Owens and Jodi A. Mindell (Marlowe & Co., 2005) is a parent-friendly book on sleep problems in kids, including chapters on sleep apnea, bad dreams, and ADHD, among others.

Chapter 11

Off to School

Preparing Your Child (and Yourself!)

After being a mom for not quite three years, I wasn't expecting to be enrolling my daughter in public education. I had envisioned two more years of playgroups, parks, and Play-Doh. But after a whirlwind meeting with the SLP and special education coordinator at the school district, I was leaving the building with a stack of papers, handbooks, and registration forms. "Fill these out and get them back to us in three weeks. You will need to schedule and complete a school physical in that time too. If the transportation department doesn't contact you within two weeks, call them. Here's their number." I painstakingly herded my two girls out of the bright and cheerful assessment room, baby Kelly on one hip, the papers on the other, and made my way home.

By 10:30 a.m., I was mentally and emotionally drained. My little girl, then two years and eleven months old, had just been confirmed as "severely apraxic," and because of this disability, she would be attending special education preschool five days a week. She would qualify for *bus* services, too! I tried to be optimistic for Kate's sake (and mine too), but I desperately needed to process the events of the morning. My husband was traveling and attending an important meeting. My fingers were itching to dial someone—*anyone*—on my cell phone, but no one was available to talk at this hour. No one who *really* understood, anyway. We drove home quietly. I held back tears. My chin wobbled as I pointed out a big yellow bus. "Kate look! You'll be riding one of those soon."

I ended up calling my dad once the girls were down for their naps. Always a pillar of strength and support, he listened to me review the morning's events and gave me his ever-reassuring words of wisdom: "Everyone wants their kids to be above average in every way, but this is the best thing for her." He told me other things, too: "It's good you caught this when you did . . . you're doing the right thing . . . how great there's a school for this."

And he was right about all of it. But it still hurt, a lot. I did cry that day—and other days too. But, I will tell you that it *does* get better, and you *will* get through this.

This chapter will walk you through the steps of having your child assessed through the school district and help you ease your child through the transition from being home with you full-time (or attending day care) to going to school. Special-needs students and their families have, well—special needs when it comes to school. We'll explore IDEA, FAPE, and IEPs . . . a bit different from your 123s and ABCs.

Think of this chapter as your "Cliff Notes Guide" to sending your child with CAS to school. I will attempt to touch on your most pressing concerns, feelings, and questions, but I know you will have questions specific to your own child. Please continue to seek out all the resources you can as you navigate the school system.

The Nuts and Bolts of This Chapter

- General guidelines for selecting a school (but keep in mind, not all aspects may pertain to your situation)
- Overview of preschool and kindergarten, as well as all of the players involved
- Some pros and cons of homeschooling
- Teaching your child's teacher about CAS, being an involved parent, and hosting an in-class lesson on CAS for all students
- What to expect from speech therapy at school
- Special education jargon such as IEP and IFSP, your role in the education process, and tips on staying organized and filing a complaint
- Theories as to why kids with CAS may have a harder time academically, plus solutions and possible interventions
- Learning styles, emotional IQ, and grade retention

Qualities to Look for in a School

When we moved from the Minneapolis area to Chicago, my husband made a nice spreadsheet comparing the new school districts of our suburban area with ones we were familiar with, even including some data on the public school system we attended as kids. I thought this was sweet but overly nerdy and systematic of him. At the time of our move, our two girls were just four months and barely two years old, and while I wanted the girls to attend a good school district, I was more interested in how I was going to baby proof the new digs than where we'd send them to school!

But my husband was on to something (as usual). Assuming you have a choice where you send your child to school—be it public or private, suburban or urban, "special" or mainstream—it's not a bad idea to be "nerdy and systematic" and carefully plan for the long haul. Here's a checklist for you to consider. If your child is just entering preschool, try not to get overwhelmed, especially when we discuss academics. This section covers the basics for all grade levels.

General Considerations:

- Find out what the school's visitation policy is and then . . .

- Visit the school during regular school hours. Did you feel welcome? Did the kids look happy?

- What were the teachers and administrators like?

- Is the school clean and well kept? Bright and cheerful?

- How are the students dressed? Do they wear uniforms? Does your child look the part?

- Does the school have a mission statement prominently displayed in the building or on its website? Was the mission reflected in your first impression?

- Does the school accurately reflect the cultural diversity in your community?

- Is admission based on chronological age guidelines, not on mastery of skills?

- What was your commute like to the school? Were you stopped by a train? Going against morning traffic? Now imagine the same drive in inclement weather . . . still doable?

- What transportation options are available? Parent drop-off, bus, before- and after-school care?

- Is transportation provided if your child must attend a school that is not her "home school?"

Teachers and Administration:

- Do teachers take part in regular professional development? How often?

- Do the teachers have experience or education in child development? Even in stand-alone preschools, and private preschool centers, teachers are required to have a certain amount of educational credit to work with the children.

- Are teachers ready to meet children "where they're at?" A big phrase in education these days is *differentiation of material*, which generally translates to: material and curriculum should meet the needs of each student and may vary from student to student.

- How accessible are teachers? Can they be reached through phone or email?

- Will teachers communicate regularly with one another and with you at home? How?

- Are the teachers national board certified? What percentage of teachers are?

- What percentage of teachers hold advanced degrees? Is that important to you?

- Are there regular school improvement days where teachers and administrators collaborate?

Social and Emotional Learning:

- Is there an antibullying curriculum in place? (More on this in chapter 13)
- Does the school support student relationships, kindness, consideration, and respect?
- Is there access to a school psychologist or social worker?
- Are social skills supported and encouraged through facilitated play, nonverbal options (PECS, visual schedules, signing/gesturing), and social skills groups?
- Do kids get outside time? How often?

Student Resources:

- Does the library have current media and technology: computers, books, subscriptions to online resources, DVDs? Does the library feel comfortable and accessible?
- Is the cafeteria clean? Are there healthy food choices? Ask for a lunch menu.
- Who provides speech services? What are their qualifications? How will you be apprised of developments? (Ask similar questions regarding occupational therapy, if that is a need for your child.)
- Where and how often do kids receive extra help (tutoring) if they need it?

Academics:

- What curriculum has the school adopted? It should have a formal name. Is it challenging, but appropriately so?
- Is there balance within the curriculum? Is it "heavy" in one content area? Does that matter to you?
- What special education classes are housed at the school, or does the school use an inclusion model?
- Is there a speech classroom, language classroom, or other special classrooms?
- How much homework can be expected each day?
- Request a copy of a progress report and a report card.
- How will your child's progress be reported? If your child has an IEP for speech, or any other special education service, the law requires regular progress reports.
- How are grades determined? What's the grading scale?
- Do yearly stats show a tendency for consistency? Is there improvement or not?
- Visit a classroom (you'll need special permission first). Are the kids actively engaged? What is the teacher doing? Is there an aide?
- What type of student work is on display?
- What is the average class size per grade? Teacher-to-student ratio?
- Is foreign language part of the curriculum? What percentage of students go on to a four-year university?

Before and After School:

- Ask for a school calendar. What types of sporting and social events are listed?
- Are there before- and after-school clubs? What are they? Do they appeal to you and your child?
- Do the hours of these events fit in with your typical schedule?
- Is transportation available to school-sponsored events?
- Is there transportation to/from daycare facilities?

Parents:

- Ask for a newsletter or classroom bulletin from the front office. Read it. What other school-home communication exists? Emails? Phone calls? Website?
- Does the school have any partnerships with the community at large? With whom?
- Does the school help connect families to the community resources to promote learning outside of the classroom?
- Are parents encouraged to volunteer in the classroom and within the school?
- Is there an active PTA/PTO?
- Talk to other parents in the same district. Parents of older kids are a great resource. Ask, "What do you love about your kid's school? What don't you like?"

Please, listen to your instincts. If something just doesn't jive with you, there's probably a better school for you and your child (assuming you are looking at private schools or deciding what neighborhood to settle in). Obviously, if you're already settled in and looking at the neighborhood public school, you may not have a choice. You may also be interested in checking out this website: www.schooldigger.com. Here you can obtain test scores, rankings, teacher : student ratios, district boundaries, etc. for more than 120,000 K-12 schools in the United States. Of course, you'll have to focus on the speech–language piece of it once you find a school district you are happy with.

Preschool

> *I am so anxious about where to send my son to preschool. I know it's a drop in the bucket compared to all of the schooling he will receive in his lifetime, but I want to make sure he is in a really good program, especially because of his CAS.*
>
> —Mom to Josiah, age three

Your child may just be three years old, but you are already thinking about her education. If you started out with early intervention services (sometimes called "Birth to Three" or "First Steps"), then your little one will be transitioning from EI to the regular school district where you reside. If that's the case for you, then consider yourself lucky. The EI program will guide you through the process of transitioning to special education services.

To qualify for preschool services through your local school district, your child will need to be evaluated just shy of her third birthday. Give yourself about three months lead to her birth date. If your child is receiving EI, your team members will let you know the steps involved. Otherwise you'll likely need to call the school district where you live, and the special education coordinator will take it from there. Granted, this process is not so simple and you may need to make several phone calls or be a bit of a pest to get the answers you need. If you have a private SLP, you will want her onboard with the plan (she may even initiate it) and for her to write a letter requesting the evaluation. If your child is seeing a private OT, consider getting a letter of recommendation from her too.

Your child will be assessed by the school personnel—an early childhood educator, a special education consultant, and a school-based SLP are likely to be part of the assessment team. If the team concurs that your child's speech and language skills are significantly delayed, then you're in. The size of the delay required varies from district to district, but often it is three to six months (sometimes referred to as "lag time" in educational circles). Sometimes children with less significant delays in speech may qualify if they also have mild to moderate delays in other areas. According to Rhonda Banford, MAT, CCC-SLP, teams sometimes also make a professional judgment if a child is "on the cusp."

Once your child is in, you will find that what "special needs preschool" consists of varies depending on your school district, your child's needs, and sometimes your own preferences. These preschools may be separate programs housed outside of a regular school, or they may be classrooms within public schools. Then again, for some children, needed services may be provided within a private preschool or daycare that you have enrolled your child in.

Blended versus Self-Contained: Your child's classroom may be either "blended" or "self-contained": A *blended or integrated* ("inclusive") classroom is one where students with different abilities are combined in one classroom. This is often done in public school settings. Your child with CAS may be in a classroom with typically developing peers as well as those with CAS or other special needs. On the other hand, your IEP team may decide that your child would be best served in a *self-contained* classroom where all students have a special need of some kind (hearing impairment, Down syndrome, congenital disorders, etc.), or where the primary concern for all of the students is speech and language skills. However, note that a 2011 study in the journal *Child Development* indicated that "among children with low initial language skills, those who were placed in the lowest-ability [preschool] classes tended to lose ground during the school year, while those placed in average-ability classes tended to improve their language skills."

Be sure to discuss what kind of classroom your child will be in at the IEP meeting and make your views known about the pros and cons of different settings. (See pages 235–41 for more information on IEPs.)

Thoughts on Blended Classrooms

"Putting our son with [CAS] in our school district's early childhood program has been the best thing we could do. It is a blended program with up to five typical kids, five kids who are considered at risk, and five kids who are considered special needs. I will not tell you this program is perfect—there is no such thing—but overall it is absolutely amazing. If you can find a blended program in your area, I highly recommend it."

—Mom to twins, one of whom has CAS.

"We live in a district that does not offer a blended ECE program, and it has been a challenge to expose my son to typical peers who will reinforce all of his language and social growth. You would think that if a child has it written into his IEP that he make gains in his social pragmatic speech, the school would be responsible for creating [that] environment. Like many families, we have been responsible for creating and paying for those experiences. As parents, we wear so many hats for our children. Adding the job of taking on the structural system of one's school district is just too much."

—Jessica K. Paganis, LCSW

Although the term *special-needs preschool* may have some negative connotations, there are instances when this is the best thing for a child—and you. Trust me, I've been there.

- Teachers at these schools (or in the special classroom) *know* kids and almost always have additional training in special needs, learning disabilities, and literacy.

- Class sizes are smaller and more manageable. Kids will receive more 1:1 assistance. Having a teacher's aide also helps reduce the teacher-to-student ratio.

- Smaller groups and individualized lessons help children adapt and make progress.

- Multiage classrooms mean kids can learn from older kids, and older kids can help the younger ones feel more comfortable in a new setting.

- It's less likely your child will be targeted by "mean kids"—making her feel bad for being "different." Everyone at a specialized preschool is struggling with a unique need.

If your child *doesn't* qualify for preschool through your school district (or the district doesn't provide it), you have a couple of options:

- ***Depending on the school, your child may qualify for itinerant speech therapy services held at the school.*** For example, Kate's school offered a "walk-in speech class" for children who struggled with speech, but on a more mild level. The class met at different times throughout the week for about an hour. Students received group instruction from a qualified SLP. It was offered at no cost for families who fell within district boundaries.

- **You may consider Montessori or Waldorf preschools.** Their educational philosophies incorporate multimodal learning, which helps with speech development. Ask specifically what the school does to foster speech and language in the classroom when you visit.

Whatever form your child's special needs preschool takes, it will be geared toward getting your little one ready for kindergarten. *The goal for your child, although she has CAS, is to be on par with her classmates by the time she reaches kindergarten.* Maybe you are thinking that's a tall order, wishful thinking, or just not going to happen, but you will be wildly amazed at the progress your child will make in the two or three years she is in preschool.

Kids Cope

Preschoolers with communication disorders are more likely to choose teachers and aides (adults) as their conversation partners than fellow students. In one study, it was found that kids with delayed expressive speech also had lower socialization skills. These kids were more likely to play with toys in unusual ways and have difficulty sharing, but were less likely to play with peers.

In my personal experience, this does seem to occur. Kids with CAS may feel comfortable with adults because they are in a position of authority and tend to be patient and give cues and assistance. Peers may not "get" the language delay and give up trying to understand kids with CAS. However, if peers are told simple things like Nora's still learning to use her words, but she's a lot fun to play with, it may help open the doors to friendship. Also, it may be wise to teach and encourage kids with CAS to play nonverbal games such as tag or chase.

Kindergarten

Transitioning from preschool to kindergarten can be worrisome, but most often the anxiety produced leading up to the first day is unnecessary. *Remember, if you are anxious, your child will become anxious.* Parents who are positive and optimistic about a new experience will produce happy, confident kids. Communicate your excitement and hopes to your child often. One more tip: avoid talking about kindergarten as the "real school" or the "big school" or any other term that may negate the preschool experience. Preschool was once very real and very big to your child. Kindergarten is just the next step.

So, what's kindergarten all about, *really?* Friedrich Froebel was the German educator who "invented" kindergarten, literally meaning "child's garden." And that is exactly what a *good* kindergarten is: a vital place for kids to grow, carefully tended by knowledgeable expert gardeners (educators) who water and fertilize young minds to blossom into eager and ready lifelong learners.

Five- and six-year-olds are busy, curious little people. It takes a skilled teacher to run a kindergarten classroom with finesse. Culturally diverse and enriched programs take into account all of the strengths, interests, needs, and cultural backgrounds of students. These curriculums offer a variety of experiences that are educational, fun, and interesting.

Besides the intellectual development (basic scientific and mathematic concepts such as problem-solving and prediction, reading and writing basics such as letter recognition and handling books), kindergartners are working on social and emotional development (sharing, cooperating, collaborating, rule following); physical development (climbing, skipping, hopping, holding pencils, manipulating puzzles and other items requiring fine motor skill); and . . . language development.

Notice I mention language *development*? Kindergarteners are not expected to be finished developing language. *It is still in progress.* Don't despair if your kindergartener's grammar and articulation are not perfect. The good news is the teacher will infuse the day with speech- and language-rich opportunities. Teachers explain unfamiliar words and actively introduce new ones through projects and assignments. Your child will soak it up. Plus, the teacher will engage her students in what they are doing and thinking. Your little learner will continue to develop language skills through problem-solving and idea sharing.

Is Your Child Ready for Kindergarten?

As a parent, you are going to grapple with this question as your "baby" gets closer to "K-Day." You are especially concerned because your child has CAS, but may also have some other concerns: difficulties with social skills, distractibility (*sometimes* associated with CAS), and decreased verbal skills. It's an individual—and difficult—decision to make, to say the least. Here's what I recommend:

- Look into your state's requirements for admission to kindergarten, as they all vary.
- Consider talking with your child's SLP the summer before kindergarten to get his or her honest and professional opinion.
- If there are concerns, try some summer interventions—additional private speech therapy or working on phonics, sequencing, distractibility, etc.
- Consider seeing an occupational therapist (OT), who can better address some of the other concerns not completely associated with CAS. Seek out social skills classes that may be offered through a private speech clinic, or ask for recommendations from your child's pediatrician.
- Try "beefing up" your child's social skills by role-playing potential social encounters at home: "How do you ask a question in the classroom? Let's practice!" or "Do you know how to sit at circle time? Let's try it out here at home."

Who Are the People in Your School? Seeking Out Allies

Remember that *Sesame Street* jingle "Who are the people in your neighborhood. . . the people that you meet each day"? Well, there are a variety of faces you will soon need to become acquainted with. Who are they?

- **Principal:** The principal is the head administrator of the school (sometimes called the "headmaster"). Typically a principal will have advanced educational degrees (MEd or EdD) and experience as a teacher. Make sure you introduce yourself to the principal—better yet if you're on a first-name basis. Otherwise, just make sure he or she recognizes your face.

- **Vice Principal:** Not all schools have vice principals, but when they are present, they often are responsible for handling disciplinary issues, as well as for serving as the principal's second-in-command.

- **Administrative Assistant/Principal's Secretary:** This individual has a tremendous amount of knowledge of the inner workings of the school and perhaps the district as a whole. Get to know and appreciate this person—he or she is an invaluable resource.

- **Support Staff:** There may be additional secretaries, teacher's assistants , computer/IT personnel, custodians, and cafeteria staff in the building who assist with the day-to-day functioning of the school. Always be polite. You never know when you (or your child) may need their assistance.

- **Special Education Coordinator:** This individual often does assessments, recommends classroom assignments for students with special needs, and generally coordinates all of the educational needs of a child with an IEP. The role may be filled by your child's teacher, a therapist, or other school staff.

- **Classroom Teacher:** He or she teaches your child according to the district's approved curriculum, makes observations, keeps records, and evaluates your child's progress.

- **Classroom Aide:** Often classrooms have an aide or paraeducator who assists the teacher. Assistance may include helping a child use scissors, complete ADLs (activities of daily living—bathroom, wash hands, zippers, eating, etc.), stay on task, or follow directions. A classroom aide is a support staff member who works within the classroom.

- **Speech-Language Pathologist (SLP):** Your child with CAS will most likely have a school-based SLP who ensures she is able to communicate appropriately in the classroom. This individual may provide group therapy, individual therapy, or run a weekly speech group for all students. She may be your child's case coordinator, if she is not receiving special services in a classroom. The SLP, your child's teacher, or the special education coordinator will lead the IEP meeting.

- **Occupational Therapist (OT):** Your child may or may not have an OT. If she does, it's likely to help her improve her motor planning skills and participate in classroom activities/academics that require fine motor skills. OTs also assess a child's sensory needs and self-help skills. In a school setting, OTs only work with children on deficits that *directly affect their ability to make progress at school*, so they don't work on skills such as toothbrushing, which are not used at school, but can help with skills such as zipping, as children need to put on their jackets to participate in recess.

- **Physical Therapist (PT):** Unless your child with CAS has additional concerns and diagnoses, it's unlikely she'll have a PT. If she does, then your PT is likely to help your child improve gross motor skills such as sitting or walking that are needed at school. As with OT, in a school setting, PT is only provided if a child's deficit *directly affects her ability to make progress at school*, so the PT wouldn't work with your child on bike riding or the like.

- **Social Worker or Counselor:** Most schools have a social worker/counselor or a psychologist, at least on a part-time basis. Some have both. Their job is to make sure students have someone they can talk to if they need it. The social worker can help with bullies, teacher-student conflicts, emotions and concerns, and mediation skills. Some may have special groups for kids coping with parents' divorce, or for help with socialization and peer interaction.

- **Psychologist (PhD):** Like a social worker, a school psychologist may be the trusted individual kids can go to if they just need to talk about a problem or a concern. A school psychologist also works with academic research, testing, and evaluation of cognitive skills (e.g., IQ tests). He or she may assist students with career placement and college entrance preparation (in high school). In many larger school districts, there is just one psychologist assigned to a cluster of schools, and most students have little to no direct interaction with him or her.

- **School Nurse:** The school nurse is usually an R.N. and administers prescribed medication, mends boo-boos, completes screenings, and maintains health and medical records. He or she may participate in health education, especially in upper grade levels.

- **Bus Driver:** You will see the driver every day. Get to know him or her. Offer a smile and a "thanks" for the important job they do each day: assuring your child's safe travels to and from school. Your school's buses may or may not be equipped with seat belts. There are safety harnesses available for preschoolers. Make sure to specify on the IEP that your child requires a seat belt or harness. Likewise, you'll want to specify when or if you are comfortable removing that safety parameter. In our case, Kate felt like it was "too babyish" to be in a safety harness (car seat) when she was in kindergarten. The driver told me, "Well, it's on her IEP. If you want it changed, you have to talk to the school." See the box below on riding the bus to school.

- **Bus Aide:** See the box below on riding the bus to school.
- **Transportation Office/Supervisor:** Make sure you have the phone number to this office in a handy location. Don't call him or her every time the bus is five minutes late, but do call if your family is going out of town during the school year or your child is very ill and won't be riding the bus for several days. Other reasons to call: your child no longer needs to ride in a restraint system (reached a weight/height requirement), you have concerns about the bus driver, you have concerns about the kids on the bus, or your contact number is changing.

Your Child on the Bus

The idea of your child riding a bus may frighten you or make you jump for joy. Likely, you're somewhere in the middle. On the one hand, it's nice not to have to do the drop-off and pickup every day, especially if you have younger kids at home. On the other, you could quickly morph into a high-maintenance worrywart following behind the bus to ensure its safe arrival at your child's school.

Bus drivers are required by law to follow a standardized set of safety rules and guidelines. Get a copy of your school district's school bus safety policy and consider adding a few transportation and safety goals to your child's IEP.

Bus drivers hold a commercial driver's license (CDL), and must have demonstrated their skills to drive a school bus and have passed a knowledge test. They must be able to read and speak English well enough to prepare daily or weekly reports. Generally, bus drivers are at least twenty years of age, but many employers prefer them to be twenty-four years old or older.

Your school transportation department might request your preschool child's height and weight measurements to ensure she is placed in the proper safety restraint. They will tell you about the route, the bus number, who your child's driver will be, and if there is an aide. (There often is an aide who greets the children at the door and helps with their belongings and gets them buckled in properly. Our aide even sang songs with the kids!)

Since your child has limited verbal communication, you worry. Of course you do. Teach her to say a few things like "Wait!" or "I'm Here!" or something of that nature. Make sure she has proper identification on or in her backpack, as described below.

There are a lot of friendly and familiar school faces ready to greet your child when she gets off the bus. Teachers, classroom aides, SLPs, and even the principal may be involved in ushering kids to their classrooms.

Riding the bus helps your child prepare for her school day (giving her a buffer between the transition of home and school), provides some downtime on the way home, and even encourages the socialization that's so important to incorporate into her day.

Homeschooling Your Child

Some parents choose to homeschool their children for various reasons. The choice is ultimately up to you. Here's a list of potential benefits to homeschooling your child with CAS:

- consistency,
- flexibility,
- ability to teach coping skills with academics,
- less academic peer pressure,
- no chance your child can be bullied or made fun of,
- ability to incorporate speech practice into lessons,
- ability to use a more hands-on learning approach,
- ability to let your child pursue individual interests,
- ability to spend extra time on a weakness area without the added pressure of keeping the rest of the class engaged.

Of course, homeschooling is not for every parent or child. It requires a huge time commitment from parents, not to mention organizational and time management skills, patience, and creativity.

A few possible downsides to homeschooling your child with CAS:

- Your child may not get the socialization and communication practice with other children so desperately needed.
- Your child benefits only from the observation and perspective of one involved school personnel (the homeschooling parent/teacher), as opposed to many at the school level.
- Your child may lack age-appropriate language models, and you may not recognize all of your child's delays if there aren't typically developing children to compare against.

Preparing Your Child for the First Day

Start early, but not *too* early, in prepping your child for school. Be sure to drive by the school ahead of time. Point it out and get excited about the place where your child will be learning and playing. Then, a week or so later, pack a picnic and head over for lunch and some time on the playground. Your child will remember that you were there with her, so when she is playing with classmates, it won't seem so unfamiliar. Teach her how to ask others to join her in play (see bullet points below).

The building may be big and potentially confusing. Be sure to go to orientation and show your child around. Remind her that she will never be walking around the school without a teacher or parent. Take photos of your child with her teacher and the classroom and some common areas of the school (ask first). Print them out and present them to her in a little photo book. Study the photos and talk about them together. Have her carry the photo book in her backpack to look at on the bus.

Speaking of which, if your child will be riding the bus, calm those fears, too, but be careful not to create new ones. Kids often worry that they will get on the wrong bus or that they won't make it home. Assure her that teachers will make sure she gets on the right bus and you will meet her at the bus stop. Kids who ride the bus are often better prepared to start the school day than if Mom and Dad do the drop-off. Why? It gives kids a chance to be introspective and prepare in their own way. It also lessens the separation anxiety from you.

A final tip is to go to the local library and check out some books on going to school. Read those books periodically in the days leading up to the first day.

Other ways to prepare:

■ **Describe the school-day routines** (get a copy of the schedule from the teacher). Discuss what happens first; where her cubby is located; the bathroom, snack, and lunch routines; and going-home procedures. Answer any questions your child may have. This helps prevent any surprises.

■ **If your school has such an event, make sure you attend the "sneak peek day" with your child before classes start.** Get to know people who may be able to help your child and point them out to your child. "If you ever need help being understood, look for this nice lady at the front desk. She will help you."

■ **Practice saying these feel-good confidence boosters:**

  • "I know you can do this!"

  • "I trust you will do well at school."

  • "You are very important to me."

  • "I will always love and care for you."

  • "If you want to talk, I will listen."

  • My youngest daughter liked this one: "Parents always come back [for pickup]."

■ **Make your own Social Story about a child going to school for the first time.** It's simple. Take photos or draw pictures (or have your child draw them) and then write a brief sentence on each page about what's happening in the picture. Page one might go like this: "This is Kate. Today is her first day of school." Page two: "She is going to kindergarten. Hooray!" Go through general steps and feelings. The book should be no more than ten pages.

■ **Address special concerns of kids with CAS.** Practice saying the teacher's name several weeks before school starts (or as soon as you know it). Depending on your child's verbal skills, you can teach her how to ask others to join her in play, "I'm Aaliyah. Want to play?" Or offer a variation. The more you model statements like these, the more equipped your child will be to try them on her own.

- **Remind your child about safety identification.** By the time children reach kindergarten, it is important they know—and are able to recite—their parents' names (first and last), their address, and telephone number. In fact, many kids are unable to do this, simply because they haven't been taught. However, your child with CAS is different in that she *can't* do it. For your child's safety, consider writing her name on the inside of her clothing, or sew on labels, attach a label to her shoelaces, create a necklace she wears, or use some other identification system. Folks will need to know who your child is and how to get hold of parents in an emergency. Teach your child how and where this special identification is if a "safe" adult inquires. See "Recommendations for Further Reading and Resources" at the end of this chapter.

- **Talk to your child about "strangers."** You don't want your child's personal identification broadcast to the world. Keep it as discreet as you can. Remind your child to only ask adults with a school name tag for help, or other individuals you specifically list and describe. Schools these days are carefully monitored, but there is always the potential someone with less-than-noble intentions is lurking around.

- **Together, create a special "'Twas the night before school" tradition for your family.** How about a family night at the ice cream stand or a back-to-school bonfire with marshmallows?

- **Plan a special way to say goodbye the morning of the big day.** Will you walk her to the bus stop? Drive her? Decorate the car with balloons? For other mornings, your goodbye ritual should be simple, yet meaningful for her. A quick hug and kiss and a reminder that you will be there when she gets home from school may be all she needs.

- Once your little sweetie is established in her school and has found activities—and friends—she likes, **have a playdate with some of her new peers.** Invite her parents and siblings, too!

Preparing Yourself

And now a piece of advice for parents: ease your fears by taking control of the things you can control. Did you read that right? *Worry about what you can control, not what you can't.* Sure, make some calls to the school if you have to, but chances are, school staff know what they are doing. Make a list of all the things your child has learned to do in the past—independently. Kids are pretty amazing and resilient creatures, and going to school is just another event. If you make a big deal out of it, your child will fear that school is scarier than it really is. So, have fun with the idea that your little one is going off to school and let that fun shine. Do you adore the fall clothes and shoes or maybe the smell of fresh vinyl school supplies? Make a date to take your child shopping for the essentials. She'll pick up on your excitement and feel good about the process.

On the other hand, it's perfectly normal to feel sad that your "baby" is growing up. Saying goodbye will get easier every time. It's also perfectly OK to be excited or relieved.

One more tip, parents: slow down. The days leading up to the first day of school can get hectic. There are last-minute forms to fill out, meetings to attend, school supplies to gather, and fall schedules to arrange. Kids feel this pressure too. They are fueled by your anxiety level, which may mean they rev up their own activity, resulting in problematic behaviors. Talk less, stretch out and play, sip lemonade, and hit the pool one last time.

Teaching Your Child's Teachers about CAS

Do you wonder what you should tell your child's teacher about CAS? Not all teachers have specific knowledge on *all* special needs. Kate's preschool teacher admitted that she didn't know much about CAS, but she was very willing to learn. She knew it had something to do with verbal skills, but that was about it.

It helped a little to give Kate's teacher the scientific explanation: "It's a motor-neurological communication disorder in which she knows what she wants to say, but just can't quite get it out." What really helped was when I said, "It's like being totally exhausted and not able to carry on a conversation." She got it then. I further explained that Kate had to work really hard to have even a *simple* conversation.

Rhonda Banford gives this explanation to parents, and you may be able to relate to it as well: "Can you wiggle your ears without touching them? Most folks say no. I then tell them that my mother can. When I ask her how, she shrugs and just says, 'the same way I wiggle my fingers. I don't have to think about it.' I go on to tell these parents that there is no way I would know what muscles to access or even how to activate them. I know what I want to do, but I just can't figure out how. That's how CAS is—these kids know what they want to say, but they can't figure out how to make their muscles move."

Other explanations from parents you may consider adapting:

- "You know that feeling of being tongue-tied, or having a thought on the tip of your tongue? Well, that's how Luna feels most of the time."

- "Ask someone how their day was, and then tell them they can't use their words to tell you. That is what my little man faces every day," says the mother of Drew in Frankfort, Illinois.

- "Aidan has a speech disorder called childhood apraxia of speech. He knows what he wants to say but has trouble coordinating his mouth to say the words," says one Naperville, Illinois, mom.

What's a Parent to Do?

Meet with the teacher as early in the year as possible and share with her specific information about CAS and how it affects your child. You might be able to find suitable letter-to-the-teacher templates via an internet search. Try keywords like "Letter to my child's teacher about CAS." You can tailor these to your own needs. The Apraxia Kids website has some free brochures about CAS written with a layperson in mind. Currently, you may request up to five of these to be mailed to you for no additional fee. Consider including one with the letter you give your child's teacher. Make it into a little "welcome to my child packet." Including a brief description of your child is very helpful too. It doesn't have to be long or fancy, just a few bullet points like this:

- Fun, outgoing child
- Likes art and being creative
- Excels at gross motor activities
- Slow to warm up, may need to be drawn into social situations with specific questions or play
- Loves books

Of course, your descriptions may be different than mine! Now, if every parent would do something like this for their child's teachers (whether or not they have CAS), it would take a lot of guesswork out of teacher's lives.

Here are some more *tips on putting together an information packet for the teacher:*

- *Give her a book (like this one).* I Want to be Your Friend by Angela Baublitz tells the story of a young girl who wants to make friends at school; it's hard because she has CAS. Both *Speaking of Apraxia* and *I Want to be Your Friend* (available at apraxia-kids.org) make excellent classroom or lending library donations.

- *Provide a list of easy ideas* that may help with speech in the classroom (refer to chapter 9).

- *Remind the teacher that* while your child sometimes has a hard time communicating or takes longer than usual to respond to a question, *CAS does not affect her intelligence.* She does not have to simplify things for your child if she only has CAS. (Of course, if she has Down syndrome, fragile X syndrome, or another disability in addition to CAS, you will want to advise her about any learning difficulties related to the other condition.)

- *Offer to create a communication notebook or worksheet that can be shared between parent and teacher.* We made worksheets on the computer. I printed out five of them Sunday night and placed them in Kate's backpack for Monday morning. Each day her teacher filled them out and sent them home with Kate. This daily report gave me some talking points for Kate about her day.

- **Be open and available.** In *The Complete Guide to Special Education*, authors Linda Wilmshurst and Alan Brue recommend that you keep your ears and mind open to new ideas from your child's teacher or other school professionals. They typically have lots of experience and ideas in working with kids that just might help yours. If you disagree with a suggestion, ask more about it. It's part of their job to explain it.

- **Consider communicating some tidbits from the home front.** For example, "Papa and Nana visited this past weekend," or "Kate really enjoys the unit on frogs—ask her what we saw last night when we visited the neighborhood pond." This gives your child's teacher something to ask her about and encourages verbalization on things that are meaningful to your child's homelife.

Parents Ask

What was on your parent/teacher communication sheet?

I wanted to know who the helper was for the day, what the snack was (did she eat it? How much?), where she played, who she played with, what songs were sung, what book was read, what the SLP did, how verbal Kate was (I used a ten-point scale), and finally—what she struggled with that day (couldn't sit still during circle time, got frustrated when she practiced writing her name).

It sounds like a lot of writing for a busy teacher, but you can streamline your worksheet by providing "circle me" options. For example, the "who did she play with?" question can be a copy of the class list. The teacher can just circle the names of the students your child played with. Do the same for snacks—that is, if they have the same snacks available day after day. Or, you could say something like, "Snack today was __. Kate ate: all / some / none." You get the idea.

Tips for Teachers

If you are a teacher reading this, then hooray! I applaud your efforts to learn more about the students in your classroom. I'd like to give you a few pointers for teaching a child with CAS.

- Read the child's IEP.

- If parents challenge your knowledge, make special requests, or argue for a special IEP meeting, remind them that you are on their side, and please don't take it personally. As parents, we just want the very best for our children and we might get a little passionate about it.

- Communicate privately with parents and never in front of other classmates, unless it is to give really good praise that will make your student feel proud. These kids often know they can't communicate as effectively as their peers, and they may feel a bit defensive about it. Help build their self-esteem in every opportunity you can find.

- Give parents advice and insight you learned from teaching their child. For example, "Kate did a great job teaching another student about how we sit at Circle Time. She loves to be in the helper role." Parents love to hear praise and stories about their child doing well.

- You may need to do a bit more preteaching when working with a child with CAS. Let her hear and practice vocabulary words ahead of time (send them home with a letter to parents indicating the upcoming unit).

- You might need to work a bit harder to engage a student with CAS in group activities. Don't take it personally if she doesn't respond right away (or at all); just keep trying.

- Each day is a new beginning. What this student struggled with yesterday could be a nonissue today.

- Be sure you give your students with CAS lots of praise. It helps their confidence level and self-esteem. While you're at it, praise her parents too. They're working really hard all day, every day, to help their child.

- Relate something special about your student to the parents. I can't tell you how happy it made me to receive an out-of-the-blue email from our teacher saying something like, "Kate was really cute today in class when she started dancing and singing 'Mama Mia!'" Small accomplishments mean a lot to us parents.

- Respond to parents in one way or another (phone, email, "I'll get back to you later"), even if you don't have an answer. Parents do not like feeling like they have been forgotten.

- Realize that we all get burned out. Parents need encouragement and motivation, just like teachers. If we can encourage one another, then all the better!

Parent Involvement at School

There's one more aspect of sending your child to school we should cover before jumping into the nitty-gritty school stuff like speech, IEPs, and all of those other intimidating acronyms. It's called parent involvement. Studies show that when parents are *actively* involved in their child's education, their children enjoy school more, get better grades, and don't have as many behavior problems. Many studies have found that parent involvement is the number one predictor of a child who does well in school. (It's actually *not* natural intelligence, parent education, or income, although those things do *influence* a child's education.)

What's a Parent to Do?

It may be as simple as helping your child with her science fair project, brainstorming with her on her essay about "what I did this summer," or reading aloud from a book each night before bed. You don't have to be the fundraiser chairperson or run the school carnival to make a difference. Little things add up. Volunteer in the media center once every couple of weeks, go to literacy night, attend parent-teacher conferences, or work the book fair for a two-hour window. We're all busy, and yes, you have your plate especially full with speech therapy and CAS-related issues, but if you are serious about your child's education, I urge you to get out there.

Here are a couple of points to remember:

- *Your involvement boosts teacher morale.* When they see you take an active role at school, teachers feel more valued.

- *Kids develop better social skills*—and isn't that the whole idea, especially with our children with CAS?

- *Kids feel supported and valued when Mom and Dad walk into their place of learning.* This develops kids' sense of self, thus increasing self-esteem and confidence.

- *You will benefit too.* It's empowering to be a part of your child's school day. You'll feel more confident about the layout of the building, plus gain confidence in parenting and educating your children.

For more information and helpful tips, see www.SchoolFamily.com.

Should You Volunteer in the Classroom?

Volunteering in the classroom offers a fantastic opportunity to see what happens there each day—a plus for parents of kids who aren't able to communicate well. But Dr. Linda Wilmshurst and Dr. Alan Brue point out a few caveats in *The Complete Guide to Special Education*. First, keep in mind that young kids who have a tendency to be clingy may find your classroom volunteering difficult. Your child may expect to see you in the classroom every day, even if it's only Wednesdays that you volunteer. Also, she may not perform as well because she just wants to play with you. Know your child and anticipate how she may react if you choose to volunteer.

Talking about CAS with Your Child's Classmates

Here's another way to increase your involvement at school, help your child, her classmates, and her teacher at the same time: go into your child's classroom and give a little lesson or presentation about CAS. This works well for kids in pre-K through third grade. It's easy, and you don't have to be a professional speaker to do it.

First, check with the teacher and agree on a good day and time. Plan to be in the classroom for twenty minutes or so. With the teacher's permission (run it by your child too), get started with your lesson plan.

You might consider reading *My Brother Is Very Special* by Amy Glorosio-May, or *I Want to Be Your Friend* by Angela Baublitz. Both authors share intimate feelings and experiences their own children with CAS experienced as a way to teach other kids about the disorder. You might consider typing up a brief letter for kids to take home to their parents explaining why you were in the classroom and what you told their children.

The lesson might focus on strengths and weaknesses: "What are you good at? What are you not so good at?" Make a list on the whiteboard. Turn the table and ask students about their classmates: "What is _____ (say a child's name) good at?" They may or may not know.

Introduce yourself as your child's parent. Explain that you are in school because you want to tell them what your child is good at and not so good at. Start with the good. Make a list. See if others can identify what she does well. Your goal is to let others see your sweetie as any other "regular" kid. Then tell them about CAS. Start with a simple explanation: "She knows what she wants to say; it just takes her longer. She has a hard time getting the words out."

Let them ask questions. Do your best to answer. You might even ask if the kids have noticed your child leaving the classroom at times (to attend speech therapy). Do they know why? Ask if the kids have any ideas on how they can make your child's day easier. I'll bet they do. The CAS lesson you present to the classroom will hit on things like diversity, sensitivity, and self-esteem.

Give yourself a pat on the back! It takes guts to go into the school and talk with a bunch of kids—your child's peers—about something so close and personal to you.

Speech at School

Make friends with your child's SLP at school. Get her contact information and use it. Consider giving her handouts and a letter (see "Teaching Your Teacher about CAS"). Let her know you are available to answer any questions about your child. Even though her expertise is in speech and language problems, she may not be an expert in CAS. Like your child's classroom teacher, she may need a little tutorial in "CAS 101."

Your child's IEP (see next section) will indicate how many minutes a week your child is to receive speech services. It may be 60 to 90 minutes—maybe as many as 120. If you get more than 60, consider yourself lucky. I know it sounds kind of puny, compared to the hour or more your child might receive two to three times a week in a private setting—if you have excellent insurance or can afford to pay out of pocket—but school is a different beast.

The school is only required to provide a free appropriate public education (FAPE) to children who qualify for special education either under the Individuals with Disabilities Education Act (IDEA) or Section 504 of the Rehabilitation Act. The laws state that school districts must provide access to general education and special education services. What that really means is "adequate" and not "superior" or even "really good." Schools really have no nationwide standard they need to meet, so that puts the responsibility back into parents' hands. We have to be proactive and advocate for services that are in our child's best interests.

Although your child may not receive as many minutes of therapy as you would like, bear in mind that CAS is best remediated in numerous short sessions, rather than one long session. Short, intensive sessions five days a week are preferable to one long session once a week. The key is "intensive," meaning lots of intervention and plenty of practice.

What you probably want is for the SLP to come into the classroom, smile and wink at your little precious, and motion for her to come to speech room for a full hour of uninterrupted therapy. Unfortunately, that's probably not going to happen. Your child will miss way too much classroom instruction (days in preschool and kindergarten are short—an hour away is too long), and the SLP has a busy caseload.

A more likely scenario is this: your child and one to three peers (also with speech or language delays or disorders) are pulled out to work with each other and the school SLP for twenty minutes or so. That counts toward your child's sixty minutes a week. The SLP may also come into the classroom a couple of times a week to work with the class as a whole. She might do some verbal exercises and games, read a book, or something of that nature. This counts too. In addition, your child *may* receive a private session with the SLP if she has goals that can't be worked on in a group.

With that in mind, it's not a bad idea to give the school SLP a few tips to help ensure his or her time with your child is as productive as possible. Type out a list of things that you and your private SLP have done that have been particularly successful. Sign any releases between the school and your child's speech clinic so the two can communicate. Please ask, if they don't offer. Our private SLP even made a school visit. Ask if yours will too (but expect to pay for his or her time). The goal is to get both professionals working on the same skills, or at least working together so that skills your child is learning from one professional are easily transferred to the other setting.

Our school SLP did a fabulous job of keeping parents in the loop. She sent home a weekly speech newsletter describing what she did with the kids (even if it was whole group work) and suggestions to try at home. Since Kate received some pull-out therapy, too, she'd often email me with progress Kate made, or she'd tell me directly when she saw me pass through the school. Ask your school SLP what communication style would work best for her. Perhaps you can develop a special speech notebook that you can pass back and forth. Or perhaps you can designate a weekly or daily email schedule.

As you get more comfortable (and confident) with your child's school day and SLP, the communication may dwindle. Don't take it personally. At the same time, your child's speech is improving, and she just might be able to share some of these things with you on her own!

> **Kids Cope**
>
> Now that Jude is in kindergarten [and no longer the speech-intensive preschool], he wonders why he is sometimes singled out to go to speech therapy. I think it kind of bothers him.
>
> What can you tell your child when she asks why she needs speech and the other kids don't? Remember, no two individuals are alike, but addressing this question is often a good place to start when discussing differences. Keep the conversation positive and as light-hearted as you can: "We all have things we need extra help with. It's no big deal." If you know the other children in the class, you may be able to use them as an example: "Layla gets reading help and Oliver needs extra help with math."
>
> You may be interested in reading Ronda Wojcicki's book, *Speech Class Rules,* with your child (best suited for ages four to eight). It's a great picture book designed by a school-based SLP in which speech therapy is introduced in a kid-friendly, "cool" manner.

Individualized Education Programs (IEPs)

I've been alluding to IEPs throughout the book, but what exactly *is* one? In short, it is a written plan developed for all children who qualify for special services under the Individuals with Disabilities Education Act. The IEP, individualized education program, is a document that is developed collaboratively with parents and school personnel during an IEP meeting.

An IEP is a legally binding contract between the school and your family. It lays out the following:

1. What your child's qualifying disability is (in this case, a speech-language disorder called CAS, though there may be other diagnoses you child is also struggling with)

2. Your child's present level of functioning (this is where assessment results are reported—are her receptive language skills at the level of a six-year-old, while her expressive language skills are at the level of a four-year-old?)

3. What goals the IEP team thinks she should work on, over and above what is covered in the regular school curriculum (e.g., goals to expand the length of her sentences, to respond to another child's greetings, or to bring her reading skills up to grade level)

4. What special services ("related services") your child needs to help her reach those goals and make progress in the general education curriculum (speech therapy, occupational therapy, social skills group, special education instruction).

5. What accommodations and modifications your child needs to access the general education curriculum (see below for definitions)

6. Where your child should receive the instruction and therapy she needs (e.g., receive all instruction and therapy in the classroom or perhaps leave the classroom for thirty minutes a week for speech therapy)

7. How the school will monitor your child's progress and report that progress to you

8. Who will provide your child's speech therapy. You may assume it's the school SLP, but that may not always be the case. Look at your IEP very closely. If it reads that speech services should be provided by the SLP, then that is a good thing (legally correct and legitimate). But, if your child's IEP says speech language services will be provided by "SLP/Staff," "SPED staff," "special education staff," or a "speech language assistant," then your child may receive speech therapy from an untrained, unlicensed individual, including substitutes, aides, and paraprofessionals or any staff member willing to do speech therapy. They are not licensed by your state Department of Education, nor are they accredited by the American Speech-Language-Hearing Association (ASHA). *Make sure your child's IEP states that speech therapy will be provided by an SLP*.

Note that the school is not required to develop an IEP that will "cure" your child's CAS as quickly as possible or provide everything you think would help her reach her potential. *The school is only required to provide services to allow your child to "access the curriculum" and not to perfect his or her speech.*

Whoa . . . what does this mean, exactly? It means that schools want our kids with CAS to be able to participate in classroom activities and to be intelligible. And if your child has another disability in addition to CAS, the IEP will address how your child can "access the curriculum" and participate in classroom activities despite that disability—but not necessarily to "fix" every single difficulty your child has.

You will be able to propose goals that will help your child "access the curriculum" and participate in classroom activities. A possible preschool goal may be:

■ Mack will use a variety of means to request items and actions within the classroom (e.g., signs, single words, two-word phrases, pictures, and gestures) 80% of the time, which will be evidenced in quarterly data charting by teacher observation.

Another might be:

■ Amelia will verbally approximate the words for common objects within the classroom setting, *without* a model, in the following categories: food, classroom items, toys, and actions with 80% accuracy. This will be measured by teacher observation and charted quarterly.

You will also get to discuss and agree upon the *least restrictive environment (LRE)* for your child. This means the classroom setting where she will have the maximum contact with typically developing children while still being able to meet her individual goals. For most children with CAS in kindergarten and above, the LRE is the regular education classroom in the neighborhood school. For children with additional disabilities such as learning disabilities, Down syndrome, or autism, the LRE may be a combination of the regular classroom plus time spent in a resource room to receive extra help in some academic areas.

Every year, you will be expected to attend a new IEP meeting to discuss your child's progress and all the issues above, setting new goals, rehashing the LRE, determining what related services and accommodations and modifications are needed. You can also request an IEP meeting at any time you think one is needed.

"My oldest son was diagnosed with CAS just prior to his third birthday. He just turned five and is speaking at an appropriate level. Early intervention and our local school district did wonders for him."

—Jennifer

Parents Ask

What's the difference between an accommodation and a modification?

An **accommodation** is a change to the way information is presented to your child, the way your child responds to that information, or the setting where your child learns. Accommodations do not affect the content of what she is learning. For example, if your child can't respond orally to the teacher's questions about days of the week, she might be given written words or pictures to use to respond instead. If your child is having trouble paying attention, she might be seated near the teacher's desk.

A **modification** is a change in the content of what a child is learning. For example, if a child struggles with spelling, she might be given simpler or fewer words to learn each week than the rest of the class.

Prior Written Notice

Before we get into the heart of IEPs, I'd like to introduce you to a term you will likely encounter on your special education journey: ***prior written notice (PWN)***. Perhaps one of the most overlooked, yet most powerful, tools for parents to keep in their special needs toolbox, PWN requires the school district to provide written notice and explanation of any changes or proposed changes to your child's IEP. The school is also required to send you prior written notice before your child's very first IEP meeting—which will probably happen either when she is transitioning out of early intervention, or when you ask for her to be evaluated before kindergarten.

These changes can include your child's identification as a student who requires special services, notice of evaluation techniques to be used, or changes in educational placement within the school, among others that may affect the school's ability to provide FAPE (free, appropriate public education).

PWN forces educators to stop, think, and write things down. It's assurance that their decision is not just an off-the-cuff remark or decision. It's formal and meaningful.

PWN provides a written history of exchanges between the school and family, resulting in a paper trail that cannot be denied.

PWN works both ways. Parents can and should write down (typing is best) their questions, complaints, compliments, and requests for clarification regarding their child's education. If you want a written response, start with a written request. This is exactly why you should know about and use PWN. Of course, you'll want to keep copies of all of the written communication between you and the school, no matter how big or small the comment (more on organizing later in this chapter).

Parents Share

What Happened with Our Family

It was the beginning of the school year for Kate (early October). She had completed one full year of special education with an IEP plus extended school year (more on that at the end of the chapter). She had just started in a new classroom with a new teacher. Her new SLP stopped me in the hall one day and told me that she thought Kate was doing great and needed a reassessment.

I was dumbfounded. We had just started private OT, and Kate was continuing with private speech therapy as well. I didn't like what the school SLP was implying—that Kate no longer qualified for services. The SLP continued: "I'll be sending home a letter with Kate indicating what we are seeing and have you sign it." Ah ha—that's the PWN! I could have not signed it. But after reading the large packet of information, I agreed that Kate probably did need a reassessment. After all, she had made a lot of progress. After Kate was reevaluated and the treatment team met with us, Kate's IEP was discontinued, as were her speech services at school. I was told that Kate's CAS was not affecting her progress in the classroom, though her speech was certainly not perfect. We celebrated the accomplishment with dinner out and a scooter Kate had been eyeing for some time. Yes, the event was filled with uncertainty and emotion, but in the long run, I'm glad things worked out as they did.

Advice about IEP Meetings

Be Prepared! Do not just show up for your child's IEP meeting expecting the school staff to handle the whole process without any input from you. Here are some guidelines to prepare for the meeting:

1. Ask to see any assessment results the school has done at least three days *before* the meeting and then review the report so you have a good picture of your child's strengths and needs. When parents have time to review results ahead of time, it strengthens the collaboration between home and school.

2. Ask your child's teacher(s) and therapist(s) to tell you what goals they are considering for your child. (In some school systems staff often go into the meeting with preliminary goals already written. If so, ask to see these preliminary goals before the meeting.)

3. If the teachers and SLPs haven't written goals about something you think is important, try your hand at writing your own. Share them with the staff before the meeting if you want their input; if not, bring them to the meeting to discuss.

4. If you think your child needs a service she isn't presently receiving, or needs more of a service she is receiving, try to articulate *why* so you can advocate for the service at the meeting. Has she fallen further behind? Failed to achieve goals set for her in the last IEP? Been bullied or become depressed due to her speech difficulties?

5. If this isn't your child's first IEP, read and review IEP progress reports, which should be sent home throughout the school year. Keep them and compare them. Bring them to the meeting, along with other supporting documents (more later on organizing the boatload of paper you have for your child).

6. Educate yourself about the IEP process. Research IEPs from trusted sources. You may want to spend some time reading *From Emotions to Advocacy* by lawyers Pam and Pete Wright. Together they have written several books, built websites, and have a blog. Their website is professional and helpful. Check it out at www.wrightslaw.com.

Do Some Classroom Reconnaissance

One parent I was in contact with while writing this book suggested that one of the best things a parent of a child with an IEP can do is to spend an entire school day observing their child at school. Look at academics, socialization, scheduling, distractions, and how your child fits into the microcosm of school—or doesn't. Then make sure all your concerns about your child's functioning in any of these areas are addressed during the IEP meeting. It's a big commitment for a busy parent to make—but doing so just may help your child's school experience.

Pointers on Writing and Evaluating Goals

An IEP is a blueprint for your child's education. It should address your child's needs related to academics and social and physical functioning. Deficits (such as in speech) are identified and annual goals are made by breaking things down into manageable steps.

Please note: ***Only goals that the SLP or teacher feels the child can achieve in a year are written.*** If the child achieves the goals sooner, new ones can be written. It is better to write achievable goals than goals your child has little chance of meeting, no matter how much you may want your child to accomplish them.

As a parent, your job is to **make sure goals are meaningful to your child, specific, measurable, and attainable.** Merely writing "Kate will learn to talk" as a goal is laughable. What will you do to get her to talk? How much talking is enough? How will we know if she's making progress? What incentives are in place to push her along? Granted, you probably won't see this written as a formal goal in an IEP, but you get the gist. A better goal is something along these lines:

> "Mason will imitate 1- to 2-word phrases to comment within the classroom." (If Mason needs a certain type of prompt or model to imitate phrases, that should be noted in the goal as well.)

Teachers are pros at "catching students being good," and often praise or otherwise acknowledge their attempts. It may work for some children to receive a sticker or token as an incentive and as a way to measure their own progress. Be sure you mention to your child's teacher what may help with your little one's progress.

Remember to separate the forest from the trees. The IEP is the trees; your child's overall education is the forest. If you are trying to figure out goals to propose for your child, ask yourself: Where do you want your child to be educationally? Work backward from that ending point and get those skills in the IEP as early as possible.

Make sure goals are addressing meaningful progress. Your little one may be talking more. But is she speaking *well*? How are her pragmatics and social skills? Can she effectively ask others to join her in play? Does she know how to stand up for herself?

Pointers on Participating in the IEP Meeting

It's overwhelming and intimidating to go into the meeting with a bunch of folks from the school staring at you. **Bring support**—your spouse, a friend, and/or your private SLP. Going with an unbiased person can help you make sense of the information later. Sometimes our emotions run high during these meetings which can cloud memory. This person might be able to point out key factors from the meeting without the emotional investment you have for your child. You might consider asking a third-party special-needs advocate to go with you (they usually charge for their services). Bottom line: don't go alone.

Be familiar with the terminology you may hear. If the teachers and staff use words you don't know like "benchmark," "goal-directed," "outcome-oriented results," ask what these things mean in plain English.

Don't just sit there. You are an active member of the IEP team. Did someone say something you don't agree with? Speak up—diplomatically, of course. You don't want to wait until after the meeting to express concerns.

Bring up everything that concerns you about your child's education and progress with communication skills. That includes such topics as making friends and preventing meltdowns.

When I was practicing nursing, it was drilled into us, "if it wasn't charted, it wasn't done." Even if I knew I did something for a patient, but I didn't chart it in the medical record, there was no proof I had done it. *Get it in writing*, no matter how small the request, idea, or action seems.

Make sure you have read all of the forms and double-checked all of the boxes. If the boxes are prechecked that you agree with something that you don't (sometimes they are), then *don't sign* it. Add a note to the existing paperwork stating that you don't agree. Sign or initial it. Then ask for a clean copy and set a date for another meeting in the near future.

Afterward, *give yourself a special treat.* Stop for ice cream on the way home or stop at a park for a little nature. While you're at it, consider giving your child an extra-special treat, too. After all, she's the one who really deserves recognition for a job well done.

Techy Tools to Help

IEPs are notorious for generating reams and reams of paper. If you're like me and don't want all of that stuff to keep track of, maybe an app is for you. The Tech Advocate has several suggested apps to consider: *IEP Goals and Objectives with Common Core State Standards*, *IEPS Action Tracker* mobile app, *Birdhouse*, and *Fastbridge*. You can learn more here: https://www.thetechedvocate.org/.

Transitioning out of Elementary School

If your child still needs an IEP when she is getting ready to transition out of elementary school, you will want to make sure everything in the document is up-to-date and ready to go from day one. Valle Dwight, a parent and disability writer, listed these pointers in her article "Getting Off to the Right Start: Ten Tips to Make Sure Your Child's IEP is Ready":

- *Meet early.* Meet with your preteen's team before school even starts so you can hash out the details of the IEP. Keep it casual, and remember, this meeting sets the tone for future conversations.

- *Talk to your child.* Ask, "What worked for you last year? What didn't? What changes would you like to see?"

- *Go to the pros.* Get to know other parents who have walked this road before. Parents of older kids can be a great resource, if you know where to find them. Start with your neighbors.

- *Make it stand out.* Make copies of the IEP on brightly colored paper for all of the teachers, even the P.E. teacher—emphasize how important it is to read it (you'd be surprised).

- *Check in.* Schedule a meeting a few weeks after school has started to chat with your child's homeroom teacher or school counselor. See if he or she has any questions about your child's IEP now that he or she has gotten to know her a bit. Explain how she learns best, offer to answer questions about CAS, and suggest ways to help. If a meeting is unrealistic, email is a great alternative way to reach all teachers that come in contact with your child during her day. This is also a springboard for continued conversations and a way for you, the parent, to document the interactions with staff.

Parents Ask

What about therapy during a public health emergency?

Children with IEPs continue to have rights to receive special education and related services during a public health emergency—unless *no* students in the school are receiving *any* education services. Your child may be required to receive services via remote learning. Specifics differ from school to school and state to state, so check to see how yours handles this.

In a remote learning environment, the SLP chooses activities to target your child's specific speech and language goals. They will likely be posted to a shared electronic platform, such as Google Classroom or FlipGrid, or Microsoft Teams. The SLP can also provide individual or group therapy sessions online, as explained in chapter 7.

Allison, the mother of Nate, age ten, says that during the Covid-19 pandemic in 2020, "Our SLP sent activities over as a link through Google Classroom. I also purchased a simple phonics book. We picked one goal to focus on one or two times a week."

Maureen Wilson, MS, CCC-SLP, says this about independent speech therapy work: "Often, we ask parents to send along a follow-up piece confirming the activity is complete." For Nate, that follow-up involved making videos of his speech work and sending it to the SLP. Nate also completed Boom Cards, digital interactive task cards (see chapter 7). His mother, Allison, says, "The Boom Cards are very 'hands-on,' and this really accelerated Nate's progress. Plus, he enjoyed sending videos to the SLP. After just a few weeks, I could see and hear the improvements in his speech."

"Remember, an IEP is a legally binding document entitling your child to the services described within it," says Maureen Wilson. "And we love seeing these videos."

You can find information about states' responsibilities to provide special education services on the IDEA website of the US Department of Education (go to https://sites.ed.gov/idea/ and search for "public health emergency"). Also check out "Coronavirus (COVID-19) Closed My School" on the Wrightslaw site: https://www.wrightslaw.com/info/fape.svcs.covid-19.htm.

- *Make a plan.* Set up a communication system with the teacher(s) or counselor to stay in touch with daily concerns, homework, behavioral issues, or social skills. Many folks do this over email or with a daily log filled out by the teachers that work with your child. You can make a habit of checking in the first of the month, or if a problem or change should occur. Whatever you decide, stick to it. Be persistent but polite!

As mentioned earlier, Kate did have an IEP in elementary school, but it was mostly for her ADHD—not CAS. She needed additional support in organizing her thoughts—especially in writing, double-checking math problems, and general check-ins from the special education teacher, whom she adored. Kate's transition to junior high was absolutely unremarkable. No IEP, no 504 plan. She flourished, finding passion in art, history, even writing. Her short story won first place in the district-wide mystery contest, and she was recommended for honors history. That might not be every child's path, but the point is, IEPs and 504 plans do help, and our children with CAS do improve.

Filing a Complaint about Your Child's IEP

Most teachers and SLPs want the best for your child, but they have to work within parameters you may not know about. Be sure to ask why they are proposing something if you do not agree with it.

If you still don't agree with something the IEP team has done, you do have the right to file a complaint. If services were decreased or changed in any way without your knowledge and you don't agree with the change in services, or if you disagree with where your child is receiving her services, then you absolutely have the right to address it. (Be aware, however, that in some states, IEP teams are allowed to make changes without the parent's permission—as long as it is not the first IEP.)

Here are the steps in filing a complaint:

- *Send a letter by certified mail or return receipt requested.* Better yet, hand deliver. To whom should you address your letter? That depends on what kind of complaint you are filing. If you are just not happy with a decision the school has made, then make sure it gets into the hands of the director of special education at the school district. If the school has broken a law, file a complaint with the state for noncompliance. To cover your bases, go ahead and send a copy to both the school and the state.

- *Find out your state's process.* Visit your state's Department of Education website, find a contact number, call them up, and ask about your state's mediation process or how to initiate a due process proceeding. The Wrightslaw website has some good information and articles on due process hearings: www.wrightslaw.com/info/dp.index.htm.

- *You may be required by your state to start with a mediation process.* You and the school staff will meet with a mediator (without lawyers) to present your sides of the issue, and the mediator will try to get you and the school to reach a compromise. Generally, it's the "nice" way to go, and hopefully you and the school can settle on a compromise.

- Otherwise, *you might have to go ahead with due process.* A due process hearing takes place in a courtroom with both sides using lawyers to present evidence, calling upon witnesses, etc. It can be extremely expensive and emotionally draining for parents. Each state has an advocate to guide you (the parent) through the process. They will help you understand the law and your rights.

- *The state will take procedural violations (violations of the right to FAPE and LRE) very seriously.*

- *You'll need to include evidence*—so review and include bits and pieces of your child's educational records, as well as speech therapy progress notes.

- *Check in periodically*—but don't be a pest—to make sure things are being monitored and implemented. You may have to do this as the due process case is underway; but continue to check in with your child's school after the case is over.

Parents Ask

Can an iPad or iPhone help my child with CAS?

Technology can be a blessing and a curse. But the parents I've heard from love the benefits an iPhone and iPad bring. One mom I know was so pleased the first time her son took his iPad to speech therapy and "read" an interactive story with his SLP. Another mother notes that the iPad was less frustrating for her son because the large size makes fewer demands on fine motor skills. Still another parent says that her son loves his iPad and was thrilled that an AAC specialist came to school to help find more apps for her son to use during peer play within the classroom.

As you explore the ever-growing world of technology, I urge you to look into a program called *TouchChat*, adapted for iPhone/iPad by Nancy Inman (creator of *WordPower* and *Picture WordPower*). Go to www.silver-kite.com/touchChat for more information.

One Place for Special Needs founder Dawn Villarreal has put together a comprehensive list of apps that may help your child with communication, among other concerns. It just may give you more information than you bargained for! Find it at: www.oneplaceforspecialneeds.com/main/library_special_needs_apps.html (link shared with permission from One Place for Special Needs).

Organizing School-Related Paperwork

There are mounds of papers and emails and all kinds of stuff you'll need to keep straight when your child is enrolled in school. Don't rely on your own brain to make sense of it all. What you need is a *system*. Don't put this off too long, like I did, or you'll really feel overwhelmed when you do get around to organizing your paperwork. Pick a system that you will use. You don't need anything cute or fancy.

Here are specific items I recommend you acquire, keeping in mind that you will need both an electronic and "real" file:

- a large three-ring binder, two- to three-inch size (my personal favorite)
- filing cabinet with carefully labeled hanging file folders
- an expanding file
- a word processing program on your computer

And here is how to organize paper and electronic documents within your files:

- Create a special folder for all letters and correspondence specific to your child's CAS-related issues.
- Create a folder in your email account for your child's speech therapy emails (cc yourself so you always have a copy of what you send), and another folder for your child's school communications.
- Ask for your child's IEP to be emailed to you, and also ask for a paper copy. You can easily send the digital copy to private SLPs or access it if you misplace your hard copy.
- Put your system in an area where you will see it and use it. (What good is a really great filing system if you can't find it or have to climb into the crawl space to get to it?)

You'll soon be receiving lots of school-related documents—newsletters, progress reports, sample pieces of artwork or assignments. Some items don't require keeping. If you have decided to use the binder method, lightly mark each "savable" piece of paper that comes out of your child's backpack with the full date written in pencil. Pop the papers in the binder in chronological order. What's on the top page of the binder will be the oldest document and the bottom page will be the most recent, that way your binder reads like a book. You can look back on the binder as a way to measure progress.

Avoid using staples or page protectors; they just cause confusion and delay. Even dividers can slow things down. Instead you may want to use those nifty little page tabs that stick to paper (but can be removed easily) for pieces of paper you want ready access to (like the most recent IEP).

Avoid writing directly on the papers in your binder. Use a sticky note if you must. You never know when you'll need to make a photocopy or scan that document. You wouldn't want the name and number of the pizza place you ordered from last weekend to appear on a letter you are sending to your child's speech clinic, would you? Questions, comments, and thoughts you have about a particular document also go on the sticky note. Once you get answers to your questions, remove the sticky and move on.

Wrightslaw has some great suggestions for making your binder work for you. Head to their website, www.wrightslaw.com, or look for a copy of the Wrights' book *From Emotions to Advocacy.*

Parents Ask

Do you combine school and private speech into one binder?
That's up to you. I combined ours into one megabinder (that's where I used dividers) and dubbed it "Kate's School and Speech Binder." I kept everything in there, even the receipts from private therapy and EOBs from our insurance company. It cost little to nothing to create and maintain.

You may appreciate *An IEP Toolkit*, a binder system that can help you get all of your child's school papers organized. It can be downloaded for free at Parenting Chaos http://parentingchaos.com/iep-toolkit-for-parents/.

How Does Special Education Work in Private Schools?

Private schools vary in their ability and willingness to accommodate children with developmental or learning differences because—unlike public schools—they aren't given funds or guidelines from the state. They are also not required to provide a free and appropriate education in the least restrictive environment for children with disabilities, as public schools are required by IDEA to do.

Here are some things worth asking prospective private schools:

- Are there other students with learning/developmental differences?
- What special accommodations does the school currently provide? What other changes is the school willing and able to make to ensure the best learning environment for students with special needs?
- Is there a care team, tutoring team, or group of specialists available? If so, are their services included in tuition?

Keep in mind that *every* child in the US is entitled to receive any therapies/support services they are found eligible for. However, *where* those therapies are given can vary from district to district and state to state. Some public-school districts may be willing to send professionals to a private school, day care, or other educational facility to provide therapies. In this case, you will need to consider and discuss with teachers and administrators the impact of removing your child from her daily schedule at the private school to receive the services from the public school specialists. In many other instances, you need to take your child to a public school district facility to receive "itinerant" or "walk-in" services. (These services may be provided during normal school hours, or possibly after school. Often public school employees are restricted from entering any "faith-based" educational setting or from traveling outside district boundaries.)

Even if your child does not attend the public school for her main educational needs, she will need an IEP if you opt for her to receive *any* services through the public school.

Parents Share

Receiving Supports for CAS in Private School

"Since my daughter's pre-K program is both faith-based and outside our district boundaries, she receives itinerant services at one of the district's early childhood centers. If she continues to need speech therapy into kindergarten or beyond, her services will likely be given at an elementary school."—St. Louis mom of a daughter with CAS

"We went from a public school to a private Lutheran school. I was extremely worried about support in the classroom. The private school is working hard to accommodate children with special needs. We attended orientations, open houses, anything that would help familiarize [my son] with the school. The director of special services had us do a walk-through of Zach's day the day before classes began. That helped immensely."

—Mother of a son with CAS

School Is Hard

I wish I had better news, but studies have documented that there are relationships between early speech-language problems such as CAS and reading/writing difficulties. Researchers have proposed a few theories for this connection:

Theory #1: Kids who aren't making many sounds (or saying the ones they do have correctly) don't have a very good mental/visual representation of the sounds. Without this, they have a harder time developing the sound-letter correspondence that helps them sound out the words they are reading and writing.

If you believe this is the case for your child, I highly recommend the *Jolly Phonics* program for teaching sound-letter correspondence. It's systematic, sequential, research-based, and multisensory. The program incorporates a body movement piece to learning the sounds as well, which we know by now is huge for these little people with CAS. If your school doesn't use Jolly Phonics, consider buying their products for home use at www.jollylearning.co.uk.

Theory #2: Kids who have speech-language disorders have difficulty reading and understanding symbols (think about it: letters are a pretty abstract way of representing sounds). This could translate into having a difficulty with manipulating numbers and symbols in math as well.

Theory #3: Kids with CAS have "differently wired" brains. Speech is one area of the brain that is affected, but other areas that contribute to learning might also be affected. This theory might explain why not all kids with CAS have the same strengths and needs: their wires are all connected uniquely.

Reading, (W)riting, and 'Rithmetic: The Three Rs

Reading might be hard for your little one with CAS. In fact, it's hard for *many* kids. The next chapter offers specific suggestions for helping your child at home and school. But since this chapter is on school, and reading is a big part of school, I want to give you a brief overview.

In the US, kids are typically taught to read in kindergarten or first grade. You can start preparing your preschooler by reading to her every day, teaching her the alphabet and the sounds the letters make, and playing word and rhyming games. The idea is to get her comfortable with written language. Your child with CAS may also have difficulty reading aloud because she skips the smaller, supportive words in a sentence—it's as though the brain doesn't register them. (*If your child has fallen significantly behind in literacy skills, it's time to look for a reading specialist. Chapter 12 covers specific reading programs.*)

One resource to consider is the Riggs Institute of Reading (www.riggsinst.org), along with Jolly Phonics, mentioned in the section above.

Handwriting is hard for kids with CAS too. No surprise there. Letter recognition, plus the motor planning piece of getting from brain to hand to paper, can be difficult due to the underlying neuromotor issues of CAS. What can you do? Ask if the program *Handwriting Without Tears* is an option for your child at school. It may need to be done with a school-based OT (if there is one and your child qualifies). Otherwise, you can work with her on handwriting at home with some of the *Handwriting Without Tears* products you can find online at www.hwtears.com. The earlier you correct those handwriting mistakes, the better off your child will be as academics get more and more challenging. Note: some children with CAS also have limb apraxia, which makes the motor aspects of writing very challenging.

Math: Kids with CAS *may* have difficulty with mathematics because symbols (numbers) represent even more abstract concepts. Plus, it involves a whole new set of vocabulary words such as "addition," "subtraction," and "factor." In addition, it's hard to draw from real-life experiences when the language of math is so obtuse (another math word)!

Kids with CAS may also have difficulty sequencing (even following two-step directions from parents and teachers can be tricky). That makes it especially hard to assess and apply problem-solving skills to mathematical problems.

Note that not everyone believes that CAS can be intertwined with math difficulties. According to Rhonda Banford, MAT, CCC-SLP, "In my experience, most kids with CAS do not have trouble with math; in fact it may be a strength!" Remember, each child with CAS is unique.

Please don't get the wrong idea about CAS. There is no reason to expect that CAS will *most definitely* cause difficulty with math! I present this to you so you can keep a watchful eye on your child's mathematical skills.

What's a Parent to Do?

There are lots of programs and curricula for teaching math. Find out what your school uses. In the meantime, consider looking at *Everyday Math* for some inspiration and tips: www.everydaymathonline.com. Its educational philosophy is to teach students to play with numbers, suggesting a variety of methods of correctly solving the problem, hoping your child will pick the option that "fits" her best. You might prefer another program called *Math U See* (www.mathusee.com), which was developed by a former math teacher for homeschooling and special ed students. It's clear, systematic, and multisensory.

Another simple thing you can do at home to help your child with sequencing is to practice digit spans (remembering increasingly long series of numbers) for "fun." What you do is this: say, "I am thinking of three numbers: 3 . . . 6 . . . 4. Do you "see" those numbers in your mind?" Then quiz your child on what those numbers were. Did she remember? Did she get them in the correct order (sequence)? You may need to start with just two numbers. Once your child can repeat the sequence correctly, add in another digit. Mix it up. Have your child quiz you.

Why bother? It's a fun game to do while you pass the time on a family walk, in a waiting room, or in the car. Plus, if you practice while you and your child are doing something active (jumping on the trampoline, walking, swinging), you activate that vestibular system that is so important in speech development *and* sneak in a little exercise. Your child will be none the wiser. Well, actually she *will* be: she'll be able to sequence better!

If your child is struggling with mathematical concepts, you may be interested in checking out this sampling of research-based programs:

- *Addition the Fun Way* (www.citycreek.com): The creators want kids to know that "math is a story to be told," so there are books, music, and even coloring pages in which addition facts are worked into stories intended to make those facts easier to learn.

- *Everyday Math* (www.everydaymathonline.com): Their educational philosophy is to teach students to play with numbers, suggesting a variety of methods of correctly solving the problem, hoping your child will pick the option that "fits" her best.

- *Math Graphic Organizers:* There are numerous graphic organizers that help school-age students learn to visualize mathematical concepts and word problems. I like understood.org, an online resource designed for children with learning and attention issues. It's not just for math, but encompasses feelings and friends, family, and community, and other academic subjects. If you search for "Jenn Osen Foss," you will find several free downloadable graphic organizers. You may also be interested in looking at programs on www.luminosity.com and Nintendo DS's Big Brain Academy.

- *Memorize in Minutes* (www.multiplication.com): This program combines stories, activities, and pictures to make math meaningful and memorable.

- *Right Start Math* (www.rightstartmath.com): Joan Cotter developed the double-sided AL abacus and then, with her husband, developed a curriculum combining visual, auditory, and kinesthetic systems to "help children understand, apply, and enjoy mathematics."

- *Touch Math Method* (www.touchmath.com) is the leading multisensory mathematical program. It involves teaching kids to recognize "touch points" on each number, adding up to the value of the number (e.g., 5 touch points on the number 5). Then children are taught to touch each touch point on the numbers that they are adding, subtracting, etc.

Parents Ask

What about standardized testing at school?

Your child will undoubtedly complete some testing in school—at the state level—which evaluates kids at their school as compared to other schools in the state and across the nation. Tests that may be used include the *Stanford Achievement Test, Iowa Test of Basic Skills*, and tests developed by your state to comply with the Every Student Succeeds Act (ESSA). You can ask for accommodations to assist your little one on these tests. For example, some students qualify for extra time, or a smaller, less distracting test-taking setting, or someone to read the tests aloud to them. Talk with the IEP team and see what might be appropriate for your child.

Helping Your Child Focus at School

You may think you've got it all figured out as far as the school system goes. Sure, you've had some bumps along the road, but you've worked them out. Then a curve ball is thrown at you: you're told your child can't focus at school. She can't keep herself organized either. Her backpack is a junky mess, and homework somehow never makes it in on time. The fancy word for all of this is "executive functioning" difficulties.

CAS does not cause a child to have executive functioning problems. A child can have both CAS and executive functioning concerns, but they are not the same thing!

If your child's teacher is concerned about executive functioning, here are some suggestions:

- *Consider requesting an extra set of textbooks for home reference.* You will be glad you have them, especially if your child gets into the middle elementary grades (3–6) and continues to struggle with CAS and executive functioning skills.

- *Consider asking for some accommodations at school.* Perhaps worksheets that have been streamlined with less clutter and unnecessary visuals would be helpful?

- *You may want to get an occupational therapist (OT) onboard*, either through the school district or privately. OTs often have a wealth of ideas for helping kids regain focus. Perhaps your child just needs some oral stimulation (like chewing gum) to help her focus at school. Weighted vests, background music, even a reminder note or image taped to the desktop might help.

- If you are truly concerned about your child's executive functioning skills, please refer to Appendix A, which covers executive functioning disorders (like ADHD) in more detail. *Again, just because your child has CAS, it does not necessarily mean she also has ADHD!*

Learning Styles

No two people learn in the exact same way. Often, kids with CAS do best when using their hands and bodies to learn, but not always. For example, kids with CAS *do* benefit from visual cues because auditory cues in speech are not enough; and sometimes just a visual cue is all that's needed without adding a tactile one.

The chart on pages 251 to 253 lists some ways to incorporate early academic skills into a fun-filled at-home activity. You can use these ideas for any child, not just a child with CAS. All of these suggestions work well with more physical learners.

Early Academics the Fun Way

Pre-reading	Writing	Math	Listening & Focus
Create a reading fort and use it for a cozy reading spot (e.g., drape a blanket over some kitchen chairs, or find another suitable area at home).	Work on writing something together, especially something "real" like a grocery list or your daily to-do list. Ask her to practice saying sounds, words, or phrases that go together with food.	Search the house for common everyday shapes like circles, squares, triangles. Throw in some tough ones like ovals and cylinders. Ask her to tell you about them or say them in unison with you.	Play Simon Says or Follow the Leader. See if she can imitate your words or gestures.
Host a book-related party or playdate. Ask her to help select the book or theme.	Use sand, glitter, glue, or Play-Doh to spell out words and names like your own and your child's.	Play with puzzles, blocks, and other building-type materials.	When you are cooking, read the recipe out loud and have your child gather the ingredients. Practice saying the word, sounds, and phrases that go with that ingredient.
Make an ABC poster or collage with your child. Ask her to practice saying the sounds, words, and phrases on your collage.	Keep a travel log of your outings and errands—stash it in the car and talk about it on longer trips, or allow your child to look at it while you drive. Ask her to talk about it with you.	Allow your child to experiment with volume of liquids and solids—think: kitchen sink with plastic measuring devices or mixing a batch of trail mix using different quantities of nuts, raisins, or other ingredients.	Suggest your child go on a household mission for you. Tell her 2–3 items you need help gathering. Have her repeat the item's name as she looks, if she is able.

Attend story time at the library or bookstore and then talk about it.	Buy a composition book for your child and encourage her to keep a journal. Even better if the book has blank spaces for drawing pictures and lines for practicing handwriting, just like at school. Talk with her about what she draws.	Look for patterns at home, or develop your own. Have your child say the pattern back to you: "Plate, bowl, plate, bowl."	At the grocery store, ask her to get very specific items to put in the cart: for example, three yellow apples; the big blue bottle of detergent on the middle shelf; the tub of butter with the red lid.
Act out a scene from a book.	Get a whiteboard and assorted colored markers for a family message board. Encourage your child to write her own messages, even if they are picture messages.	Stage a math game at snack time. "You have five grapes. If I take away two, how many do you have?"	Ask your child to help you remember a list of objects for a shopping errand, e.g., "paint, sandpaper, and string."
Use or make finger puppets to go along with a story.	Encourage your child to talk about and make a list of her daily activities.	Categorize and talk about small objects such as rocks or hair clips.	Ask your child to repeat a series of numbers you make up. Start with the numbers in your address.

Serve a meal from a book such as *Green Eggs and Ham.* It is fun to connect books with everyday experiences. Target words like "ham," "green," "Sam," as well as work on rhyming activities, which can be challenging for kids with CAS.	Have your child practice writing and saying her name *at the same time.*	On the road, add up all the school buses (or other type/color of vehicle) you see on an outing. "I saw one bus on ___ road plus (+) two buses on ___ road, which equals (=) three buses total." See if your child can say a target word/phrase from this activity ("bus," "two," etc.).	Say a variety of words you know your child knows (e.g., "hi," "park," "sun"). Tell her to remember them; you'll ask again what they were. Quiz her on those words in a few minutes.

What about IQ Tests?

I don't really believe in formal IQ testing. The tests can be frustrating and can unfairly affect how children are perceived and others' expectations for them. Plus, they tell parents of kids with special needs little about their child's long-term learning potential. Why? These tests are scored according to the mean performance of children *without* disabilities.

Some school districts insist on administering standardized IQ tests when children are being evaluated for special education eligibility under IDEA. If your school insists on an IQ test such as the WISC (Wechsler Intelligence Scale for Children) or the Stanford-Binet, then you may be stuck with it. Just keep in mind that the results may not be an accurate assessment of your child's abilities now or in the future. The standardized IQ tests that schools routinely use are *language-based* and require children to respond verbally to the test questions. That's a tall order for any child and obviously "penalizes" kids with CAS from the start.

One option is to pursue IQ testing through an independent evaluation, not from your school district. An independent evaluator—child psychologist or neurodevelopmental psychologist—is unbiased and won't make specific recommendations that could affect your child's education. He or she will give you a long list of ideas you can take to the school. A thorough psychological evaluation will cost several thousand dollars, though, so make sure the results are worth the financial investment to you.

Any IQ test given to a child with CAS should not require a verbal response. Consider the TONI-4 (Test of Nonverbal Intelligence, for kids six years and older), the Leiter-R (Leiter International Performance Scale-Revised, best for ages two to twenty), or the UNIT (Universal Nonverbal Intelligence Test, ages five to seventeen, or K-12).

Extended School Year (ESY)

Just because you made it through the school year successfully doesn't mean you and your child are home free when it comes to summer vacation. IDEA mandates an extended school year (ESY) for students at risk of losing their skills during the summer break. It is *not* a program to increase skills or develop new ones. Participation in ESY is determined by IEP team recommendations. It must be documented in the IEP. Generally, these programs are held for a portion of the summer—maybe six weeks of half-day reinforcement.

The Wrightslaw website (www.wrightslaw.com) discusses a federal court case (Ruesch v. Fountain) in which eligibility standards for ESY were determined. These factors are what the educational team should consider when determining whether or not students are eligible for ESY:

1. **Regression and Recoupment:** Is the child likely to lose critical skills or fail to recover them in a reasonable time after a break from school (regression in life skills)? If you want your child to be included in the ESY program for the upcoming summer, start making a list of any and all regression noted over breaks from school, especially the longer ones like winter and spring break. Give specific examples if you can (e.g., forgot how to say "st" blends).

2. **Degree of Progress toward IEP Goals and Objectives:** The team needs to look at how the child has progressed on established goals. If the child is having difficulty keeping up, then ESY may be necessary.

3. **Emerging Skills with Possible Breakthrough:** If formal instruction is halted or interrupted, will there be a problem, regression, or future difficulty, especially with significant skills like reading?

4. **Interfering Behavior:** Does the child have ritualistic or self-injurious behavior (SIB) that may prevent her from benefitting from her IEP? If so, ESY may be appropriate.

5. **Nature and Severity of Disability:** Does the child's educational team believe that the nature and severity of the disability warrant summer services?

6. **Special Circumstances:** Are there situations beyond your control that interfere with your child's ability to participate and benefit from special educational services?

Your child may *not* qualify for services, and that may be a good thing. It means she is progressing and doesn't need reinforcement over the summer—at least, according to your IEP team. To learn more about the requirements for ESY, open your favorite search engine and type in: *your state name + extended school year regulations + students with disabilities.*

The results will help you understand how your state generally handles ESY. Keep in mind that CAS occurs along a continuum of severity, and kids with moderate to severe CAS will be most likely to qualify. If you feel that your child really would benefit from ESY, be prepared to state your case and come with supporting documents to any meeting held to discuss the issue.

Our Experience with ESY

When Kate didn't qualify for ESY one summer, I was a bit perplexed. She had in the past, and it had been good for her. Her teacher and the rest of the team pointed out that she could receive ESY if I really wanted her to, but I needed to be aware that she would probably be the highest functioning kid in the program. At the time, I thought that might not be such a bad idea. Perhaps it would boost her confidence, as she might be able to help other kids. After more thought, we ultimately decided against it. If Kate was to continue to progress in speech and social communication, she needed to be surrounded by typically developing peers to serve as motivation. See Appendix C for some guidance on selecting a summer program for your child.

Grade Retention (Being "Held Back")

A big concern for parents who have a child with CAS is when and whether a child should be retained in a particular grade level. Hopefully, you will receive guidance from school staff if things get to this point. You will also have some IEP meetings where you can discuss the pros and cons. Here are some questions to discuss:

- What do you (and school staff) believe will change in the school environment that will address your child's needs, if she is retained?

- What changes in your child do you think will improve her progress (social maturity, academic maturity, better communication)?

- What, if anything, are you and the teachers willing to do to assure that things move along at the "right" pace if she spends another year in the same grade?

- How would it affect your child socially and emotionally to stay behind while her classmates are promoted?

Many school systems actively discourage grade retention, even if children have very significant disabilities. So, even if *you* believe your child would benefit from being held back, you may not be able to convince the school to do so.

I should mention here that not all kids with CAS continue to struggle with speech and language issues for their entire school years. CAS is a *dynamic* (ever-changing) disorder specific to the *childhood* years (up to about age ten). Sure, remnants of speech/

language issues may resurface at times, but for the most part, if you are aggressive in getting your child the appropriate speech therapy and she doesn't have another disability that affects communication, your child will be a typically speaking tween, teen, and adult.

Say That Again?! Chapter Summary

We've certainly covered *a lot* in this chapter! From what to look for in a school to navigating an IEP, this chapter was loaded with tips, ideas, and resources I hope you have found helpful. Of course, I can't possibly include everything you may want or need to know about your child's education. I urge you to do more research on your own so that you can develop an individualized educational guidebook for your child. Remember, each individual is unique, and we all learn in our own unique ways. I'll leave you with this favorite quote from William G. Spade:

"All students can learn and succeed, but not all on the same day in the same way."

Recommended Resources

- Your child may like these books: **First Day Jitters** by Julie Danneberg (Charlesbridge Publishing, Whispering Coyote Press, 2000) and *JoJo's First Day Jitters*, based on the Fancy Nancy series by Jane O'Connor (Harper Festival, 2012).

- Other children's titles that may help ease the separation and anxiety are: **It's O.K.— Tom's First Day of School** by Beth Robbins (DK Publishers, 2001) and **What to Expect at Preschool** by Heidi Murkoff and Laura Rader (Harper Festival, 2003).

- If your child is a fan of the Maisy storybook character, then look for **Maisy Goes to Preschool** by Lucy Cousins (Candlewick, 2010). The simple illustrations and text are a sure way to comfort and pave the road to a successful first preschool experience. And if you're a fan of *Daniel Tiger's Neighborhood*, you might like **Daniel Goes to School** by Becky Friedman (Simon Spotlight, 2014).

- Read **Choosing a School for a Child with Special Needs** by Ruth Birnbaum (Jessica Kingsley Publishers, 2009).

- You may find the **Homeschooling Catalog Site** helpful for additional resources, even if you choose *not* to homeschool: www.rainbowresource.com.

- When seeking **safety awareness** for your child, check out Safe Kids Worldwide (www.safekids.org), an organization dedicated to preventing injuries in children. The website offers many tips on school, home, and pedestrian safety.

- Rich Weinfeld and Michelle Davis present an excellent and information-packed resource on what you can do to help influence your child's education in **Special Needs Advocacy and Resource Book: What You Can Do Now to Help Advocate for Your Exceptional Child's Education** (Prufrock Press, 2008).

- ***The Complete Guide to Special Education: Expert Advice on Evaluations, IEPs, and Helping Kids Succeed*** (Jossey-Bass, print version 2010, Kindle version, 2018) by Linda Wilmshurst and Alan W. Brue. Includes tools, checklists, forms, and advice.

- ***The Complete IEP Guide, 7th edition*** by Lawrence Siegal (Nolo, 2011) explains the intricacies of IEPs in a clear, concise way; includes sample documents and pull-out forms.

- The All About Adolescent Literacy website has some tips for ***summer programs***. It indicates it's for grades 4–12, but you can glean something for younger kids too: www.adlit.org.

- ***The Discovery Center in the UK*** offers a website by Professor Amanda Kirby that may provide you with valuable advice and ideas for home and school: www.box-ofideas.org.

- ***Kiz Club*** has some great free resources for parents and educators alike. Check them out at www.kizclub.com.

- Looking for ***parenting articles and fun ideas for home and school?*** Check out www.PreschoolRock.com.

- Check out ***Dr. Jean Feldman's website:*** www.drjean.org. She has been in education for five decades and is the author of many books on topics ranging from transitions and games to self-esteem.

- Older kids with more homework and projects to keep track of may benefit from a ***graphic organizer*** such as those available at www.eduplace.com.

- ***Lost at School: Why Our Kids with Behavioral Challenges are Falling Through the Cracks and How We Can Help Them*** by Ross W. Greene (Scribner, 2014) is a nice resource for kids with social, emotional, and behavioral challenges who lack important thinking skills.

- ***Taming the Recess Jungle: Socially Simplifying Recess for Students with Autism and Related Disorders*** by Carol Gray (Future Horizons Press, 1993). Although this book focuses on kids with autism, it can be applied to just about any child. It discusses transitions at school, how to ask the "right" questions, and how to help a child who may have delays in social skills.

- ***The Anti-Bullying and Teasing Book for Preschool Classrooms*** by Barbara Sprung and Merle Froschl with Dr. Blythe Hinitz (Gryphon House, 2005) is a nice resource for teachers, but may also give parents a peek inside teasing within the classroom.

- ***The Mislabeled Child: How Understanding Your Child's Unique Learning Style Can Open the Doors to Success*** by Brock Eide and Fernette Eide (Hyperion, 2006) may be useful if your child has additional concerns with vision, attention, sensory processing, or autism.

- *Different Learners: Identifying, Preventing, and Treating Your Child's Learning Problems* by Jane Healy (Simon and Schuster, 2010) discusses current changes in education, the case of difference vs. disability, and genetics vs. environment, all with a research-based background. She writes in a straightforward, no-nonsense way busy parents can appreciate.

- Laura E. Berk's *Awakening Children's Minds: How Parents and Teachers Can Make a Difference* (Oxford University Press, 2004) includes lots of good information on why and how children talk to themselves, learning in classrooms, and helping children with deficits and disabilities.

Chapter 12

Phonological Awareness

Learning to Read and Reading to Learn

You know the scene well: your child is sitting comfortably on his bed or the floor and "reading" a favorite book. I remember walking into Kate's room one day when she was about four and seeing her in a similar situation. I proudly remarked, "Oh look—you're reading!" In her broken language, she replied, "No read, Mom. Look pictures." I was doubly proud. My little girl with CAS was able to string a few words together to tell me she wasn't really reading, but instead just looking at the pictures.

This wasn't the *first* time she was able to say more than a few words together, but she was doing several things I was especially pleased about: looking at books and studying their pictures (a prereading skill), giving herself (and me) some down-time, exhibiting insight (she knew she wasn't really reading), *and* communicating that insight to me. Of course, I had to give her a hug, lie down on the floor, and join her for a little mother-daughter book reading.

In fact, what we were doing is what researchers and educators refer to as strengthening "children's memory for words and literacy." Think back to your own childhood for a moment. I am sure you have some favorite books and literary characters that really stand out in your mind. Who and what were they? What did you love about them? Do you remember where you read those books? Who read with—and to—you? Do you look back on those memories with fondness and delight?

Those memories shaped your childhood, and they continue to shape your adult reading life as well. Other memories may not have been as positive when it came to reading: the material selected may have been too challenging, you may have been bored, or perhaps the story lacked imagination.

- An overview of why kids with CAS tend to have more difficulty learning to read—and how you can help
- Research-based interventions to give you specific ideas for enhancing literacy at home
- Suggested books to read with your child and activities to promote excellence in reading
- Handwriting and story-writing tips and ideas to help your eager young reader write on her own, without frustration
- Potential reading concerns for children with CAS, and when to bring in a specialist
- Types of home-based reading programs available

Essential Terminology

Before we get started, let's get a couple of definitions out of the way.

Phonological Awareness: This term was first used in research in the late 1970s and early 1980s. Simply put, phonological awareness is an individual's awareness of the sound structure of spoken words. It includes the ability to recognize rhyming words and to identify how many syllables there are in a given word. Without the awareness of sounds in words, it's much harder to learn to read and spell correctly. That's why phonological awareness is an important and reliable predictor of later reading ability.

Phonemic Awareness: A phoneme is the smallest unit of sound that influences the meaning of a word, regardless of how that unit of sound is spelled. For example, the phoneme that we perceive as a /k/ sound can be written as a *k* in *kitten* or a *c* in *cat*. Phonemic awareness refers to the ability to hear and manipulate the individual sounds in a word (for instance, to recognize that *soup* and *sand* begin with the same letter, or to understand that if you take the /n/ sound and put it in the front of the /o/ sound, you get *no*. When we speak, listeners aren't saying to themselves, "I hear the /r/ and the /i/ sound." Instead, they blend those sounds into syllables; they have learned to *perceive* the phonemes in spoken language. In the English language, there are 41 phonemes (25 consonants and 16 vowels).

Phonemic awareness is a component of phonological awareness. They are not the same thing, but the terms are often used interchangeably.

Children with CAS and Reading

Many kids with CAS *probably* will have *some* difficulty with phonological and phonemic awareness—the precursor skills that are needed to understand how speech sounds translate into written words on the page. In addition, kids who have persistent speech difficulties such as CAS and no other medical cause are at risk for related literary problems such as trouble with reading comprehension (Puranik et al., 2008; Stackhouse, 1997). Some more proof:

- The following researchers concluded that a "large percentage" of kids with a speech pathology diagnosis in the preschool and kindergarten years encounter difficulty learning to read and spell: Lewis, Freebairn & Taylor (2002), Catts, Fey, Zhang & Tomblin (2001), Larrivee & Catts (1999), Johnson et al. (1999), and Boudreau & Hedberg (1999).

- Kids with speech-language impairment are four to five times more likely to have reading difficulties than children from the general population (Catts et al., 2001).

- Of course, not all kids with spoken language impairment have reading problems. But those with a *specific speech-language impairment* just may.

- In addition, 50 to 70 percent of kids with spoken language impairment will have some academic difficulty in their school years, according to several researchers (Felsenfeld, Broen & McGrue, 1994; Shriberg, Tomblin & McSweeny, 1999).

I don't mean to be all gloom and doom, but I do want you to have the facts. There is a light at the end of the tunnel. Follow along in this chapter and I think you'll start to see it.

Why Is Reading Difficult for Children with CAS?

We touched on this a little bit in the last chapter. To review, here are some reasons kids with CAS may have problems related to reading:

- Kids who aren't making sounds accurately (or at all) may have a decreased visual representation of what letters look and sound like.

- Kids with speech-language disorders may have a distorted sense of what the symbols (letters) represent (letters are symbols that represent words).

- Kids with CAS may have "differently wired" brains, affecting the way they read, learn, and interpret information.

- Children affected with CAS may have a decreased ability to consistently sound out words.

When it comes to *reading comprehension*, researchers say that some kids with CAS and other learning difficulties lack the appropriate strategies to allow them to understand what they just read. It's complicated. Reading requires a lot: decoding words, visualization, understanding context, activating prior knowledge, a large vocabulary, and the ability to comprehend what you just read. For example, if a kid has to work really hard to understand (decode) the words on the page, then he may not have much energy left over for defining an unfamiliar word.

In a 2009 study published in the International Journal of Communication Disorders, researchers compared the phonological awareness and reading development in twelve children with CAS and twelve kids with speech sound disorder (SSD), and twelve other "typically developing" kids. They found that kids with CAS had "inferior" phonological awareness (letter-sound knowledge and decoding) compared to the ISD and typically developing kids.

Parents Ask

What's a Speech Sound Disorder (SSD)?
Kids with SSD have a high degree of variability (40 percent or more of the time) in the way they say a word. For example, a child with SSD may say "rabbit" like "wabbit" one time, "babbit" another, and even "tabbit" another. See the similarity it shares with CAS?

This research supports that **kids with CAS need early intervention in learning to read**—because they are more likely to develop a reading delay. It also suggests that parents, caregivers, and educators really ought to help these kids develop underlying skills to improve their written and spoken language, as well as the words they read on a page. Of course, we can't base a claim on just one research study with twelve kids with CAS. Just know that there is a correlation and this study helps support that correlation.

What Can We Do?

Research can give us great insights, but we need some clear guidelines as to *what to do right now* with our struggling kiddos. If your child is at reading age (five to eight years old) then I *know* you are curious as to what to do. What do you consider to be realistic for a "typical" child at this age? How might you need to adjust your expectations for *your* child?

Here are a few suggestions to stoke the fire:

- Aim for your child with CAS to read at a level that is appropriate for him, even if he is considered "behind" when compared to his peers.
- Improve his sequencing skills in activities of daily living (ADLs) such as getting dressed, bathing, and eating. After all, being able to follow steps in a sequence has a lot to do with reading.
- Work with your child to make sure he is up to speed on prereading skills such as rhyming words, alliteration, sound segmentation, and isolating sounds.
- Incorporate some of this preliteracy work into speech therapy, school, and home environments.

Spend a few moments jotting down your goals on your child's reading and writing life. Go ahead, dream a little. Now, brainstorm about how you can help your child with the resources you already have (consider time, effort, and your own special skills and talents, not just money, books, and tutor centers as resources).

Want to know what educators say the real goal is? The real goal is getting the child to break the code from sounds to letters (writing the correct letters that represent the correct sounds) and from hearing what is said to reading what is written (auditory to visual). I know, it sounds daunting. This next section will focus strictly on working with your child with CAS on reading.

Breaking the ABC Code—Reading with CAS

As discussed above, some researchers say that kids with CAS have difficulty understanding the abstract idea that letters represent words. Sometimes these kids don't even have a good visual of what a particular letter looks like. Finally, kids with CAS may have "differently wired" brains altogether and process information in a totally different way. That doesn't mean it's impossible for them to learn to read; it just means you need to take a different approach.

The approach that is most beneficial to all kids is simply this: read to them and read to them often. That's not all, of course—if you want to raise a reader, then you need to read yourself. And your kids need to *see* you reading for this monkey-see, monkey-do approach to work. I know you likely don't have the luxury of time to plop down with a great novel while your children quietly play at your feet. Here are some ideas:

Pick up something quick and easy that you can do within the eyeshot of little ones. Glance at the headlines, flip through a magazine, bring a book along to a waiting room, and establish a fifteen-minute reading time at home for everyone.

Beyond reading to your kids and setting a good example, there are two other winning strategies, according to Joy Stackhouse's text *Persisting Speech Difficulties in Children: Children's Speech and Literacy Difficulties*. Teach phonological awareness skills and add strong literacy skills (reading strategies) and then you've got a kid ready to learn to read.

Phonological Awareness + Reading Strategies = Ready to Read

How do you do that? Well, there are five specific learning abilities necessary for reading:

1. **Phonemic Awareness:** awareness of the individual sounds in a word (syllable knowledge, sound manipulation, onsets, and rhymes).
2. **Phonics:** sound-syllable correspondence, invented spellings.
3. **Text Comprehension:** ability to decode symbols and sounds, understand syntax (grammar), vocabulary, and semantics (word meanings).
4. **Vocabulary:** expressive, reading, and writing vocabulary.

5. **Fluency:** the ability to read a text smoothly and accurately, to be able to understand what one reads without having to stop and decode words.

Check out this chart to understand what this really means. The top of the chart depicts skills that are typically more advanced, while the bottom of the chart shows earlier literacy skills.

Building a Foundation for Reading

Learning Ability	What It Is	Example	What You Can Do	Check Progress
Phonemic Awareness	Knowing linguistic sounds. Having the ability to hear different sounds by the way letters are grouped together.	Knowing the difference between the /p/ and /b/ sounds in *pat* and *bat*; being able to distinguish between the /sh/ and /s/ in *show* and *sow*	Say, "Is *show* and *sow* the same word?" Ask your child to listen carefully as you emphasize the unique sounds. Can he tell you the difference?	Look at words in print that are similar in spelling— *mat, pat, cat, sat*— and ask if your child knows what's different and the same about them.
Phonics *(Not to be confused with phonetics, which is the range of possible sounds in languages, and not used in teaching and education-land)*	The *instruction* piece of building on kids' phonemic awareness. Knowing that letter symbols have sounds.	Knowing that when the sounds of /b/, /a/, /t/ are put together, they make *bat*.	Word-Slam! Sit with your child and with one hand say, "I have a /ba/ sound." With your other hand say, "I have an /at/ sound . . . put them together and you get *bat*!" Clap your hands together (with the different sounds "in" them) for a slamming sound.	Ask your child to do some word-slam activities with you. He may be able to make up some of his own. Accept it even if it is a made-up word.

Segmentation and Blending	Pulling apart and putting together different combinations of sounds and letters.	Think phonics in reverse. Knowing that the word *bat* can be broken down into /b/, /a/, /t/.	Cover part of a printed word and ask your child to sound out what he sees. In the word *jump*, you can cover up the /ump/ and have your child sound out the /j/ sound, add in /ump/, and make a word.	"Hey, look! Here's a *b*. Tell me what sound a *b* makes." Then ask, "If we add the *at* sound to the *b*, what word do we make? That's right— *bat!*"
Letter Identification	Knowing that the letter "names" of the letters in the alphabet correspond to symbols. There are also blends of two letters, called "digraphs" (*ch, sh, br, bl, fl,* etc.). Diphthongs are the vowel combinations, such as *ow, aw,* and *oy*.	You know that *a* and *s* have different names and sound different.	Talk about the letters whenever you see them. Environmental print on signs, stores, etc. (out and about in the community) is great for this.	Quiz your child when you see a letter on a coffee cup, at the newsstand, while driving. Ask, "What letter(s) do you see? I see an *m*—do you?"
Letter Sound Identification	Knowing what sound each of the letters in the alphabet makes.	Awareness that the letter *i* can sound like *i* in *pit* but sound different in *ice*.	Sing a little jingle with all of the different sounds one letter makes. "*E* makes the "ee" sound; it also goes like "eh." Now you say it!	Practice and listen carefully to your child!

Visual Discrimination	The ability to discriminate between letter shapes and words.	Being aware that *b*, *d*, and *p* are different, even though they kind of look the same. Also, recognizing that *h* and *z* are quite different because they appear so unalike in structure *and* sound.	Buy or make some alphabet flashcards and present two at a time. Ask, "Are these two letters the same?" You're just looking for "yes" or "no" at this point. Do the same with other print material.	Kids love to see parents make mistakes! So have your child play teacher and see if he can trip you up. Let him win sometimes!
Print Awareness	Knowing that printed text has meaning.	When your child brings you something and says, "What does this say?"	Read whatever your child brings you. "Oh, that's an invitation to Luna's party. It says . . ."	Show your child a book or scratch paper with words on it. Ask, "What does this say?" Let him elaborate or talk nonsense. He will make a connection to print, regardless.
Book Knowledge	Knowing how a book "works" (cover, spine, how to hold, left-to-right orientation, page-turning).	Hold a book by first looking at the cover. Talk about what you see. Turn the book page by page and follow from left to right.	Show your child the parts of a book. "Here is the spine. It tells us the title and author's name." Point to the words as you read them. Let your child use a finger to follow along with the words. Ask him to turn the pages for you.	Get goofy. Hold the book upside down and see if your child can correct you. Start reading from the back of the book. Read a few pages out of sequence and see if he notices.

Adapted from *The Young Child's Memory for Words*, Daniel R. Meier (Teachers College Press, 2004).

Lisa Circelli, an early childhood educator, advises parents, "Focus on letter sounds rather than letter names. This helps children correlate and discriminate letter-sound recognition."

Encouraging Phonological and Phonemic Awareness at Home

Now that we've covered some of the nitty-gritty of how kids learn to read, here are some activities you can do together in the comfort of your own home.

Read, read, read, and read some more. Books are multisensory learning media. Think of your senses when you read a book—you can hear the dialogue, see the scenery, feel the emotions, and almost taste the salty sea air. Frequent practice of hearing, saying, and seeing words in print in familiar books can help kids with CAS.

Start out with repetitive books. According to speech-language pathologists Michelle Soloman and Lavinia Pereira, creators of the First Sounds Series, repetitive books are an effective therapeutic tool for kids diagnosed with CAS. That's because repetitive books are usually highly predictable. This helps kids grasp the sense of the story early on, and there is less to think about and more opportunity to verbally express their thoughts and the actual words from the book. So, if you are reading a book that has the same phrase page after page, pause occasionally and see if your child can "fill in the blank." Be sure to give your child enough time to respond. Also do this with words or characters' names. This lets your child participate more in story time, allows for more turn-taking opportunities, and possibly decreased frustration. Read favorite repetitive books repeatedly. Redundant? I know. It helps, I promise.

Some Repetitive Books to Try

- Boynton, S. *Red Hat, Yellow Hat* and *Snuggle Puppy*. If you like this author, you're in luck—she has many to choose from!
- Brown, M. *Goodnight Moon*. This classic is sure to hook your child, as is *Home for a Bunny*.
- Campbell, R. *Dear Zoo: A Lift-the-Flap Book*.
- Carle, E. *Have You Seen My Cat?* along with *123 to the Zoo*.
- Carlstrom, N.W. *Jesse Bear, What Will You Wear?*
- Christelow, E. *Five Little Monkeys Jumping on the Bed*.
- Eastman, P. D. *Are You My Mother?*
- Guarino, D. *Is Your Mama a Llama?*
- Kalen, R. *Jump, Frog, Jump!*
- Katz, K. *Where Is Baby's Mommy?* among others. Great lift-the-flap fun, illustrations, and repetition.
- Rosen, M. and Oxenbury, H. *We're Going on a Bear Hunt* and variation, *We're Going on a Nature Hunt*.
- Williams, L. *The Little Old Lady Who Was Not Afraid of Anything*.
- Of course we can't forget about good ol' Dr. Seuss books as well! Lots of his stories not only repeat but rhyme. Both are skills needed to help kids learn to read. Check out classics such as *Green Eggs and Ham* or *Hop on Pop*.

Read wordless books. Wordless books are important in getting kids to be the storyteller. Each time a child "reads" a wordless book, the story changes slightly. Of course, this may be harder to do if your child isn't saying much. But the more you present the book, the more he will attempt. For kids who are more verbal, you will see their creativity, vocabulary, and knowledge grow as they add to and elaborate on the story. Some wordless titles you may want to look for: *Pancakes for Breakfast* by Tomi dePaulo, *The Surprise Picnic* by J. S. Goodall, and *Good Dog, Carl* by Alexandra Day, as well as books by these authors—Emily Arnold McCully, Mercer Mayer (the author of the Little Critter series), Peter Spier, and Nancy Tafuri.

Engage in dialogic reading. What this means is you stop and ask your child questions about the book you are reading. "Oh, look. I see a little girl who is ready to go to school. She has a backpack. Can you say *backpack*? What else do you see?" You don't have to do this type of reading on every page, but once in a while as you read. Plan for extra reading time so you can point out things in the illustrations and allow for your child to engage with you.

Read riddles. Riddle books are great for long car rides or an after-dinner family activity. Riddles provide good exposure to, and practice with, the nuances of language. Kids have to really listen to the story and hear that some words have multiple meanings. Riddles also help develop a rich vocabulary and improve reading comprehension.

- Talk about the structure of a riddle. It's a question/answer "story" in which words "play" with one another.
- The answer makes silly sense if you understand the multiple meanings of words.
- Share your thoughts on how the words work together so your child can understand the riddle more clearly.

Keep in mind that riddles are tricky. It may be best to wait on these until your child is developmentally more mature. Generally, kids who are in kindergarten to second grade find them hilarious.

Explore letters and sounds. Develop a "Letter Center" at home if you have the space. Supply it with magnetic letters, alphabet puzzles, sponge letters, foam letters, sticker letters, rubber letter stamps, clay or Play-Doh and cookie cutters shaped like letters, and apps or software or web-based programs focusing on the alphabet. It may be a nice extension to offer different types of literacy materials: catalogs, labels, newspapers, empty cereal boxes, recipe cards, junk mail, and greeting cards. If it has print on it, it counts!

Clap it out. You may want to start with a simple adaptation of clapping out syllables. Say, "I am going to clap my hands in a pattern. Repeat after me." Then clap out a simple little sequence. Your child is listening to the rate and pattern of your claps. He should repeat it back to you. Make them more complex as he grasps the idea. Then, add in clapping out syllables to words. Remember, a syllable will always include one vowel. "Momma" becomes "Mom"-clap-"ma"-clap. Do this often with words you and your child say. Have your child try it. You can vary this activity by stomping or jumping.

Try body cues. Rhonda Banford shares this idea for teaching about syllables: "I like to have kids put their hands on their heads for the first syllable, shoulders for the second, waist for the third, knees for the fourth, and toes for the fifth. I find this helps more than clapping when I ask them how many syllables there are. It is easier for some kids to remember which of these different movements they made when they count the syllables than remembering how many times they clapped."

Play the "Letter a Day" game. Pick a letter and have it be the focus of your day. "Today we are going to focus on the letter *B*. Let's see how many *B*s we can find. Let's try to say words that begin with the letter *B*. But first, let me show you what the letter *B* looks like." Everywhere you go, point the letter out in its uppercase and lowercase form. Practice making the /ba/ sound. Make a collage with the letter. Play ball and say *B* words as you bounce or roll it to each other. Practice writing the letter *B*. Rhonda Banford suggests: "Make the activity multisensory in other ways too. Write it in pudding, construct it out of Play-Doh, trace it with the finger on a piece of sandpaper you've cut into the letter shape, paint the soles of the feet and have the child walk the shape of the *B* on a large piece of butcher paper (available at craft supply stores)."

Shop at home. Give your child a shopping bag. On the bag, write or attach a letter. Tell him to go around the house and collect things in his bag that begin with that letter sound. Talk about what he shopped for together.

Make a name collage. Start by writing your child's name on a large sheet of construction paper. Then look in old magazines and catalogs for items that start with the sound of his first name—e.g., Steven = stove, stop, stick, stone, stay, story. Let your child do some of the work.

Match letters to toys. Grab a few of your child's favorite toys. Spread them out on the floor and make your own alphabet cards, making sure that you include some "correct" as well as "incorrect" cards. For example, say your grouping of toys consists of ball, doll, car, puzzle, and jump rope. Your alphabet cards would include the letters *Bb*, *Dd*, *Cc*, *Pp*, and *Jj*. Throw in a couple of random letters as well, such as *Rr*, *Zz*, *Hh*. Have your child match the correct card to the correct toy. Practice saying the name of the object, as well as the sound the letter makes with your child.

Does this rhyme? Play this simple game in the car, in a waiting room, or even in the grocery story. Say, "I am thinking of three words. They are *cat*, *bat*, and *ball*. Which words rhyme?" This works on short-term memory as well as rhyming skills. You may first have to describe what a rhyme is. Your child will get good at this and begin developing his own list of three rhyming words. Praise your child for attempts at creating a rhyme, even if it isn't 100 percent correct. A simple and fun book to read to your child that uses rhyme is *There's a Wocket in My Pocket* by Dr. Seuss. Don't forget about your classic nursery rhymes too!

Play with your food. At snack time, consider playing with your child's food. Pretzel sticks, carrot sticks, or any other sticklike foods work well. You can create many letters this way—*M*, *N*, *E*, *K*, to name a few. If you need the circular part of a letter, try using bendable foods like licorice or string cheese. Consider making pancakes in the shape of different letters. This may be the perfect breakfast for your letter day fun!

Find letters in nature. Go on a hike and look for natural formations that look a bit like letters. Need a little inspiration? Check out *ABCs Naturally: A Child's Guide to the Alphabet through Nature* by Lynne Smith Diebel and Jann Faust Kalschuer. You can start with the letter *a* and work your way through the alphabet by having the first person find something that starts with *a* (acorn, anthill), the next person something that begins with *b* (bug, bluebird), and so on. To make it harder, you can have each successive person list the words that the other players have already said (so the third person might say, "Anthill, bug, crow"). This helps with observational skills, recall, and phonological awareness. Of course, modify if this recall portion is too tricky.

Making Reading Fun

While some kids love to read, others may grow to dread it. Here are a few ideas that you might consider adopting as you try to impress upon your child(ren) that reading is fun:

- *Pick books that are easy for your child to read.* Give him some success early on, and he will find that reading really isn't as difficult as it seems.

- *Sit with your child as he reads a book for the first time.* I know, we're all busy— who possibly has the time? Your child needs to know that you value reading, and may need help with some of the more difficult words

- *Find—and help your child find—different kinds of books.* That means wandering into the children's section at the library. Let him peruse the shelves for something that piques his interest. Consider poetry, mysteries, biographies, nonfiction, among others.

- *Read harder books to your child than he could read himself.* Researchers and educators have found that kids can understand stories about three to four grade levels above their reading level. It introduces them to the story structure of more complicated tales, along with vocabulary, plus it's motivation to continue reading on one's own.

- *Make connections to books and real-life experiences.* Reading the Little House on the Prairie series? Visit one of the historical centers that honors Laura Ingalls Wilder's life or a pioneer village in your area. Other examples could include visiting the bakery in your grocery store after reading a book about cookies, or touring the pizza parlor. Call ahead, of course.

- *Suggest having your child read books aloud to practice expression and inflection.* Hard skills for anyone to master, but even more so for kids with CAS.

- *When your child comes across a word he doesn't know, have him predict what it could be.* "What makes sense in the story?" This not only teaches prediction skills, but also the concept of context.

- *Extend reading activities* by suggesting your child create a play around the story with neighborhood friends, draw a picture of what you just read (especially helpful if mom and dad are reading to a child from a chapter book), or make your own book.

- *Host a book playdate.* Decide on a theme based on a book, book series, or character your child is particularly drawn to. Send out an appropriately themed invitation to the guests. Decorate accordingly and prepare food that the storybook character might also like (green eggs and ham, anyone?). Have a reading of the book, followed by a short discussion, throw in a few book-related games and crafts, then call it a day.

- *Create a parent-child book group in your neighborhood or school.* Depending on your child's grade level, you can read all kind of things—start with picture books, pick a favorite author, or go with a theme (animals as the main character or books that focus on feelings and self-esteem, for example), then set a schedule—say once a month. Everyone reads the same thing—or picks from a few titles—then comes together and shares what they learned.

What Is Guided Reading?

Guided reading helps kids develop important concepts as they read and helps lay the foundation for writing stories of their own. What is it, exactly? Guided reading is the process of supporting reading in a small-group setting by first introducing the book and story in a prereading exercise. Our teacher called this a "book walk." It could simply mean talking with your child about the author and title and identifying the spine, table of contents, etc. Next, you might introduce characters, new vocabulary, and prediction-making skills. Supporting your emerging reader with context clues, letter-sound recognition/relationships, and word structure would be the final step. It's not as easy as it appears, but this is a very important part of learning to read.

You'll also want your child to be able to retell a story (narrative skills) and follow the general structure of a story. You can practice and build these skills by asking the right questions after a reading session. Try this: purchase or repurpose a beach ball and write questions about books in general on each of the colored wedges with a marker. Examples may include: Who is the author? Is there an illustrator? Who is the main character? My favorite part was ____. The story was about ____.

Mention the beach ball activity at the beginning of the book: "We're going to read a book and then play this game with the ball. The ball will 'ask' some questions about the book we just read. Some questions will be ____ (read them). Pay attention as we read so you are prepared to answer the questions." Read the story, then sit in a circle (with multiple kids) or across from your child. Toss or roll the ball back and forth. Answer the question on the part of the ball your hand touches first.

What Should Schools Be Doing?

Is your child's teacher doing the right thing when it comes to teaching his or her students the basics of reading? Here are a few pointers to keep in mind. You can find answers to these questions by asking directly during a conference, sending an email to your child's teacher, visiting the classroom, or asking to review the school's reading curriculum.

- Does the teacher read aloud frequently?
- Are favorite stories read again and again?
- Is "pretend" reading encouraged? Do kids have the opportunity to do so?
- Does your child have access to a variety of books in the classroom?
- Do kids practice writing? Is there a writing center in the classroom?
- Does the teacher teach phonics? Does she teach that there is a relationship between letters and sounds?

In elementary school, teachers will likely keep a portfolio of your child's literacy growth over the school year and talk with you about this at conferences or whenever you inquire. Generally, teachers are looking to see if your child

- can handle books properly (e.g., knows when a book is right-side-up, "reads" from left to right, etc.);
- is aware of story sequences;
- recalls details from familiar stories;
- expresses a preference for a specific story;
- uses pictures to "read" a storybook;
- is aware that print has meaning;
- recognizes his own name in print;
- records ideas (by using drawing as writing, then pictures and scribbles for writing);
- makes letter-like forms for writing;
- uses random letter forms for writing;

- practices with invented spellings;
- finally uses conventional spellings.

Teachers in formal preschools (as opposed to daycare centers) also often keep a written record of students' literacy awareness, which they pass on as children are transitioning from preschool to kindergarten. This gives your child's kindergarten teacher a sense of "where he's at" in terms of literacy growth. Modifications, special assistance, and instruction, if needed, can be made from there.

Reading Problems? Programs That Help

If you think that your child has a reading disorder, or a difficulty with reading, by all means, bring it to the teacher's attention. The good news is that most schools have a reading specialist who can home in on those skills. Plus, many reading issues can be addressed by your child's SLP, especially in the case of moderate-severe CAS. If you are interested in specific reading programs for your child, here are some well-known and researched programs:

Visual Phonics. Originally developed for kids who are deaf or hard of hearing, this program can be used in a range of settings from the classroom to a speech clinic. Visual Phonics is a method in which kids can *see* the phonemes in action. It's quick and easy to learn, can be used with any reading curriculum, and is multisensory and interactive. Visit www.seethesound.org for more information.

Lindamood-Bell. Do you ask yourself or your child, "What do the words help your mind see as you read?" If so, then this program may be right up your alley. Patricia Lindamood and Nanci Bell have been helping kids and adults read, spell, comprehend, think critically, and express language since 1986. Their model encompasses three "rights": "the right evaluation, the right instruction, and the right environment." It is often used for children with significant dyslexia (diagnosed reading disabilities). For more information: www.lindamoodbell.com.

LiPS Program. Part of the Lindamood-Bell program for reading, the LiPS program targets phoneme sequencing for reading, spelling, and speech. It can be especially helpful for kids to *feel* the mouth movements involved in the decoding process of speech sounds. See Lindamood-Bell above. Look for the LiPS manual and DVD at www.ganderpublishing.com/LiPS.

Immediate Intensive Intervention. This program is designed for customized reading instruction in small groups or 1:1. It's systematic and explicit, requiring ninety-minute reading blocks and calls its approach "balanced literacy."

Florida Center for Reading Research (FCRR). The FCRR presents a multimodal series for beefing up reading skills. The three modes consist of the following: (1) Core (all kids, comprehensive, small group, reteaching methods); (2) Supplemental (like the Core program, only these kids need a bit more instruction in vocabulary, phonics, and strengthening of existing skills); and (3) Intervention instruction (kids who are lagging behind their peers in critical reading areas). For more information, visit www.fcrr.org.

Phonics Faces. Phonics Faces is a nice program for kids who are still working on basic sound and alphabet skills. This collection of flashcards focuses on phonemic awareness, rhyme, letter-sound association, phonics, and articulation. There is a clip on YouTube that shows a child with CAS working on this program. Look for it at www.youtube.com/watch?v=70AoRIUOjHc. For more information: www.elementory.com.

Directed Reading Thinking Activity (DRTA). A strategy that guides kids in asking questions about a text, making predictions, and then continuing to read to see if their prediction is correct. DRTA helps produce active, thoughtful readers. For more information, see: www.readingrockets.org.

The DuBard Association Method. This is a phonetic, multisensory teaching-learning strategy for children with language deficiencies that was originally designed by the late Mildred McGinnis, a teacher at Central Institute for the Deaf in St. Louis. It has been successful for children with severe CAS. See www.usm.edu/dubard/what-dubard-association-method for more information. Your child's SLP may be familiar with this program.

Fast ForWord. Fast ForWord (www.fastforword.com) is an expensive software program for home computer use that has a series of fun, engaging games. These games are meant to "retrain" the brains of struggling readers to improve attention, memory, and the ability to process the sounds in words. To be effective, this program must be used consistently for a long period of time (ninety minutes a day for weeks). The website www.scilearn.com has many studies about its effectiveness in helping children with disorders of language and reading. Other studies suggest Fast ForWord may be an effective treatment for kids with auditory processing disorder. However, according to research, it is not a cure-all, and other programs were just as good, as was direct therapy. For more information see www.gemmlearning.com.

Earobics, Step 1. Earobics is a fun-to-play interactive computer software program designed to teach the fundamental listening and sound awareness skills that research has proven are the best predictors of reading success. For more information, see www.hmhco.com/classroom-solutions/early-learning.

Wilson Reading Program. Like the Lindamood-Bell program, the Wilson program is frequently used by schools to help children who have a diagnosed learning disability in reading. It is a very rule-intensive, multisensory program for kids of all ages who are not progressing in reading skills. Teachers ideally should be formally trained in the method. Check the program out at www.wilsonlanguage.com.

ABeCeDarian Reading Program. This is a multisensory decoding program that focuses on phonemic awareness, phonics, and fluency. This program has an easy instruction model for parents and teachers to use with their children, but it can also be used for adults who have reading difficulties. It's less expensive than many other programs. For more information: www.abcdrp.com.

Lexia Core 5 Reading for Pre-K-5. Lexia is one of the most rigorously researched, independently evaluated, and respected reading programs in the world. Lexia's products are designed according to the latest scientific findings in education and offer

276   SPEAKING OF APRAXIA

differentiated literacy instruction for students of all abilities in grades pre-K–5. Lexia's research-proven program provides clear, systematic, personalized learning in six areas of reading instruction, targeting skill gaps as they emerge, and provides teachers with data and student-specific resources needed for individual or small-group instruction. Visit the Lexia website for information about their products: https://www.lexialearning.com/.

> *My son Joey utilized the Lexia program at school and at home with me and had great success. As a special education teacher and reading specialist, I highly recommend it.*
>
> —Renee Mindy, MSEd

Keep in mind that not all of these programs can be used by a parent at home. They may require training and certification to implement. You can start with asking your SLP about them, research them online, and then determine if your child will benefit.

In addition, these programs aren't cheap! If you have a network, group, club, or Facebook group you frequent, consider posting a message to see if anyone has an older program you could purchase. If you're lucky, someone may allow you to borrow their copy or just give it to you! We borrowed *Earobics* from Kate's preschool teacher. It never hurts to ask.

Determining If Your Child Needs a Specialized Reading Program

Hopefully, your child won't. But if you have concerns, you'll want your child to have a comprehensive and accurate evaluation. Your child's school may do one for free if they suspect your child has a learning disability in reading. However, they will likely put off evaluating your child while they try various types of "response to intervention." RTI is a procedure detailed in IDEA that requires schools to gradually provide more individualized, intensive help to students who *may* have learning disabilities before actually labeling them as having a learning disability.

If you don't want to wait while the school is trying RTI and you have the funds, get an evaluation outside of school by an educational psychologist, if possible. SLPs don't typically evaluate children formally for reading problems, although they may do informal assessments with phonological awareness skills. Independent evaluators typically have no other motivation for doing the assessment and evaluation. Schools, on the other hand, might. Funding and teacher and evaluator availability, and other resources may all come into play.

Here's a sampling of tests that evaluate reading skills:

- Gray Oral Reading Test/Gray Silent Reading Test (GORT)
- Test of Phonological Awareness (TOPA)
- Test of Early Reading Ability (TERA)

- Test of Word Reading Efficiency (TWRE)
- Woodcock Reading Mastery Test (WRMT)
- Kaufman Test of Educational Achievement (KTEA)

Your own thoughts on your child's reading progress should also be an important part of any evaluation.

There is no single test that measures reading skills comprehensively. Different reading tests measure different types of skills. It is up to the evaluators and educators to synthesize the results into an individualized package. They assess your child's passage comprehension, word comprehension, ability to read nonsense words, letter identification, decoding fluency, and word recognition. Even if your child is not communicating well verbally, you can still have his reading skills evaluated. There are many nonverbal components to these tests. Keep in mind, however, that not every diagnostic test is given well or appropriately.

One more thing about any evaluation: don't interpret it as a "label." Use the results of an evaluation as a baseline. You need to know where your child started before you can begin to assess any progress.

Visual Tracking

Another thing to keep in mind is that young readers with CAS may have difficulties learning how to track visually. That is, your child may have a hard time following the words on the page because he is unable to track where he was reading, even in a short paragraph. Or he may have difficulty switching from looking at the chalkboard or Smartboard to looking at the paper on his desk (reading print from far and near). It all has to do with convergence of the eyes, the inward movement of both eyes toward each other at the same time. By no means will all children with CAS have difficulty with visual tracking. There is no known connection between the two, although it *can* occur in children with CAS.

What's a Parent to Do?

A pediatric OT can help with some simple visual exercises. Tracking, for example, can be practiced by having your child follow a fingertip back and forth. Convergence can be practiced by having your child follow a light source (such as a penlight) from two or three feet away from his face to his nose. Do it several times in a row several times throughout the day. Another idea is to have your child follow an object around the room with his eyes only. It doesn't count if he has to move his head or body to track the item. Move the item up, down, right, left. Keep him guessing. Let him test you too. It's fun for kids when they can play at being an SLP.

Tell Me Something That Makes Me Feel Good

The key to working with your child with CAS on reading is to remember that he will get it!

It might be challenging at times, but you'll both get there. Treat him as though he is any other kid in terms of how you go about teaching it, and try not to get too hung up on the CAS piece.

Here's another "warm fuzzy" to keep in mind as you travel down the road less-read: in many other countries, kids don't learn to read until the third grade. For some reason, the US seems to think we need to be ahead in this area, often attempting to teach kids to read at an earlier-than-ready age.

I leave you with this analogy: You are in an intense exercise class but your knee is killing you. You can't do lunges and squats as your instructor would like, so you modify. You do something similar that still gives you the benefit, but with less strain. As a parent, and as an educator, *you may just have to modify how you teach your child with CAS to read.*

Write On!

Learning to write is a complicated process. First you need a basic understanding of the alphabet and the fact that letters represent sounds and sounds make words, and then you need to know how to order those letters so that they spell recognizable words. Here are some more steps that need to happen for the "write" stuff:

- Lots of reflexes need to come together to control the rate and rhythm of writing. Your child's body needs to be anchored in time and place.

- Your child will need to be able to cross the midline of his body with his dominant hand—the one that holds the writing utensil.

- He should understand that his fingers are controlling the writing utensil—sort of an abstract concept, but important nonetheless.

- Eyes must focus and move along the paper he is writing on.

- He must be able to control the fine muscles in his fingers.

- He will need to have the motor planning to draw the letters correctly.

- Most of all—he needs to have the ability to sit still.

I present this information to you because some kids with CAS also have limb apraxia and fine motor delays. Not all children with CAS will exhibit the above concerns.

Where to Begin

It may be helpful to start by teaching large arm movements. Have your child swing his arms in big circles, flap them like a bird; get creative and have fun (this is because large motor movements come before small motor movements in typical development). You don't even have to tell your little one what you're up to. He'll be none the wiser.

Some folks recommend starting to write up and down on a vertical surface (like a chalkboard or easel), rather than on a traditional horizontal writing surface such as a table. Again, this strengthens those large arm movements of the body, trunk, arms, and shoulders.

Try taping paper to a wall, having your child write on an easel or the fridge—just make sure you are using washable markers or dry-erase materials. Another fun activity is to use "window markers." Just as they sound, these markers are safe to use on windows and patio doors. Look for them at craft stores or the kids' art aisle at your favorite discount store. In fact, my kids enjoy using dry-erase markers on windows and mirrors, and they wipe clean.

Kids can "paint" the house with a bucket of water and a paintbrush when the weather's nice. Sidewalk chalk presents similar opportunities and works the whole body.

Try "writing" in various outdoor settings such as on a gravel driveway or mud using a stick, a shoe, or your finger. Your kids will think you are very cool if you do this with them. They love to get down and dirty while at the same time being instructional. "Sneaky" parenting, but it works!

To work on fine motor control, seek out toys and manipulatives that your child can squeeze and twist (fidget toys), as well as small toys common in many households, like Polly Pockets and Transformers. Wikki Stix and Bendaroos might also appeal and can be found at craft and dollar stores.

What You Can Do at Home

Assuming that all is "good to go" after a period of warm-up writing activities as outlined above, then it's time to jump in to printing. Most kids learn to print their names first. Start by encouraging your child to write his name with a capital letter followed by lowercase letters. Uppercase letters are easier to master, but don't let your child get into the habit of writing in all caps. It's a hard one to break. When he's in kindergarten and first grade, lowercase letters will be encouraged, if not required.

Once your child learns to write his name in upper- and lowercase letters, you can move on to the alphabet in all capitals. But here's something you may not know: it's not best to go in order. Start with straight letters and then work into curvy ones. That's the order of progression from easy to difficult. You'll want to give your child some success early on, right?

Here's a chart to refer to as you move through the ABCs, in order of difficulty (adapted from our experience with the *Handwriting Without Tears* program):

Sequence of Difficulty in Forming Letters

FIRST (easiest to master)	SECOND (moderate)	THIRD (most challenging)
E, F, H, I, L, T	B, C, D, G, J, O, P, Q, S, U	A, K, M, N, R, V, W, X, Y, Z

You can also encourage your child with some tracing exercises. It doesn't necessarily matter if he's tracing letters—although that could be part of your approach. Sneak it in by starting first with those coloring books with tracing paper. Move on to tracing dotted line pictures and letters, which you can make yourself. Other prewriting skills include mazes and dot-to-dots.

Handwriting and CAS

A lot of components come into play as our kids learn to write—visual-motor coordination, motor planning, strength, sensory processing (proprioception), and cognitive processing, to name a few. You know your child best, so observe and see if you can determine where in that process things are breaking down. For my daughter, I would bet that it is visual-motor coordination and motor planning. Your child may also have something amiss in this sequence (but not always). Not all kids with CAS have motor planning problems beyond verbal or oral apraxia, but they *could*.

Think about how you deal with the motor aspect of speech. You'll need to apply similar principles to helping your child lay down the motor pathways to handwriting. *Verbal cueing* and *verbal feedback* may be just the ticket, "Big line down, big line up, little line across the middle . . . that's it—you got it!"

Of course, just as with speech, **you'll need to provide many repetitions of the writing movements so that they become automatic.** Also, be sure to provide lots of positive feedback in the form of results: "I like the way this letter looks," and knowledge: "To make an /o/ you need to connect the top of the circle."

Need Some Handwriting Intervention?

Your child may require some 1:1 writing intervention that you alone—at home—can't accomplish. Teaching handwriting is complicated and time-consuming, and it will test your patience. Don't lose heart and try not to feel like a failure if you can't help your child be successful. You may need an occupational therapist (OT) to step in and evaluate your kiddo's writing abilities. Writing evaluation tests include the following:

- The *Print Tool* by Jan Olsen, which is part of the *Handwriting Without Tears* program
- *Diagnosis of Remediation of Handwriting Problems*
- *The Minnesota Handwriting Test*
- *Children's Handwriting Evaluation Scale-Manuscript*
- *Evaluation Tool of Children's Handwriting-Manuscript (ETCH)*

- *Test of Legible Handwriting*
- *School Function Assessment* (looks at *all* school-related skills and functions)
- *The Miller Assessment of Preschoolers* (can be administered to kids up to age 5.8 years)

Most of these evaluation tools look at the eight basic handwriting skills:

1. Memory—remembering and writing letters that are dictated by another person
2. Orientation—ensuring all letters face the same direction
3. Placement—putting letters in the right direction
4. Size—how big or small a child writes
5. Start—where each letter begins
6. Sequence—the order and stroke direction of the letter parts
7. Control—the neatness and proportion of letter parts
8. Spacing—the amount of space between letters and words

As you go about seeking an evaluation and interpreting the results, keep in mind these very important pieces: how the test was administered and the scoring, reliability, and validity of the tool. Ask questions, seek answers.

If your child needs the help of an OT, get to it as soon as you can. Our OT used *Handwriting Without Tears (HWT)* for Kate and it was quite helpful. The basics behind this program is that most letters can be "drawn" with straight lines, with a few exceptions (P, O, C, and D, for example). Initially kids work with a group of wooden sticks that look a bit like twelve-inch rulers to "make" letters. Next, they draw them on a small chalkboard. It's whole-body and multisensory—something our kids with CAS can appreciate and excel at. See www.hwtears.com for more information.

Loops and Other Groups: A Kinesthetic Writing System helps kids visualize and feel the movements in writing. It's good for those who require more attention to detail, and kids learning cursive handwriting.

Scribblenauts may be more up your child's alley. It was designed for Nintendo DS to get kids to work on bringing their writing to life. It's a game in which one can "Write anything. Solve everything." It may just be what your child needs to motivate him and improve his writing. Plus, it sort of disguises work as fun.

You may want to try *Mead Writing Fundamentals: Learn to Write with Raised Ruling*, a notebook containing paper with raised lines. It may provide enough of a tactile cue for your child as he learns to navigate the intricacies of print. Look for it where school supplies are sold.

Finally, Kid-O makes a product called the *A to Z Magnatab Magnetic Writing Tablet*. This fun, multisensory tool may help your child focus on forming letters correctly and consistently. The magnetic stylus pulls metal balls to the surface, snapping them into place to form the letter. To reinforce the "feel" for each letter, kids can lightly trace over the letters with the tip of their finger, pressing the metal balls back into the base. Look for it online or where educational toys are sold.

Writing to Communicate: Stories

At some point, your child will move into more independent storytelling and story writing. I know, it may seem eons away from the here and now, but before you know it, his imagination will be taking him to "far, far away land." Look for ways to promote writing for fun.

Provide him with notebooks and pens. Have a time of day that you let your child experiment with "writing" books, cards, newspapers, diaries, journals, letters, checks (old, out-of-date), grocery lists, to-do lists, whatever you can think of. It's an important step in teaching kids to learn to love writing for a purpose.

Children with CAS may have a harder than usual time getting their thoughts from their brain to their hands and out of their writing instrument. It's just like the underlying neuromotor issue with verbal communication. Only now it's with written communication. There are some software programs that can help your child get his internal narratives out of his head and onto the paper or screen and organize them. (See the resources at the end of the chapter.)

Remember, if your child still struggles with correct syntax and morphology, it will show in his story-writing abilities. "Encourage him to read what he has written aloud. This will help him catch missing and extraneous words," says Rhonda Banford. Again, your child's classroom teacher, reading/writing specialist, or SLP can also assist with these skills.

What about Spelling?

So, you finally got your little one to progress from scribbles to more meaningful letter development; maybe a few words or two have emerged. But there seems to be one little problem: your child isn't spelling correctly! No worries. What your child is doing is referred to as "invented spelling." It's a term that was coined by linguist Carol Chomsky and used by many others, even the prominent child development psychologist Jean Piaget. It's the young child's unpressured efforts to write words his own way before learning the correct spelling. Invented spelling enables self-expression and is not something to stress about.

Invented spelling reveals how your child *thinks* words are spelled. It's actually a step in the right direction. It's like putting phonics on paper. Your child is using the symbols he knows or makes up to "write" words. Invented spelling gives children a window to their own awareness. Your child will spell correctly when he is cognitively ready. Look at this period in his writing life as inquiry, experimentation, and growth.

Say That Again?! Chapter Summary

I hope you found this a jam-packed source of information and encouragement when it comes to helping your child succeed in reading and writing. These are two skills he will undoubtedly need in his academic career and beyond. Please don't give up. These skills are extremely difficult and time consuming to teach for the parents of any child, with or without CAS. They will test your patience. But you don't have to go it alone. Remember, you can always call on the assistance of your child's school, his SLP, his OT, or an educational psychologist. And remember, your child will be successful in his own way.

Recommended Resources

- While it's a huge book, *The Mislabeled Child: How Understanding Your Child's Unique Learning Style Can Open the Doors to Success* by Brock and Fernette Eide (Hyperion, 2006), covers a lot of good information on learning and memory, autism and giftedness, handwriting and dysgraphia.

- A book you may find helpful in your journey is *Different Learners: Identifying, Preventing, and Treating Your Child's Learning Problems* by Jane Healy (Simon and Schuster, 2010). It does a great job of discussing current changes in education, the case of difference vs. disability, and genetics vs. environment, all with a research-based background.

- If you'd like more nitty-gritty reading research, look for *Phonological Awareness: From Research to Practice,* 2nd edition, by Gail T. Gillon (Guilford Press, 2017).

- *The Young Child's Memory for Words: Developing 1st and 2nd Language Literacy* by educator Daniel R. Meier (Teachers College Press, 2004) is a good resource for getting a grasp on literacy development, teaching, and learning.

- *Miss Brooks Loves Books (and I don't)* by Barbara Bottner (Random House Children's Books, 2010) is a fun and adorable book that even the most resistant reader will appreciate.

- *The Teacher's Guide to Getting Started with Beginning Writers, Grades K–2* by Katie Wood Kay and Lisa B. Cleaveland follows two teachers in their quest to help teach writing to their students (Heinemann, 2018).

- *Mosaic of Thought* by educators Ellin Oliver Keene and Susan Zimmerman (Heinemann, 2007) offers a step-by-step approach to developing thoughtful, independent readers.

- *Learning to Read and Write: Developmentally Appropriate Practices for Young Children* by Susan B. Neuman, Carol Copple, and Sue Bredekamp (NAEYC, 2000) gives concrete examples of how to teach reading and writing to kids before third grade. It's mostly geared toward early childhood educators, but parents can glean something from it as well.

- The First Sounds Series by Michelle Soloman and Lavinia Pereira was written and designed by two SLPs, one of whom is PROMPT trained. It is an interactive series of children's books that foster the growth and development of speech and language skills. You'll help your child discover functional vocabulary and familiar phrases through repetition. For more information, http://www.firstsoundseries.com/.

- *Over 1000 Games, Activities, Tongue Twisters, Fingerplays, Songs, and Stories to Get Children Excited about Reading* by Pam Schiller and *The Complete Book and CD Set of Rhymes, Songs, Poems, Fingerplays, & Chants* by Jackie Silberg and Pam Schiller (Gryphon House, 2006) suggest some great ideas for things to do at home to build phonological awareness.

- I really like Language during Mealtime, the website and podcast of Rebecca Eisenberg, MS, CCC-SLP. She's a parent, certified autism specialist, and author whose passion is children's literature, special needs, and evidence-based research tips for reading with your child. Her Kindle book, *Improve Your Child's Language and Learning in 20 Minutes: Evidence-based Tips for Reading during Mealtime: A Parent's Guide* might be helpful along your journey. Look for it here: https://languageduringmealtime.com/.

- The Zaner-Bloser website is dedicated to *early literacy*. The site includes information on reading, leveled books, vocabulary, spelling, and handwriting: www.zaner-bloser.com.

- *A Fresh Look at Phonics: 7 Causes of Failure and 7 Ingredients for Success* by Wiley Blevins is informative and hands-on (Corwin Literacy, 2016).

- Lakeshore Learning has some great products for teaching *phonemic and phonological awareness* skills. My favorites are *Rhyming Big Book, Phonemic Awareness Activity Card Library and Chart, Match a Sound*, and *Rhyming Sounds Basket*. Visit their website at www.lakeshorelearning.com.

- Here are *some great books* you may want to read with your children. They have been recommended by parents of kids with CAS:

  - *If You Give a Mouse a Cookie* and any other *If You Give* books by Laura Numeroff
  - Cornelius P. Mud series by Barney Saltzberg
  - *Dinosaur Roar* by Paul and Henrietta Strickland
  - *Polar Bear, Polar Bear* and *Brown Bear, Brown Bear* by Bill Martin Jr.
  - *Pout-Pout Fish* by Debra Diesen
  - *Something from Nothing* by Phoebe Gilman
  - *Mr. Brown Can Moo, Can You?* by Dr. Seuss

- *It Isn't Easy Being a Bunny* by Marilyn Sadler
- Curious George books by H. A. and Margaret Rey
- *Go, Dog. Go!* by P. D. Eastman
- *Runny Babbit* by Shel Silverstein (best suited for older kids with CAS)

- Pam Allyn's **What to Read When** (Avery Trade, 2009) may be helpful in your search for the perfect books to entertain and motivate young readers.

- **Reading Magic: Why Reading to Our Children Will Change Their Lives Forever** by Mem Fox (Mariner Books, 2008) is a fantastic book written by an educator and reading specialist. It provides lists of books to consider reading to and with your children, and does a great job of surveying the literature.

- **Reading Together: Everything You Need to Raise a Child Who Loves to Read** by Diane W. Frankenstein (Perigee Trade, 2009) has great tips, tools, and suggestions for raising a reader.

- **The Read Aloud Handbook** by Jim Trelease (Penguin, 2019) is a classic book (now in its 8th edition) that recommends books that are fun for parents to read and engaging for kids.

- If you're looking for software to **help with the writing process**, I really like Snap and Read, an online resource with several options that may appeal to you and your child. For example, *Text-to-Speech, Screenshot Reader, Simplify, Translate,* and *Capture* all work to streamline reading. There is a nominal fee for the service: https://snapandread.com/. For older children, Google Read & Write and also Grammarly may prove beneficial.

Coping & Hoping

Chapter 13

CAS Affects Us All

Coping with CAS as a Family

It was a stressful time when we learned about Kate's CAS diagnosis. We had recently relocated to the Chicago area from Minnesota. My husband was starting a new job that involved considerable travel. I was in charge of getting the new house in order and unpacked while raising two young girls. Kate was only two and a half years old and baby Kelly was nine months.

I was also adjusting to the demands of being a full-time at-home mother, a change we'd made out of necessity. I'd considered going back to work as a psychiatric nurse, even interviewing for a job or two. But who would watch the girls in a strange new city while I worked? Plus, Jim's travel schedule made it nearly impossible for him to keep regular hours. Meanwhile, the housing market was going south, and our Minnesota home was not selling. We were making two house payments on one income. And Kate wasn't talking.

When I was growing up, my dad always said, "Worry about the things you can control, not what you can't." His fatherly advice resonated at this point in my life. The move, the house not selling, my husband's travel schedule—they were all out of my control. What I could do, though, was get Kate evaluated at a speech clinic. My spirits started to lift.

While it was hard to hear the diagnosis, it was also a relief. I could at least check one thing off my list—"help Kate learn to talk"—by getting her to and from speech therapy. And the ironic thing was, hearing the SLP say Kate had CAS wasn't nearly as stressful as hearing, "I'm sorry but the buyer of your home backed out at the last minute and now you have two house payments." Everything is relative.

Of course, my example is extreme. I don't want to imply that it's no big deal that you suddenly have been thrust into this world of CAS. It is very real and very challenging. But you *will* get through it. This chapter will help.

- A discussion of how it is still possible to develop a healthy, happy family life when your child has CAS
- More on the grief process (it was covered briefly in chapter 4) and ways you and your family can work through your feelings
- Differences in reactions and coping styles
- The unique stressors of raising a family in which one member (or more) has special needs, plus tips on remaining strong and developing positive coping strategies
- How to look after your own physical and emotional needs

Happy Families Struggle at Times, Too

The previous chapter talked about how we just want our kids to be happy. Well yes, that is true. But even the happiest of families can hit some bumps along the road. Everyone will be affected in some manner by the CAS diagnosis.

This chapter will break it down by family member, but generally you will all feel a sense of loss. Why do you feel this way? Well, it's as though you are grieving the loss of the child you thought you would be raising, a normally chatty kid who doesn't have to struggle to put her words together. It's akin to moving away to a new city or state, the loss of a job, the loss of a marriage through divorce, or the loss of a loved one through death. The stages that parents go through in coping with a child's diagnosis have been compared to the stages of grief identified by psychiatrist Elisabeth Kübler-Ross. Not everyone who experiences a loss goes through these stages in order, but you can expect to go through *some* of these stages at *some* point along your CAS journey, even if the amount of time you spend in one stage or another is variable.

Denial: You may be experiencing denial if you are "waiting and seeing" in regards to your child's lack of communication. Deep down inside, you *know* something's amiss, but you aren't ready to hear it. After you hear the diagnosis, you may question the competence of the evaluator or seek a second opinion because "they don't know what they're talking about."

Anger: You've heard the news—your child has CAS. And now you're just plain angry. Next, you're picking a fight with the receptionist at the front desk of the speech clinic, your husband (because it's his "bad" genes, after all), and your mom because she doesn't know what CAS is and therefore thinks it must not be "real."

Bargaining: You promise you'll do anything and everything if the CAS will just go away.

Depression: You're overwhelmed, you feel powerless, you feel vulnerable and drained. You may even feel guilty. ("It was my speech problems she inherited." "It was because I had that glass of wine when I was pregnant.") You may begin to feel uncertain about your child's future or your ability to pay for speech therapy, and that can be downright depressing.

Acceptance: You have allowed yourself to feel your emotions and process all the new information, and now you can accept the new diagnosis. The good news is, you are in the very best position to help your child when you enter this stage. And since we all want to help our kids be their best, you can finally feel empowered. It's time now to hop on the internet and join online support groups so you can offer advice and ideas to other parents. It's time to join local groups on CAS. You might feel compelled to start a blog, write a book, or attend a conference. You've got the power!

Don't get discouraged if you periodically go through feelings of anger, depression, sadness, or bargaining even though you've reached the "acceptance" stage. It's perfectly normal to regress at times. When Kate had to go back to therapy after a six-month break, I felt cheated in some ways. When her little sister, Kelly, started talking a mile a minute, I felt a sense of loss—I'd never heard Kate's sweet little voice at that age because she wasn't talking. Although Kate is older and has had more experiences than her little sister, I often felt protective of her when she couldn't keep up verbally. I felt it especially necessary to build up her self-esteem by acknowledging her other strengths when she faltered in communication: "You are a really smart girl, Kate. Let's try saying that again."

What's a Family to Do?

Realize that you are in this together. How much, what, and when you share with your other children about their sibling's CAS is a personal decision based on lots of variables—how old they are, their maturity level, how much involvement they are expected to have in the day-to-day aspects of CAS. We'll get into more specifics later in this chapter. The bottom line is to let your other children know you love them and you'll always be their parent too.

Use coping strategies that worked for your family in the past. What did you all do when Dad lost his job several years ago? You made it work somehow. What can you draw on from the past to help you in the present?

Teach your family about CAS. Hold a family meeting or two. Get out a whiteboard or make a PowerPoint presentation. If your kids are old enough, assign them some internet searches on CAS that they can present to the rest of the family. Younger kids may appreciate reading Amy Glorosio May's book *My Brother is Very, Very Special* or Angela Baublitz's *I Want to Be Your Friend* or watching movies on accepting differences (see Resources at the end of this chapter). Allow family members to ask questions. Give them the best answers you know or promise to follow up when you have the information.

Appreciate the little things. Instead of focusing on the "big news" that your child has CAS, look for the little things in life that make your family fun. The bike ride you all enjoyed, the family hike, the trip to the county fair. I will never forget the first time I heard Kate say, "I love you." That was a small moment in the grand scheme of things that we all celebrated as a family.

Remember that all members in your immediate family (and perhaps your extended family) will go through the stages of grief. It's common to feel like you are the only one. Be alert to the stages of grief and help your children and partner work through them.

The Care and Keeping of Mom

"When Momma's happy, we're all happy." I know you've heard this saying before. Is there any truth to it? Yes!

It was no surprise that I was particularly stressed in the time surrounding Kate's diagnosis. I wanted to crawl under a rock and stay there. I wanted to scream. I wanted to pull all of my hair *and* eyeballs out. Interestingly, I wasn't the only mom who felt that way.

Researchers in Germany thought that the emotional state of mothers of kids with speech impaired children would make an interesting research study. So, they designed and ran a study, "Anxiety and Depression in Mothers of Speech Impaired Children" (see references). Fully 11 percent of mothers of speech impaired children (unknown whether these kids had CAS or not) met criteria for depression and anxiety, whereas only 2.5 percent of moms in the control group (children who were not speech impaired) met those criteria. The researchers also found:

- Mothers often take on the largest part of the extra care a child with speech or language problems requires (arranging therapy, transporting to therapy, communicating with therapists).

- To take care of those special needs, mothers often have to give up their personal interests and their job.

- Mothers often feel additional pressure and strain because they now have the responsibility of supporting speech therapy at home.

- Moms worry that their children with speech impairments won't be socially accepted.

- Mothers fear that their children with speech impairments will develop other disorders such as ODD, ADHD, depression, and anxiety.

- Finally, moms worry about their child's future and whether he or she will ever be able to talk "normally."

That's not to say that dads don't feel this way too. When I asked my husband how he felt about all of this, he said something like, "Sure, I think about those things too. But I'm not overly worried about it. I don't lose sleep over it. I know Kate will get the help she needs. She's going to speech [therapy]." And he was right. She did get better. It's the way of a woman, and particularly a mother, to process these events differently than a man. Men are typically solution-focused ("she's going to speech therapy"), whereas women are more concerned with immediate feelings and understanding the "whys" of the event ("Why did this happen to Kate? Aren't you worried too?")

I should point out that while 11 percent of moms in the study meet the criteria for anxiety and depression, the majority (89 percent) did not. Don't feel you are bound to be diagnosed with anxiety or depression just because this study says you *might*. It's a good idea, though, to keep your antennae up should you start to feel a little "off," especially if you have a family history or a personal tendency to develop depression or anxiety.

It's downright hard work to be a mother. Some say, "It's the hardest job I ever loved." If you're a mom reading this, congratulate yourself. It's a great step towards understanding and educating yourself on CAS so you can be even better at the important job you already do: being a mother.

The road of parenting is spotted with bumps and potholes. There will be others in your parenting journey too. Understanding and helping your child with CAS is just one of those bumps. Go ahead and whine and cry about CAS if you need to. I know you weren't expecting it. But know, too, that there are ways to cope.

Are You Depressed? Anxious?

Curious as to what some symptoms of depression/anxiety are?

- Lack of interest or enjoyment in things you previously enjoyed
- Eating too little or too much (appetite changes)
- Weight gain or loss
- Jittery feeling; heart feels like it's beating "too fast"
- Feeling as though you are always holding your breath
- Sleeping too much or too little (restless sleep)
- Headaches or other bodily aches and pains that are new for you
- Excess worry or guilt
- Poor concentration
- Loss of energy

If you find yourself saying "yes" to more of these points than not, it may be time to see your physician. You are not alone. An estimated 14–18 million folks in the US suffer from depression and anxiety. Many physicians are comfortable treating your symptoms. (Family practitioners and internists are becoming more comfortable discussing mental health.) It never hurts to share your concerns with your doctor. He or she is there to help.

What's a Mom to Do?

Amy Baskin and Heather Fawcett, authors of *More Than a Mom: Living a Full and Balanced Life When Your Child Has Special Needs*, offer a multitude of helpful suggestions:

Get the most out of life. Even though moms often bear the brunt of the work involved in raising special needs kids, they need to have a happy and fulfilling life for themselves. Ask yourself: what's important to me? Make a list. Keep a journal. Write down what it is you want out of life. Most folks will divide their lives into these categories: friends, marriage/intimate relationship, physical/exercise, sleep, work, volunteer work, church/spirituality, housework/maintenance, education/knowledge, and health.

Draw a pie chart of the things in your daily life, add a percentage to how much time you think you spend on them. Are some pieces of the pie too small? Too big? How about making a chart with two columns: "Before we knew about CAS" and "Now we have CAS." Then compare and contrast what has changed. Determine your new priorities (getting your child to and from speech therapy, home practice) and find places where you can make compromises (I'll take her to therapy, if you [husband] can pick her up).

Determine how you keep your pitcher filled. We all need to fill our personal well from time to time. How do you do it? What do you need to feel energized and ready to go? It's different for everyone. For you, it may be a morning jog, an afternoon nap, time on Facebook, a crafty enterprise, a phone call to a good friend, or daily prayer. You need to find and make the time to keep your pitcher filled.

Know that you need breaks too. You will feel better if you schedule a break for yourself. Did you know that employers are supposed to give employees a fifteen-minute break for every four hours of work? Even if you are an at-home mom, you are still working and you deserve a break.

Reclaim past hobbies or explore new ones. Perhaps before you had kids, you loved to make handmade cards. Then kids came and you no longer had time or a place to store your craft supplies. Find them. Dust them off and start working on a card for your friend who just had a baby. Always wanted to learn about spelunking or knitting? Why not absorb yourself in learning about something new? You may find that you become less focused on the problems (of CAS) and more interested in something that revs you up.

Schedule time away. It doesn't have to be a trip to the Virgin Islands, but go somewhere, even if it is just to the hotel down the road for a night (or your parent's or friend's home). Put it on the calendar. You are that important.

Connect with your friends. No doubt you will meet others who have a child with CAS or other speech-language needs. That's great. Share stories and feelings about your unique experience, but remember that you have other friends too. It's like when you first had a baby and all you wanted to do was hang out with other new moms; your childless friends felt jilted. Connect with friends who aren't all about CAS, too.

Join a Support Group. You may want to look into a support group for parents and caregivers of children with CAS. You'll learn a lot, connect, commiserate, and have a unique bond with others. You can start by joining online support groups. Apraxia Kids has official Facebook groups you can join. Go to www.apraxia-kids.org and find the community drop-down menu. You'll find support groups there. There may be a group in your local area like the Apraxia Connection (www.theapraxiaconnection. org) in the Chicago area. For help finding a support group, ask your SLP or early intervention team or even consider starting your own (see chapter 16).

Remember that you are not alone. Ask friends and family specifically for their support. Try something like this: "I know you and I don't always respond to stress/ change in the same way. But right now I really need you just to listen to me as I work through Kate's diagnosis." Periodically, check in with your partner; ask what he or she needs/wants right now in the CAS journey, then share your needs/wants. We'll cover more relationship/marriage concerns later in this chapter.

Learn about CAS and terminology that goes along with the diagnosis. You may want to seek out more information than this book provides. Go for it. If you don't understand something your child's SLPs says, ask. You will uncover lots of terminology and abbreviations. Don't ever think your question is "stupid;" it's stupid *not* to ask for clarification.

Use coping strategies that have worked for you in the past. Whatever it is—getting a massage, heading to the gym, eating a bucket of popcorn at the movies, or reading a juicy new book—it's important that you take care of yourself.

What Stage Are You In?

We're often so concerned about what "stage" our kids are at, but moms have stages too. According to Ann Pleshette Murphy in her book, *The Seven Stages of Motherhood: Making the Most of Your Life as Mom* (Knopf, 2004), they are:

Stage 1: Altered States—Pregnancy, Birth, and the 4th trimester

Stage 2: Finding Your Footing—Finding Yourself (months 4–12)

Stage 3: Letting Go—The Toddler Years, One and Two

Stage 4: Trying to Do It All—The Preschool Years (ages 3–6 years)

Stage 5: Reading the Compass to God-Knows-Where (years 6–10)

Stage 6: Living in the Gray Zone: The Preteen Years (10–13 years)

Stage 7: It Gets Easier…and Then They Leave: The Teen Years (13–18 years)

Can you see how there are some parallels between these stages and Elisabeth Kübler-Ross's stages of grief? Can you see how sometimes you vacillate between several stages at once?

Dads Cope Too!

Since I'm not a dad, I can't give you a blow-by-blow account of how it feels to be a dad who's just heard that his child has CAS. I can recall, though, how blasé my husband seemed to be at hearing Kate's diagnosis, "Oh, hmm . . . well, now we know." I cocked an eyebrow and looked at him like, "What?! That's all you're going to say?" Just as the German study on mental health mentioned at the beginning of the chapter found, mothers often take on the lion's share of the work in caring for a child with speech and language difficulties.

But that's not to say dads never do. There are househusbands and dads who decide to quit their full-time jobs-for-pay to tend to the daily needs of such a child. There are families who make a conscious decision to co-parent—literally in a 50/50 fashion, job-share, and other arrangements.

Dads worry too. Their list of concerns may differ from a mom's, though. Dads often worry about the financial costs of speech therapy. They may be concerned about insurance issues and logistical problems such as who will take your little one to and from therapy. They may fear for their child's future—but they haven't gotten as far as visualizing her socializing in college. Their fears may be more immediate—like whether she'll be reading at an age-appropriate level or attending kindergarten with her peers.

I don't want to stereotype here; there are all kinds of people out there. Generally, though, men don't share their emotions as freely as women. Men typically aren't as chatty as women. Men often like to *solve* problems. Women often enjoy *talking about* problems. Men may gather their information differently than women. Not all men will go to their friends first for information about CAS. They will likely go to the internet. Men may shut themselves off from the family (playing golf, working longer hours) while processing information about CAS. Men care just as deeply as women but need time to absorb it all.

If you are a father reading this, take your time to process the information in your own way, but please discuss it at a later time with your spouse/partner. If you are the mother, give your husband or partner some breathing room. You might try scheduling a time to talk—e.g., "After your workout, I'd really like to talk about Treyvon's CAS."

Your Marriage—Seeing Things Eye to Eye

You knew it was coming. We can't talk about Mom and Dad in separate sections and call it done. Not if you are married—or in a partnered, live-in arrangement. As a joint force behind your child's success and rearing, it's important that we not ignore the marriage relationship.

By now, you know just how hard it is to be a parent *and* be a couple. Having kids puts a strain on your relationship (constant care, finding private couple time, finances, and equitable division of "work"). Add in a kid with CAS, and it's *really* no walk in the park. You can do it; you just may have to try a bit harder and use creative tactics.

In *Married with Special Needs Children: A Couple's Guide to Staying Connected*, authors Laura E. Marshak and Fran Pollack Prezant identified these common stresses on relationships:

- **Lack of diagnosis:** In the early stages, you just knew your child wasn't communicating like she should be. I bet you argued about this in some fashion. Now that you have a diagnosis, do you argue about that? "She does. She does not!"

- **Information overload:** You may be hearing conflicting information from specialists, other parents, or your relatives. This ultimately leads couples to confusion and delay, and sometimes anger.

- **Financial issues:** One parent may feel the CAS burden more than the other and may have had to quit work. The family is now unable to draw on that income. Plus, products, books, resources, testing, and therapy all cost money. With less income, it's no surprise that financial stress can come between couples.

- **Time constraints:** You need time to do the basics in running a household like paying bills and cooking. If your children are school-age, factor in time for assisting with homework and communicating with teachers, as well as IEP meetings. Now that you have a child with CAS, there are therapy appointments to keep and speech practice at home. You may have to rearrange your work schedule or negotiate with daycare providers for a flexible schedule that will accommodate therapy.

- **Mental and physical fatigue:** Exhaustion can bring out the worst in marital partners. You're cranky and your needs aren't getting met. Who *wouldn't* snap?! Take turns being "on," look for respite care (Grandma and Grandpa, family friends— see later section in this chapter), teach independence skills for your child so you don't have to do *everything* for her.

- **Dealing with reactions from others:** Others may tend to identify the CAS and not your child. You may deal with pity, curiosity, rude comments. It's completely natural to feel stressed by these comments and figuring out how to deal with them. Come up with a joint plan with your spouse/significant other so you're on the same page. Refer to the section "Do You Need to Justify Your Child's CAS?" in chapter 14 for additional guidance.

> **Parents Share**
>
> "I felt the need to justify speech therapy so much. I had to decline play dates often. 'No, we can't because we're at speech therapy [at that time].' I wondered if apraxia [CAS] was in his school record and how that would affect how teachers looked at him. My anxiety level just kept going up."—Small Talk: All About Apraxia parent participant

A study in the *Journal of Health and Behavioral Science* (March 2009) reported that parents of children with disabilities face more daily stress. Through a parent survey and a clinical measure of stress (measuring the amount of cortisol—the stress hormone—in parent's saliva), researchers found that 50 percent of their days are considered "stressful" as compared to 40 percent of the days for parents who did not have a child with a disability. *Stress* was referred to as time, daily hassles, positive events, and physical symptoms of fatigue. The disabilities in this study did not include CAS specifically, but did include ADHD, Down syndrome, and bipolar disorder, among others.

Parents Cope: What's a Couple to Do?

Know that you and your partner may deal with emotions differently. How do your coping styles differ? Do you even know *your own* coping style? Be honest. How does your partner cope? If you don't know, ask.

Let your spouse hear the information about CAS from someone other than you. Whether your spouse hears something about CAS from your SLP directly, or from a book or online, it gives him or her some control in your child's progress. You might try printing out an article or forwarding it to your partner's email. Set aside a day and time discuss it. Consider learning about your child's CAS together as a way of bonding.

Schedule a Date. Put it on the calendar, secure a sitter, and go on an old-fashioned date. It doesn't have to be fancy or involved, just alone time with your partner. Go on a walk, see a movie, chat at a coffee shop, have a picnic. Make it something you two enjoy doing together. Try not to talk about the kids, if you can help it.

Have a "date" at home. You can schedule a weekly date night right at home after the kiddos have gone to bed. My husband and I have a standing agreement that every Saturday night we don't do anything but hang out with each other. That means no laundry folding or internet surfing. Instead, we may get takeout and play a game of Scrabble. Have a fire, watch a movie, try a new wine. No chores and no kids.

Dream build. One mother whose daughter has CAS mentioned she and her hubby like to "dream build"—talk about future ambitions and family goals. Your version of dream building may be walking the aisles of a local home improvement store and dreaming of the projects you'd like to tackle. Or you may enjoy thinking about retirement plans or how you're going to create that tree farm you've always wanted.

Know when to say "enough." We all need time alone. Find time to pursue your own interests independently. Believe it or not, parents who connect well when they are together have other emotional and social outlets besides one another.

Laugh! Humor is the balm to a stressful or worrisome situation. Laughter increases endorphins (feel-good hormones) and opens the nasal passage so your brain gets more oxygen. Even smiling has a similar effect. Look for situations in your life—be it "CAS moments" or not—and laugh at them. I'll never forget the day when Jim took then four-year-old Kate to the mall for a cookie. They were sitting in the café area of a bakery that opened to the mall. It was spring, so the Easter Bunny had replaced Santa. Kate's eyes got as big as saucers as she pointed to the bunny hut and exclaimed, "No Ho Ho . . . Big Hop Hop!" We still laugh about it to this day.

Leaving Your Child with a Sitter

You desperately need a date night, but Grandma and Grandpa aren't available. You need a sitter you can trust and feel at ease with. Make sure you tell your babysitter about your child's difficulty in communicating. You don't even have to call it childhood apraxia of speech. Simply say something like, "Aleena has a hard time using her words. She can understand everything you say to her; she just might not be able to respond—right away, or at all. Just have fun with her and if you get stuck, ask her to show you [lead you to] what she means—that usually works for us." Of course, tell the sitter what works for *your* child.

If you are "shopping" for a babysitter, consider asking at your speech clinic for a student who may be interning, or a local college's nursing, education, speech pathology, or child psychology department. Most college students appreciate the extra money, and if you start with these departments you're almost sure to find a sitter who likes kids.

> ### Could You Benefit from Couples' Counseling?
> That's a tough decision involving lots of emotions. Generally, couples' counseling can provide you with these benefits:
> (1) new perspectives, an unbiased approach, a third person's point-of-view;
> (2) help in questioning your assumptions, goals, and intrapersonal dynamics;
> (3) ways to break dysfunctional patterns in your relationship.
>
> (From *Married with Special-Needs Children* by Laura Marshak and Fran Prezant)

The Logistics of Parenting Your Child

Let's go ahead and hammer out some boring, household maintenance things that need to happen before we jump into how the rest of the family (other children, grandparents, etc.) are dealing with your child's CAS. First of all, you will need to take stock of your family goals, schedule, and routine at some point in this journey. You may formally sit down and hash this out with your partner. Or you may need to deal with it on the spur of the moment. For example, your child needs to get to speech therapy at 3:00 p.m. on Mondays. Getting her there may be relatively easy if you are a stay-at-home parent, but what if you're not?

Consider changes to your job. It's an important part of who you are and helps keep the family living the lifestyle you've chosen. You may find that the only way you can give your child the time and attention she needs, however, is to cut back on your work. In my case, I wasn't working because I was on maternity leave, and then we relocated to a new city. When we learned of Kate's diagnosis, I saw it as a "sign" that I needed to be home with the girls. I didn't go back. But I missed interacting with adults; plus I had a hard time understanding just how important my being home was for Kate. Look for ways to make it work: cut back to part-time, work a condensed week so you can have a three-day weekend, job-share, work evenings or weekends if you can, telecommute, or start your own business.

Map out household chores. What goes into running your home? Make a chart. Who usually does what? Add in your new duties: schedule therapy appointment, drive to therapy, observe therapy sessions, read and learn about CAS and therapy techniques, research and purchase products to help your child with communication, follow up with therapists/SLPs (in-person, over the phone, via email), connect with teachers and special education specialists at the school. Now, determine how these things will be divvied up.

Maximize your peak energy time. Learn to manage your time better by finding your peak energy times. It may not be a specific time of day like 2:00 to 5:00 p.m.—instead, it may be more like two hours after you wake up, or after you've exercised. Tackle the things you hate to do first and then reward yourself with something more pleasurable. Don't deliberate on the task. Just do it!

Document everything! You will be making more phone calls, sending more texts and emails, and seeing more paper come through your door. Keep notes on any communication in a file or binder. Keep a journal or blog on your child's progress and day-to-day changes, because it gets difficult to recall specifics later. Even just marking things on the kitchen calendar can trigger a memory: "Said a 3-word sentence today!"

Keep your eyes peeled for fine and gross motor development. Children with CAS may also have global apraxia (a.k.a. dyspraxia, developmental coordination disorder, limb-kinetic apraxia). You may get so focused on communication issues that you fail to recognize that your child is having difficulties in other areas of development. If so, your child may need occupational or physical therapy.

You and the Family Medical Leave Act (FMLA)

What It Is: A federal law that protects parents' jobs if they need to take time off to tend to a child with a health concern, including a speech-language disorder.

How It Works: Parents can take an unpaid leave of absence (LOA) for as little as a few hours to as much as three months and be guaranteed a job to return to. If you need to take regular time off to get your child to speech therapy a couple of times a week, your employer has the right to make reasonable job reassignments. However, they must maintain your current salary and benefits.

How to Qualify: You must have been working in your current position for at least 12 months, and also must meet these additional conditions: you have worked at least 1,250 hours in the last 12 months and your employer has at least 50 employees within a 75 mile radius, and you intend to return to work at the end of your LOA. (A few states and the District of Columbia have passed laws enabling employees of smaller companies to qualify.) Talk to your manager or HR representative about securing the proper paperwork.

Your Other Kids

It's hard enough to parent your children equally anyway. It's even more challenging when one of them has CAS. It's hard not to think about CAS when you are interacting with your child. You wonder what it is (again). What caused it (will we ever know)? What can you do? How can you help? And the granddaddy of all questions, will she ever be okay? So, you cater to your child with CAS. You try to make life easier for her. And in doing so, your other kids may get—or feel like—they get the short end of the stick. It's not intentional; it just is. The bottom line is this: sibs worry too. They need support and a peer group and they need time with their parents. Specifically, though, siblings are struggling with lots of questions, concerns, and feelings.

Debbie Feit, author of *The Parent's Guide to Speech and Language Problems*, advises parents to look out for feelings of confusion and worry, anger and jealousy, embarrassment and guilt, and protectiveness and pride. The examples and descriptions of common sibling feelings below were adapted from her book.

Confusion and Worry: When we learn of our child's CAS diagnosis, we're confused and worried, but have skills in place for coping. Our other children may not. Try to keep discussions about CAS between you and your spouse or partner. Little ears hear a lot. If you feel comfortable—and your other children are at an appropriate age—share with them a bit about what's going on: "Arianna has a hard time using her words. We go to speech so she can get better." Consider taking your other children to the clinic so they can see what's happening. You may or may not want to label the disorder by referring to it as childhood apraxia of speech, depending on your other child(ren)'s age(s) and maturity level.

Anger and Jealousy: Even though you've explained your child's CAS to her siblings and told them why it's important for you to spend extra time with her, they still may think it's unfair. That's completely normal. Talk to them about their feelings: "I know it's hard for you to see me working with Grant on his speech issues all the time. I wish things were different too. I love you very much too." Make a date to spend with your other child(ren) on something important to them—studying for a science test, shopping for new school shoes.

Embarrassment and Guilt: Your other children may not know who to turn to when they want to talk about their sibling's CAS. Sometimes siblings are embarrassed when their friends make fun of their sister who "doesn't talk." Other times, they may feel guilty when they lose their patience with their sibling because they just can't understand what she's trying to say. Let your other children know that this is normal, and give them the opportunity to talk to you about it.

Protectiveness and Pride: Some siblings, especially older ones, may become protective of your child with CAS. They may become good "speech therapists" to your child with CAS, quizzing her on words or reaching her in a way you or your child's SLP may not be able to. For example, a mother in Illinois named Courtney shares this:

My daughter is three and a half and a little "advanced" in terms of speech development. She will help her five-year-old brother when he says something incorrect. For example, "No, Ryan. The 'p' comes from your lips. Say 'up' with your lips." Or, "'Go' comes from your throat," and she points to her throat. It's cute and helps some of the time; but sometimes Ryan won't have anything to do with it.

Coping Corner for Sibs

■ Let your other children know you love and value them.

■ Talk about how everyone in the family has strengths and weaknesses. List them for each family member.

■ Be open and honest about your child's disability and how it affects the family. Give concrete examples: "We'll have to spend an hour or so each week at Ms. Jen's office. You can bring your homework, and we can work on it together while we are there."

■ Teach your children about CAS. As mentioned in the beginning of this chapter, you may want to hold a family "in-service" on CAS. Enlist older kids to do a little research on it and present it to the family. You may be surprised how eager they are to participate.

■ Give them an explanation to share with others, should they ask. Practice saying something like, "My brother has childhood apraxia of speech. It's a speech disorder. He can't say what he wants to say because his brain and mouth have a hard time working together."

■ Role-play what they may say if someone says something hurtful. For example, your other children are taunted on the playground: "Oh, your sister is dumb. She can't even talk right." Yikes! How can your children respond in a diplomatic way?

■ Suggest they connect with other kids who have a sibling with special needs. It doesn't have to be CAS, but they can validate and share feelings anyway.

■ Your child's school counselor may offer a group for kids who have a sibling with special needs. Look into it.

■ The Sibling Support Project is an online resource your child(ren) may find comfort in. It's a national program with goals to promote peer support and education. Check it out at www.siblingsupport.org to see available workshops or participate in an online group, among others.

■ Ask around—your speech clinic, your parent-friends, and online support groups may know of a special sibling group in your local area.

Here are some resources for additional guidance:

■ ***Siblings of Children with Disabilities: Enhancing the Lives of Siblings of Children with Disabilities*** by Avidan Milevsky (www.psychologytoday.com/us/blog/band-brothers-and-sisters/201406/siblings-children-disabilities).

- ***Views from Our Shoes: Growing Up with a Brother or Sister with Special Needs,*** edited by Donald J. Meyer (Woodbine House, 1997) is a collection of 45 short essays written by kids ages four to eighteen who share what it's like to be a sibling of someone with a disability.

- ***The Sibling Slam Book: What It's Really Like to Have a Brother or Sister with Special Needs*** edited by Donald J. Meyer (Woodbine House, 2005). This book includes eighty teenagers' views of what it's like to have a brother or sister with special needs in the vein of a "slam book" passed around school. It tackles tough questions such as "Do you like hanging out with your sib?"

  Younger siblings will find comfort in these titles:

- ***My Brother Is Very, Very Special*** by Amy Glorioso May (Trafford Publishing, 2004) doesn't mention CAS by name, but is a great introduction to speech and language disorders for preschool through school-aged children. Written by an "apraxia mom."

- ***I Want to Be Your Friend*** by Angela Baublitz (Apraxia Kids, 2019) was also written by a mother whose daughter has CAS. This book includes photographs of young Emma as she does normal, everyday things in addition to working with her SLP on her CAS. (Available only from the Apraxia Kids website/store.)

- ***Billy Gets Talking: A Preschooler's Journey Overcoming Childhood Apraxia of Speech*** (2019), written and illustrated by Mehreen Kakwan, MA, CCC-SLP, this book follows Billy, who has difficulty moving his lips, jaw, and tongue to clearly say the words in his head. But Billy finds his words with the help of his SLP and his family.

- ***Something to Say about My Speech*** (2018), by Eden Molineux, MS, CCC-SLP, is all about understanding speech and language differences, self-advocacy, and embracing diversity. Characters' strengths and interests are highlighted, and readers gain a better understanding of how to support communication.

- ***Hooway for Wodney Wat*** by Helen Lester (Sandpiper Books, 2002), a picture book for kids aged four to eight, stars a rat who can't pronounce the letter *r*. Thanks to his speech problem, he's able to outsmart the class bully.

- ***Charlie Who Couldn't Say His Name*** by Davene Fahy (Limerock Books, 2004) focuses on a little boy who has a hard time pronouncing his own name. With the help of his school SLP, he is able to overcome this obstacle.

- ***It's Okay to Be Different*** by Todd Parr (Little, Brown Books for Young Readers, 2009) is not about speech and language issues per se, but it does let readers know that different is okay.

- ***Ruby Mae Has Something to Say*** by David Small (Dragon Fly Books, 1999) is about Little Ruby's dream of talking to the United Nations about "universal peace and understanding." At first, she's tongue-tied, but she overcomes her problem.

- Finally, refer to the previous chapters' resources and recommended reading. You may find that what helps your child with CAS cope will also help your other children.

Extended Family and Grandparents

Grandparents care and want to help. In one of my CAS 101 groups there was a grandmother who attended right along with her daughter. They both wanted to hear the information so they could both support their (grand)daughter. I was thrilled to see her support.

Like parents, grandparents worry when a child does not seem to be learning to talk according to the regular timetable. Sometimes, before a child is diagnosed with CAS, it is a grandparent who urges the parents to find out what is wrong. For example, it was my parents who urged me to get things checked out with an SLP. They continued to pester me, "So is she talking yet? Any new words?" Other grandparents may take longer to key into what is wrong, or may think their role is to reassure you that everything is all right. For example, they may tell you that "Einstein was a late talker," "She's just waiting until she can say it perfectly," or "It's no big deal."

Once you have a diagnosis, you will want to choose how to break the news to the grandparents. How you approach this may depend on whether they were the ones urging you to get an evaluation or the ones telling you that everything would be okay. Usually it is helpful to start slowly by telling them what CAS is all about. Give them some resources. Print them out if your child's grandparents are not internet savvy. Let them soak in the new information.

Follow up with them by phone, text, or email: "Have you had a chance to read that information on childhood apraxia of speech yet? What did you think?" Just like you, they may have a hard time believing the diagnosis. It is not unusual for grandparents to feel stunned and have numerous questions—what does it mean, what will happen, where did it come from, and how can they help? Grandparents will likely hear terms they have never heard before and will need support and understanding, just as the rest of us do. For example, "Grandma Gloria" shares: "I had never heard of CAS. I asked a lot of questions, there were moments that my daughter seemed to be upset by all of my questions. So, I took the bull by the horns and googled websites so I could understand the 'whys' and 'how comes.'"

One mother in my Small Talk: All About Apraxia group said that she received quizzical looks when she shared her son's CAS diagnosis with her own parents. "Are you sure, honey?" her mother asked. She went on to explain that she thought her mother's response was to make her feel better: "I think my mom was probably trying to suggest that it might not be as serious as it sounds."

Another parent spoke up and said, "I had a hard time trying to explain what CAS was to my parents. Once I finally started relating it to Uncle Bob's stroke, they totally got it." While the treatment of CAS is similar to the rehabilitation following a stroke, it's not exactly the same. True, kids with CAS need to learn how to use the motor system to articulate correctly and intelligibly, but CAS *starts* in childhood and is typically not a result of a stroke. However, if you and your family have had a close connection with someone who has had a stroke, then this can be a good metaphor.

Sometimes grandparents really don't "get" it, even after you've explained what CAS is all about. One Small Talk participant relayed: "I hated it so much when my father-in-law mimicked my son's grunting. He [the grandfather] thought it was funny and would laugh, thinking he'd get my son to say something eventually. It doesn't work that way. I finally had to say something to my husband so he'd talk to his dad. It was demeaning."

In my experience, grandparents are much more likely to be understanding and helpful once the diagnosis has sunk in. For example, one mother told me that her parents were particularly helpful with the new diagnosis: "They would call me up out of the blue to check in. They wanted to know how speech was going. Once, they even sent me a newspaper clipping about CAS. I thought it was really sweet."

Here are some simple ways to help you might consider suggesting to grandparents:

- Repeat and emphasize words they say in conversation with your child: "**Park** . . . let's go to the **park.** Can you say **park**?" (Part of what you are doing here is modeling.)
- Wait for a response.
- Practice sounds: "*P* makes the 'puh' sound. Can you say 'puh'?"
- Remind them how to praise: "That's it . . . you're getting it. Now try making your lips look like this." They may have to watch you and your child in action a few times to get the dialog down.

Tip: Your child very much wants to imitate and mimic you. But when you suggest or demand that your child say *park* (or *water* or *ball* or whatever) in order to receive a trip to the park (a glass of water, the ball), it might foster frustration or resentment—on your part and your child's. It's not that your child *won't* say it; it's that she *can't*. Please be patient and know she's just as eager to speak as you are to hear those sweet words.

Emphasize that your child is just like any other child. Just because she can't communicate well doesn't mean she isn't as much fun to be around as their other grandchildren. Tell them what your child enjoys doing. Maybe Grandpa can take her fishing? Or Grandma can bake cookies with her? There are numerous activities they can do together that don't involve talking. Think specifically of your child's grandparents, interests, and activity level and compare them with your child. You may find that they have a lot in common!

Distinguish between difficulties speaking and difficulties understanding. Finally, remind grandparents that your child can understand almost everything and is smart and capable. It will just take longer to hear her sweet voice. Grandparents should not talk down to your child or talk about her as if she's not there; instead, encouraging active and engaging communication is key.

Depending on your relationship with your child's grandparents, and how far away you live from them, the ways they can support your family through CAS will vary. Here are some ideas to get you started:

- Phone calls, Skype, or FaceTime can prompt and encourage your child's developing speech. Keep a "question and comment" pad handy so you can jot down ideas of things for Grandma and Grandpa to talk to your child about when they call. You'll likely answer the phone first, so fill them in on the list before handing the phone over to your child. My own father once confided, "When a grandchild has apraxia [CAS] and lives out of state, it's hard to have a phone call with them. You want to hear their sweet little voice, but you can't. Grandparents miss out on that."

- If internet access is available, see if your child and her grandparent(s) can exchange daily or weekly emails, or try communicating with Skype.

- Ask if your child's grandparents can give you some respite care: for example, a sleepover at Grandma's or an outing to the movies, park, or library.

- Inquire whether driving duty to and from speech therapy can be shared.

- Remember, speech therapy is important. Please do not cancel speech therapy because grandparents are coming over.

- If there are opportunities for grandparents to be involved at your child's school, make sure your child's grandparents are aware of them. "My dad read a book to Emma's class, and he has such a great reading voice. It made his day—and Emma's," shares a mother from my Small Talk group.

- Encourage grandparents to practice reading and sight words with your child.

You may or may not feel comfortable hitting up Grandma and Grandpa for financial assistance with the extra costs of CAS, but if they offer, have a few things in mind:

- Assist in paying for private education or a tuition-based preschool.

- Help pay for the cost for testing that's not covered by insurance.

- Reimburse you for co-pays and therapy deductions.

- Make a charitable contribution to a group that offers resources or conducts research on CAS, such as Apraxia Kids (www.ApraxiaKids.org) or ASHA (www. asha.org).

- Offer a "scholarship fund" that parents can use to set up their own group for CAS, or pay membership dues to various special need resources.

- Pay the tuition for a parent to attend a conference on CAS.

- Help pay for family, marital, or individual therapy, if needed.

- Pay for a subscription to a speech journal for Mom and Dad, or a children's magazine for your grandchild.

- Assist in covering the costs of products, educational toys, equipment, and pricy software or apps.

Grandparents need to be reminded not to focus too much time, energy, or resources on one grandchild. All grandchildren have specific and unique strengths, weaknesses, and interests.

Say That Again?! Chapter Summary

For most parents, getting a diagnosis of CAS sends them on an emotional roller coaster. You may have experienced even more ups and downs as you read through this chapter. As you deal with the initial diagnosis, and then move through a variety of stages in coming to terms with your child's diagnosis, it's important to keep the big picture in view: you will survive and so will your child. I hope you found some of the suggestions in the "coping corners" helpful. Please review the section on resources and recommended reading for additional support and guidance. But remember—most of all, you can help your child by taking care of you.

Recommended Resources

- *Going Solo While Raising Kids with Disabilities* by Laura Marshak (Woodbine House, 2015). While not specific to speech/language disorders, this empathetic book has good suggestions for single parents who don't have a spouse/partner to lean on for support.

- *All Joy and No Fun: The Paradox of Modern Parenting* (Ecco, 2015) by Jennifer Senior. Hailed as one of the most important books on parenting, this title explores how parents are more invested in their children's lives than before—participating in day-to-day lives, attending to details with more thought—and yet, we aren't particularly happy.

- *Nurturing the Soul of Your Family: 10 Ways to Reconnect and Find Peace in Everyday Life* by Renee Peterson Trudeau (New World Library, 2013) helps you reclaim yourself with tips on relationships and self-care.

- You may also appreciate *A Different Kind of Perfect: Writings by Parents on Raising a Child with Special Needs* by Cindy Dowling (Trumpeter, 2006), a book in which multiple families share their stories, all very eloquently written, with a focus on the stages of grief. Easy to read in short segments of time.

- *The Life We Never Expected* by Andrew and Rachel Wilson (Crossways Press, 2016). With two children with special needs, this married couple honestly shares what it's like dealing with the daily struggles and how their faith colors their relationship.

- In *The Sea Is So Wide and My Boat Is So Small: Charting a Course for the Next Generation*, Marian Wright Edelman (Hyperion, 2008) writes an inspiring letter to parents about how difficult it is to be a good parent, but how important it is to be the person you want your kids to emulate.

- *Perfect Madness: Motherhood in the Age of Anxiety* by Judith Warner (Riverhead, 2006) This is a haunting, bold, in-depth look at intensive parenting: its structural and societal causes, and what it means for mothers in particular. But why are mothers today suffering from such an unprecedented degree of anxiety? A thought-provoking and meaningful read with sociological undertones.

- If you are looking to find more hours in the day, you may like this book: *168 Hours: You Have More Time Than You Think*, by Laura Vanderkam (Portfolio, 2010).

- *Things Good Mothers Know: A Celebration* by Alexandra Stoddard (Collins Living, 2009) may give you some insight and ideas on parenting.

- *Being the Other One: Growing Up with a Brother or Sister Who Has Special Needs,* by Kate Strohm (Shambhala, 2005).

- *The Other Kid: A Draw It Out Guidebook for Kids Dealing with a Special Needs Sibling* by Lorraine Donlon (Llumina Press, 2017). Siblings of a child with special needs often receive a smaller share of their parent's time, energy, or financial resources, and may experience jealousy, guilt, sadness, anger or embarrassment. But siblings may also develop positive traits, such as empathy, tolerance, insight and loyalty.

- *Speech Class Rules!* by Ronda Wojcicki, SLP-CCC, is a children's book about speech therapy that can help a youngster accept speech therapy as part of life.

Chapter 14

I Am More Than CAS

Tending to Your Child's Feelings

Of course *you* know your child is more than a diagnosis, but does your child? With speech therapy (ST) appointments, home drills, and intensive pre-schooling, it may be difficult to tease out "typical kid versus CAS kid." Socialization and fitting in with peers can be particularly tricky for these speech-challenged kids. Because this part of childhood is difficult, your youngster may have trouble coping or relating. He may come home in tears because the mean kids called him a name or because he wasn't accepted by the cool crowd. Of course, these types of heartbreaking scenarios can happen regardless of whether your child has CAS. Fortunately, there are things you can do to ease the hurt.

The Nuts and Bolts of This Chapter

- What parents can do to ensure—or at least assist with—their child's happiness
- How to have the "You-have-childhood-apraxia-of-speech" discussion with your child
- Helping your child engage in social situations and make and keep friends
- Dealing with and managing bullies, aggression, and other mental health issues
- Helping tween girls navigate the complex social climate
- Exercise and recreational activities as an outlet for coping and developing friendships

---

Well-Being versus Happiness

If asked their number one goal for their child, many parents would answer, "I just want him to be happy." When your child is diagnosed with CAS, however, you begin to fear that happiness may be elusive for your child—whether because he is constantly frustrated when he can't make his wishes known, because other kids might tease him, or because he may have trouble making friends. I want to help smooth this process for you.

In reality, you don't *just* want your kids to be happy; you want a lot more for them too. Sure, you want them to achieve what most of us think of as happiness—the state of mind encompassing the ideas of contentment, love, satisfaction, joy, and pleasure. But you also care about their well-being as a whole—and happiness is only part of that. Here's what authors Aaron Cooper and Erin Keitel say you really mean when you say, "I just want my kids to be happy" in their book by the same title (Late August Press, 2008):

- Good physical and mental health
- A life of meaning
- A closeness with others
- Acts of loving kindness
- A sense of gratitude
- A sense of spirituality
- An optimistic outlook
- Gratifying pursuits
- A "fine" character

The book explains that happy people create gratifying and challenging goals to pursue. They get caught up in the "flow" or the "zone," which psychologists believe leads to happiness. As a parent, we can help our kids—whether or not they have CAS—get into that happiness zone by encouraging and supporting their natural talents through hobbies, classes, after-school activities, and specialized camps. We can also encourage not just sports and academics at home, but respect, compassion, empathy, and courage among others.

Dr. Stanley Greenspan, MD, offers another take on qualities needed for a happy, healthy life in his book *Great Kids*:

1. Engagement: Relating to Others*
2. Empathy: The Ability to Care
3. Curiosity: An Inquiring Mind
4. Communication: The Transforming Power of Language*
5. Emotional Range: Passion and Balance
6. Genuine Self-Esteem: The Importance of Self-Awareness
7. Internal Discipline: Perseverance and Self-Control
8. Creativity and Vision: A Rich and Internal Life
9. Logical Thinking: Making Sense of the World
10. Moral Integrity: A Matter of Heart

I placed an asterisk next to the two qualities that made me cringe as I read through this book. It's not that I disagreed with Dr. Greenspan, but at that time I didn't feel my daughter could engage and relate to others (essential quality #1) or communicate clearly and effortlessly (essential quality #4); therefore, I felt she was doomed to become a non-great kid. Of course, that is not at all how this list should be interpreted. Kids with CAS can and do become "great kids" in spite of their communication skills. But it takes extra effort on their part, as well as ours, to develop and keep those skills alive.

What Can You Do?

Be empathetic. Have you ever been to a foreign country? Do you remember how nerve-wracking it was to try to communicate with the people in their own language? How stressed and isolated you felt at times? Your child may be feeling this same way—but in his own country, in his own language. Remind yourself and your child that he is still learning to-talk and that you are going to help him.

Don't let him get too frustrated. It's a fine line between having your child "reach" to say a word, or just accepting his attempt as "good enough." You can ask your child to repeat himself only so many times before you both get frustrated. Know when to stop and divert your child's attention before it all ends in tears or worse.

Build his self-esteem. Everyone is good at something. Find out what it is for your child: taking care of the dog/cat, being a good friend, sports, art . . . . The key is to mention these traits to your child often. Of course you don't want to sound like a broken record, or you risk taking away that good feeling your child gets each time he hears it. Catch him being good: "I really like how kind you are to your little sister. That makes me feel good."

Be honest about his weaknesses. Consider talking frankly about your child's difficulty with speaking: "I know sometimes it's hard for you to get the words out. It's just not fair. That's why we go see Miss Jen. She's helping you, and you are doing a good job." Or, you may want to try something like this: "I am sorry it's so hard for you to talk. If I could make it easier, I would. Do you know that everyone has something they aren't very good at? I am not good at baking, and Daddy isn't very good at gardening. We all have things we struggle with. But if we work hard, we can get better."

Find other ways to have fun with him. You don't always have to talk to enjoy each other's company. Look for opportunities to be together that use other skills. Take a walk together, play tag, draw, paint, or color. Create something with Play-Doh or clay. Bake cookies. Work in the garden. Ride bikes. Explore the local library. Go to a kid-friendly movie. Go wading in a creek. These kinds of nonverbal activities strengthen your bond with your child and let him know you love and accept him, regardless of his CAS.

Support him socially. Your child with CAS is busy with appointments, therapy, and preschool or school, but it's just as important to get him involved with activities to develop his social skills. He needs time to *just be a kid.* Make sure he has opportunities to be with other kids—playing with neighbors, hanging out at the park, attending a library story hour, or taking part in a parent-tot class. As your child gets older, consider enrolling him in a class on his own, even if his verbal skills aren't developed as much as you like. Some kids actually do better when they are on their own with peers and a facilitator/teacher.

(Some of these ideas were gleaned from *A Parent's Guide to Speech-Language Disorders* by Debbie Feit.)

Parents Share

A Glimpse of What It's Like to Have CAS

One night at bedtime, I was reading *Adventures at Shelby Stables* by Julie Driscoll (Battat, 2009) to seven-year-old Kate. A passage we came across reminded me so much of CAS. Whether or not the author has any knowledge of CAS, I am unaware. However, I was so struck by something that Lily Anna, the main character, said, that I wanted to share it:

> "Sometimes, at lunch, I'd hardly say a word—not because I didn't have anything to say. Oh no! I have lots of stuff going on in my head—lots and lots. But something happens from the point where I have a thought to where it should then come out of my mouth. It never does. And on occasion, when I do speak, I feel very awkward. I feel like running away, like one of the wild horses on my pajamas—running and running, never looking back."

I used this passage as an opportunity to ask Kate if that's how she sometimes feels. She nodded and got a little tearful. "Not everyone has apraxia, you know," she told me. Whenever I glimpse what it must be like to have CAS, it makes me that much more determined to support my daughter, boost her self-esteem, or make sure she knows she is loved.

Do You Need to Justify Your Child's CAS?

This is a huge question and not to be taken lightly. Do you ever feel the need to tell others about your child's difficulty communicating? How do you bring it up? In what circumstances? Following are some suggestions to get you thinking. Remember, just as no two kids with CAS are the same, neither are their parents. You have your own style of relating and communicating with others, so do what comes naturally.

The extent to which kids are accepted by peers (and often adults) depends partly on how parents manage the situation. Therefore, we have always presented Kate as "any other kid" in social situations.

That's not to say that there have not been hurtful times. Here are a few examples:

- When Kate didn't readily answer questions, her friendly and well-meaning great aunt said, "What's wrong? Cat got your tongue?" At first, Kate regressed and retreated, and I felt helpless and defensive. But after I calmly explained why it was hard for Kate to talk, everyone felt better.

- Sitting on Santa's lap at the mall was challenging for Kate, even at almost four years of age. She couldn't tell Santa what she wanted, so I had to jump in when I saw that Santa's prompts and attempts at rephrasing the question were bringing Kate close to tears.

- The professional photographer was trying to get Kate to smile by having her say "stinky feet," but she was pouting instead. At the time, her /s/ blends were a challenge. Kate knew she couldn't say "stinky feet" and was looking to me for guidance.

- Birthday parties may cause added stress and anxiety for you and your child. Kate had a hard time at a party when her peers wanted to play a game of tag. Kate wasn't sure how to play, let alone able to say, "Tag! You're it!" She was unable to ask for clarification and became tearful, clinging to my leg. Fortunately, I was there to understand what the problem was, but it didn't hurt any less.

- We also dealt with friendly neighbors who just wanted to ask Kate typical getting-to-know-you types of questions: how old are you, what's your name, where do you go to school? When Kate was unable to answer these questions, I worried that the neighbors might think she wasn't friendly, hadn't been taught any social skills, or worse.

There are countless other social situations that can be problematic for a child with CAS. It's impossible to anticipate all of them. You may want to consider having a few answers in your toolbox for situations such as these. Here are a few of my favorites:

- "He's still learning some words, but I think he's doing a great job."

- "He has a hard time talking sometimes. It's called childhood apraxia of speech. But he's really getting better."

- "Sometimes his words get stuck. Maybe you can help him out by saying, 'show me.'"

If you don't make a big deal out of it, others won't either. Privately, you may want to talk to your child about why it's hard to get the words out. You don't have to go into detail, but you can tell him that it's hard for him to talk because he has a condition called CAS. Remind him that CAS is the reason he goes to speech therapy, that he's making lots of progress, and that you love him regardless.

When you acknowledge that talking is hard work, or you say to your child, "Yes, that *is* a tricky word," you are likely giving him validation and relief that you understand. Consider sharing some of your own childhood experiences with speech issues, if you had them. My husband shared with Kate that he had speech therapy in school as a kid. She brightened, "You did?!" I told her that I get nervous when I need to speak in front of a group of people, and sometimes I just don't want to be social (introverted by nature).

How Other Parents Feel about This Topic

Here's a snippet of our discussion one evening during Small Talk: All About Apraxia:

"I absolutely hated when we all got together for a playdate at one of those bouncy places. We showed up a little late that day because my son had speech [therapy] first. The other mothers looked at me like they wanted an explanation," said Jill, mother of two-and-a-half-year-old Miguel. "They looked at me like I was the problem. Then they looked at Miguel and said, 'Why? He seems to talk fine.'" She then had to define CAS for these other mothers while supporting her son at the same time.

Another mother chimed in and said, "Yeah, it's like one big competition. I feel like I am competing with all of these other parents about whose kid is talking more or has a bigger, better vocabulary. Sometimes I just downplay the whole thing and don't even mention it."

A third mother said, "I cringe when they ask such probing questions—when, why, how . . . those questions really get to me. It's like [other parents] feel like CAS is contagious."

Another parent joked that she wished she had a card to hand out to people who ask. "If I could just shove a piece of paper under their nose about what apraxia is all about, then maybe they would stop asking so many pointed questions. I don't think people realize how sensitive this topic may be to parents [of kids with CAS]."

Talking to Your Child about CAS

When you talk with your child about why he has difficulty verbalizing his thoughts, feelings, and requests, try a little role-play. You'll know when the time is right. It may be after he comes inside feeling left out when other kids were organizing a sports team or when he couldn't verbally participate in a karaoke video game. Have a little dialog ready when the time comes. It may go something like this:

PARENT (from dad's perspective): We all have things we are good at doing and not-so-good-at doing. Let's see . . . you are really good at building things out of Legos. Your sister is really good at riding her bike. Mommy's really good at organizing. But there are some things we aren't so good at. For me, it's golf. Mommy's not very good at singing. Your sister, well, she's not very good at sharing. And you have trouble using your words.

CHILD: May or may not say much. Ask for his thoughts, anyway. Just because your child is having a difficult time communicating, doesn't mean you should avoid asking for his opinion or feelings. *Always present information to your child with CAS as though you are expecting an answer.*

PARENT: The reason you have a hard time using your words has a special name. It's called CAS. [Use the long formal name, childhood apraxia of speech, if you don't think it will confuse your child.] You've probably heard us say that word, haven't you?

CHILD: [Will likely nod his head].

PARENT: Well, CAS is the reason we go to speech therapy [see Miss Jen]. She helps you use your words better. Lots of kids need to go [to therapy] to learn to use their words better. What do you think about that?

CHILD: Let your child answer. Be prepared to answer some questions or hear that your child doesn't want to go to ST.

PARENT: You do know that we love you very, very much and are doing all we can to help you! [End with a hug.]

Sometimes kids just need to know what the big hoopla is all about. It helps to put things into words your child can understand. Doing so can validate your child's feelings and clear the air. Of course, kids don't need to know *too* much. Avoid getting into adult concerns such as how much therapies cost, evaluation results, insurance issues, and your own frustration. Share those things with your child's SLP in private or with a trusted friend or your partner. If you really find yourself struggling, you might consider seeing a professional counselor.

When you have a discussion with your child about CAS and why he needs to go to ST, he realizes how important it is to go to ST. He may feel special and empowered. It's always best to be upfront and honest with your kids when you can.

I should point out that not everyone agrees about sharing this information with their child. A father who attended my Small Talk: All About Apraxia group said: "This may have been one of the times my wife and I argued about CAS. I knew she was ready to tell our son [about CAS], and I stopped her. I feared that if he got wind of this information he might start thinking that something was wrong with him; he might stop trying."

In my opinion, it all comes down to these careful considerations: Is your child overly frustrated because he can't speak as well as others—or communicate his needs, wants, and desires? Do you feel he is at the point where he can understand that it's not "wrong" or "bad" if he has CAS? It could be that your child is not developmentally mature enough to understand—or care—why he can't speak well. The fact that your child sees a speech-language pathologist really is just *his* "normal."

Here are some ***don'ts*** when talking to others about your child's CAS:

- Don't share unless it is really necessary (teachers and caregivers need to know; neighbors might, strangers don't).
- Don't label him in front of others.
- Never make fun of or belittle your child's attempts to speak.
- Don't refer to your child as "mute" or "dumb" or "different," and don't allow others to either.

- Don't act like it's a big secret or that you are embarrassed by his inability to communicate well or clearly; kids pick up on that quickly.

Being Honest with Your Child

You may be wondering how—or if—I told Kate about the book I was writing. She knew I spent a lot of time on the computer. She knew she was going to ST because she couldn't communicate well. I didn't really have to sit down and say, "Mommy's writing a book about why you can't talk as well as the other kids your age." Kate's a smart cookie and pieced it all together. But we used the label "apraxia" when we talked about her speech problem. She knew she had CAS. We never kept it a secret from her.

It is important to be as honest as possible. Children sense dishonesty. Kate knew how important the book was to me—and to her. In turn, my efforts to connect with others and learn all I could about CAS helped Kate and our family.

Educating Others

Why not make a written handout about CAS? Keep these parameters in mind:

Format: Decide how you'd like to communicate this information. A plain note card with a computer printout with CAS specifics glued on it works great and is cheap. If you want to do a little more, you can print personal calling cards by going to a site such as www.shutterfly.com or www.snapfish.com and adding information on CAS directly to the card. Or try a hybrid approach: using your home computer, make small informational tags or labels and stick them to the back of a calling/business card. You might include a blurb about CAS in your annual holiday letter or card. Many people share information about their CAS journey on social media too. It's up to you how—or if—you do.

What to Say: Start by giving a simple definition of CAS such as this: "a motor-neurological speech disorder in which kids know what they want to say but can't coordinate the movements to do so." You can give a couple of specific examples: "You may have noticed that Henry has a hard time asking for what he wants—that's why he grunts and whines." Let them know that your child is seeing a speech-language pathologist/attending preschool and is making wonderful progress! Suggest a couple of ways others can help: "You can help by asking Henry to show you what he means/wants when he gets verbally frustrated. He knows what you are saying. It just takes longer for him to respond." End with something positive: "Henry is a fantastic kid and a great friend!" You may want to mention a website or book that has been particularly helpful to you. If you blog or have a website about your experience with your child's CAS, list it.

Reaction(s) to Expect: The majority of folks will be supportive and sympathetic. Some will be very appreciative and will enjoy the opportunity to help and get a glimpse into your life. Don't be surprised, though, if you get an "Oh-sorry-I-asked" sort of response. Some people may be very surprised that you actually have a prepared answer and may be taken aback. Good for you—you are being your child's advocate! Some may see handing out informational cards as bordering on rude. But then again, who's being rude—you for giving a detailed (yet concise) answer, or acquaintances for asking probing questions?

Helping Your Child Make and Keep Friends

We all want and need friends. But some kids—especially those with CAS—have difficulty initiating and maintaining friendships simply because they can't communicate as easily as their peers. It can lead to hurt feelings and feelings of exclusion, isolation, and frustration. You may want to sit down with your child—regardless of his age or verbal ability—and talk about what a good friend is. Generally, a good friend is someone you enjoy being around, shares common interests, and cares about you. Friendships don't always fall into place naturally or easily. They need to be cultivated and tended to. They need maintenance.

You may want to think about your own attitude toward friendships, status, and social structure. As a family, sit down and make a list of qualities you like in a friend on poster board or some other media. Consider doing some role-play to teach social skills. Scenarios may include the following:

- How to ask a friend to play
- How to decide on/negotiate what to do together
- How to ask questions
- How to listen without interrupting
- How to be a host or hostess
- How to end play

Most of these skills are learned informally by modeling. For kids with CAS, they may be harder to grasp. Try going to www.modelmekids.com for ideas and inspiration. This site has videos of social behavior acted out by kids. Have your child pay close attention to body language and facial expressions. Teach your child about those concepts with specific examples you can act out at home.

Social nuances can be tricky for kids with CAS, as well. They may not "get" jokes, sarcasm, or snide remarks. It's a part of life and growing up—there will always be rude people. You can practice role-play for these types of situations, too. In fact, your kids may really enjoy this type of exercise! Work also on comprehension and self-monitoring skills here. While you're at it, teach your child some kid-friendly jokes he can remember and recite in social situations. Look for a joke book at your local library.

If your child is struggling to make and keep friends despite your best efforts, consider looking for a social skills group—otherwise known as a "friendship circle," "lunch bunch," or something along those lines. Your child's preschool, day care, or church may offer something like this. If those places don't, your speech clinic likely does (or knows where to find them). These groups may be run by an SLP, a psychologist, or a social worker. It's a safe environment where kids can learn social skills such as introducing oneself, taking turns in conversations, listening, asking questions, working with others, problem solving, playing "nice," and reading social cues. Some clinics offer a combination-type class in which arts and crafts or eating/dining skills are worked on together with social skills. Participants are often matched based on skills, abilities, and goals. Classes generally run for four to six weeks and may meet once or twice a week. They can be pricey. Some insurance companies may cover these groups, but it's usually an out-of-pocket fee. Call your member services folks to find out what's covered.

If you just can't afford to enroll your child in a social skills group with an SLP, you have options. If you know of other families like yours, consider pooling your resources and doing one of two things:

■ Chip in to pay for a retired or part-time SLP, special/early education teacher, or grad student to help run a similar group. To find someone who may be interested and qualified, ask at your child's speech clinic, his school, a local university's speech-language or education departments, the county health department, or place a want ad in a local paper or community bulletin board.

■ Just start working with an interested group of dedicated parents. You can create a social skills co-op in which each family hosts the "class" at their home on a rotating basis. Each parent takes turns being the facilitator. Develop a curriculum first, make a schedule, develop your class list, and get going. The best thing about this scenario is it's free or low cost. Again, you can gain interest by creating flyers and posting them on community bulletin boards or talking with other parents at your child's speech clinic.

Emotional, Behavioral, and Mental Health Concerns

Despite your best attempts at easing your child into social situations and assisting his communication, you may still have concerns and worries about his emotional and behavioral health.

Kids with CAS may have difficulty regulating their emotions. It's hard to express them, because it's hard to talk. Kids who keep their emotions bottled up are called internalizers. They are at high risk for depression and anxiety—which can take the form of generalized anxiety disorder (GAD), obsessive-compulsive disorder (OCD), separation anxiety, social anxiety, or selective mutism in extreme cases. Those kids who "let it all out" can get very angry and frustrated, resulting in aggressive behavior and mood swings.

Having been a child and adolescent psychiatric RN, I present this information to make you aware of the possibilities you may encounter. I also know that with the right intervention (various therapies, including ST, social skills training, medication, etc.), these conditions can be managed quite well.

There is no way to tell whether your child will have a mental, emotional, or behavioral health issue. However, just as I advised you to look at family history for speech- and language-related concerns, you can do the same for mental, behavioral, and emotional health and use it as a gauge. Does anyone in your family tend to be a bit unstable in any of those realms? By gathering this information now, you may be better able to identify and treat any future behavioral problems as they crop up.

Several studies have suggested that some kids with psychiatric disorders may have had undiagnosed speech-language disorders or impairments. For example, E. B. Brownlie's 2004 study in the *Journal of Abnormal Psychiatry* found that there *may* be a correlation between what she terms "late adolescent delinquency symptoms." This is not to say that your child with CAS is going to grow up to become a delinquent! I present this information only so you can be alert for any red flags signaling the need for help as your child becomes more independent. These are the "delinquency symptoms" Brownlie refers to:

1. **School Functioning:** Negative school experiences, due to a variety of reasons, could lead to poor academic performance. Poor academic performance could be a sign of a learning disorder, and not delinquency.

2. **Executive Functioning:** Executive function is also known as self-regulation. It's the cognitive ability that allows one to plan, monitor, and change one's own behavior. Executive functioning relies heavily on the ability to self-talk (talk to yourself—usually silently—about what you should and should not do). It can be assumed that our children with CAS have difficulty with self-talk; therefore they *may* have difficulty with executive functioning. If it's compromised enough, it's possible the problem is related to an attention-deficit disorder.

3. **Social Functioning:** Because hanging out with friends often involves talking with them, kids with CAS may not interact with peers as often as other kids do. They may give up, or slink to the back of the room. Even at home, kids with CAS may not be able to communicate with their parents as openly as their siblings do, causing an unnecessary rift between family members. If social functioning gets too difficult, social anxiety may develop.

4. **Empathetic Functioning:** This is a fancy term for the ability to understand and relate to the feelings of others. Brownlie calls this a child's "social competence and moral development." Oppositional defiant disorder (ODD) can potentially develop from a child's inability to be empathetic.

If you are concerned about your child's behavior, contact a child psychologist or psychiatrist. You have nothing to lose. Ask around for a recommendation.

Each of these potential concerns (learning disorders, ADHD, social anxiety, and ODD) is addressed in Appendix A.

Dealing with Teasing and Bullies

No one is immune to the "mean kids." I bet you remember who the mean kids were when you were younger. They found anything and everything to be snarky about—your shoes, your braces, your bigger-than-average nose, your academic abilities—good or bad—and athletic inability. Nowadays, kids also have to contend with cyberbullying (nasty email, texts, Facebook, etc.), but much has remained the same. Kids get made fun of for all sorts of reasons, sadly even for speech impediments and other special needs. It's not fair and it's not right, but it happens. As parents, we need to be equipped to help.

First of all, let's clear the air: not all teasing is bad. A lot of kids—and families too—may engage in playful or good teasing. Everyone is having fun, laughing and smiling, and it can be seen as a sign of friendship. Kids know when this is happening because they notice the playful smiles, winks, and tone of voice. It's all about bonding and sharing a similar experience with peers.

Bad teasing, on the other hand, happens when your child is belittled, degraded, and left feeling upset. It comes in many forms: ridicule, name-calling, put-downs, verbal insults, and gesturing. Other kids may make fun of your child with CAS because he can't say words as effortlessly as his peers, or because he can't easily engage in make-believe play.

Perhaps the sting is worse if your child is being made fun of due to a speech-language issue, because it's something he can't really do much about. It hurts because it's devaluing and because your child feels unaccepted by his peers. All kids are constantly comparing themselves to their peers. Remember to acknowledge that your kiddo (and other children) have things they are naturally good at and not-so-good at.

A 2010 article in the *Journal of Clinical Child and Adolescent Psychiatry* explains that kids who get teased may have an inability to pick up on and respond to nonverbal cues by their peers, plus they may find it hard to understand the social meaning, and come up with solutions for resolving a conflict. All of which have some underlying connection to speech and language.

> *Today, [my son] is sixteen and a half years old and has many friends and is quite popular. This is a complete 180 from the little boy who was chronically bullied as a child. But, I won't kid you. It has taken a lot of work for him to be able to speak clearly and fluidly. I think when he was about fourteen or fifteen, his speech became pretty normal, but you could still tell.*—Janice, Edmonton, Alberta

What's a Parent to Do?

- *Stop, look, and listen.* Give your child some time and validation while at the same time reviewing your own behavior. Has your playful parenting humor crossed the line?

- *Don't overreact.* When your child first reports being bullied or teased, approach it neutrally and be supportive.

- *Support your child.* Let your child know that if the bully/teaser makes him feel bad, he can—and should—spend time with kids who make him feel good.

That's the easy part. Here's the nitty-gritty:

1. Teach self-talk. We all participate in self-talk all day long. What can you teach your child to say in his mind that will take the sting out of teasing? "I'm more important than that." "That's not true—I'm good at ___." Start by listing your child's positive traits. Do this together as a family at dinner: "You are fun, smart, a great artist, creative. . . ." Make a habit of bringing up your child's qualities and strengths often, and he will begin to internalize it. Then self-talk will come easily.

2. Ignore. My mom used to tell me, "Make like a duck and let the teasing roll off your back." Some kids don't really know what it means to ignore. You have to define it for them. Walk away, don't make eye contact, make the bully invisible/disappear. Role-play it at home—this ought to be fun and easy: "I'm going to pretend to ignore you. Let me show you how it's done" (smile).

3. Agree with the facts. "You're right. I am short (have a big nose, red hair)." Leave it at that. The bully will be dumbfounded.

4. Respond with a compliment. "I am amazed that you notice how I'm dressed every day. You are very observant." Or if the teaser notices a bad grade on your kid's math test: "You're right—I'm not loving math right now. You're good at it, maybe you can tutor me?"

5. Visualize mean words "bouncing off." This goes along with the adage, "I'm rubber and you're glue; whatever you say bounces off of me and sticks to you." Can you teach your child ways of "seeing" the cranky words get squashed by a sneakered foot or hit by a tennis racket?

6. The I-message. Start teaching your child to identify feelings at an early age by giving descriptions of them (e.g., "I can tell you are angry because your face is all red"). Next, pair the feeling words with a statement to end the offending behavior of another person. It works like this: "I feel ___ (angry) when you _____ (correct my speech). Can you please stop?" Teasing is a part of growing up, but if we start teaching our kids positive coping skills at an early age, they will be ready for whatever curveballs life throws at them.

(Some of the above suggestions gleaned from Judy S. Freedman's *Easing the Teasing: Helping Your Child Cope with Name-Calling, Ridicule, and Verbal Bullying.*)

Managing Your *Own* Child's Aggression

It may be that your child isn't the victim of some mean kid's lashing out. Your little angel may actually *be* the bully. What's going on? Your child may be hitting, punching, screaming, and throwing tantrums at home and school because he gets frustrated with his communication skills. Some kids may be cognizant of these behaviors: "I am getting frustrated because I can't communicate my ideas well, so I'm going to scream." But most kids aren't introspective enough to understand their poor reaction in a social situation.

Kids who are less efficient at using and understanding language may be more likely to deal with frustration inappropriately. That's not to say that poor communication and frustration are the *only* reasons a child becomes aggressive. There is often more than one reason for a negative behavior. I urge you to explore the situation in depth with a child psychologist, psychiatrist, or psychiatric nurse practitioner if you are truly concerned. In the meantime, here are some suggestions for managing your child's aggressive tendencies at home:

- *Take a break.* Encourage your child to "take a break" (this word choice often works better than "time out") when you notice your child getting revved up.

- *Make a "no hitting" rule.* Tell your child that there will be no hitting at home or school, even if someone hits him first. Remind him that there are consequences for hitting (time out or removal of privileges). Suggest alternatives to hitting another person: hitting a pillow, pounding on clay, stomping on the floor.

- *If your child does hit,* help him make apologies. Don't allow him to go on as though nothing happened. Accept an approximation of "I'm sorry" if your child has a hard time getting those words out (due to CAS or stubbornness). When kids learn from their mistakes, they are learning consequences from action.

- *Help your child identify feelings.* You may want to do this when he is not angry or frustrated. Once children have a better grasp of what they are feeling, they can better manage it. Feelings of anger are often masked as sadness, frustration, or fear. Describe those feelings to your child. Act them out together. Talk about other feelings too: loneliness, jealousy, and happiness, to name a few.

- *Help your child identify cues about feelings.* For example, when someone gets angry, he may get a red face, tense his muscles, scowl or groan, breathe faster, and have a pounding heart. How does your body respond? How does that compare with your body's response to happiness?

- *Tell him it's okay to be angry.* Recognize that we all get angry sometimes; it's what we do with anger that makes it "good" or "bad."

- *Teach problem-solving skills.* Identify that you are angry. Count to ten or take a deep breath. Walk away if you need to. Think about what you can do: ignore or talk to the person in nice words about why you are feeling angry.

- *Allow your child to make choices at home.* In other words, pick your battles. When kids are given appropriate choices, they feel a sense of ownership and empowerment.

- *Model good anger management skills at home.* Children learn what they see. If they see you get angry and throw things or hit others, they will think it's OK for them to do the same. If they see you taking a deep breath, walking away, and later explaining what made you angry, they will be more likely to follow your good example.

- *Develop a behavior management system.* It sounds fancy, but all you need to do is make a chart on poster board or on your computer. Make a column on the left-hand side with behavior you expect, and on the right side make lots of columns for the stickers your child earns for doing the good behavior. Once your child reaches a predetermined number of stickers on his "sticker chart," he earns a prize. Your child's chart may look something like this (those asterisks are stickers/stars):

No Hitting	*	*	*		
Use all of your words	*	*			
Share toys	*	*			
Clean up	*	*			

Catch your child being good. You can start a program like this without any hard-and-fast rules. Just say, "Let's keep track of how well you can use *all* your words. Each time I notice you doing a good job, I will give you a sticker on your chart. It will be fun to see how many stickers you can collect. We'll try the same thing for not hitting, sharing, and cleaning up. What do you say?" It may be enough of a reward to just do the stickers, especially for a younger child. But if your kiddo is older, try attaching a prize for adhering to the behavior plan. "Once you get twenty-five stickers, you can _____." Remember, not all prizes have to be tangible or cost money. One-on-one time with a parent, a trip to the park, or a bike ride can still be a major incentive. If it's not, keep prizes manageable for your family. Look in the dollar section at many stores, take your child out for ice cream, buy a new book, etc. Just be sure the prize is something your child actually likes and wants.

For more information on this topic, check out the website of the National Association of School Psychologists at www.nasponline.org. I was able to find a variety of resources by using the search field at the top of the website. For example, the key words *reward systems* brought up "Understanding and Fostering Achievement Motivation" by Laurie McGarry Klose.

Special Concerns for Girls

Girls have an intricate world incorporating play and socialization. Not being able to speak as well as their peers can definitely put a crimp in their ability to get along with other girls.

When Kate was about three, she tried really hard to fit in with the neighborhood girls, who were just about the same age. It saddened me to see just how discriminating these other little girls were. Kate couldn't keep up with them verbally and was left behind. She often came running back to me in tears because she was frustrated and discouraged in trying to play with them. And let's face it—girls play by communicating with one another. Little girls playing dollhouse, babies, tea party, and other typical girl-style play use words to differentiate roles and routines. For example, "You be the mommy. I'll be the daddy." Or, "Here's your tea, Mr. Bear, and here's your cookie, Miss Bunny." Kate ended up feeling more aligned with the little boys in our neighborhood. She would run and jump, kick, and ride bikes with them. It was easier for her because she didn't have to communicate as much verbally. The boys accepted her and helped her along. Until of course, they got "too big" and developed the "girls are yucky" view.

At five years, Kate was speaking better but still struggling to keep up with her female peers. We continued to work with her through role-play and modeling. It made my day—and hers—when a group of little girls rang our doorbell one afternoon and asked her to play. In fact, according to a 2009 study of the perceptions of children with speech-language concerns, "making friends and having them come 'round to see me" is one of the best indicators of a good quality of life for kids with expressive communication delays.

What's a Parent to Do?

- *Accept your daughter for who she is.* If she wants to play with boys, who cares? If she enjoys hopping around the driveway instead of playing dolls, let her. Once you learn what type of play drives your daughter, stock your toy collection with products you know she'll like. Jump ropes, scooters, sidewalk chalk, and balance boards have all been winners for us, as were Thomas the Train toys, movies, and books.

- *Offer to host 1:1 playdates with other girls.* Often, when girls are together in a group, things are intense. Try having just one other girl over at a time. It will be easier to bond and develop friendships than if your daughter is competing with lots of other Chatty Cathies. Many girls with CAS feel more comfortable with younger typically speaking girls. When Kate was five, she often connected best with her three-year-old sister's friends. Having a playdate with a younger girl is okay. Her speech abilities may be right on target.

- *Practice Role-Playing.* At home, practice what to do when your daughter is in the company of other girls. "I know you have been invited to Alexis's sleepover this weekend. The other girls might want to talk about their American Girl dolls, nail polish, and their favorite music. What can you add to conversations like this? Let's practice. I'll be Alexis, and you just be yourself, okay?" Knowing your daughter and the current girl culture will help you both at these times.

■ *Ask your daughter for ideas.* Parents get used to feeling like they have to always be the answer person. Try going to your daughter and voicing your concern about her friendships. But use caution—don't be accusatory, or you'll risk putting her on the defense. Try something like this: "Hey, I noticed it's hard for you to break into the Sophia-McKenzie-Emma group next door. What are your ideas?" You may get an earful!

Special Concerns for Boys

Each gender has its own challenges in dealing with friendships. Boys, by nature, are often more activity driven than verbally driven. As a result, they may not have to deal with as many of the difficult friend situations that confront girls. But they have their own unique concerns. A boy with CAS may appear more immature than his peers because he sounds younger than he really is. Boys may gradually begin to exclude him from their play because he seems like "a baby." Of course, you know different, so help set the record straight. Losing your temper won't help. Instead, keep a close eye on the group of boys. When you see your son being "babied" by the others, step in. Redirect the group by offering an activity that is more appealing to your son and may get the other boys to stop the babying and engage in something else.

You may also see older girls take your son under their wings and play the role of nurturing big sister. Personally, I see this as a good thing, but being overly nurturing or treating your son as though he is "too young" is not. Use your best judgment; if it feels wrong, it probably is.

Most of the girl strategies above can be applied to your son as well. Continue on for tips developed for both boys and girls.

Social Pointers for Both Girls and Boys

■ *Find ways to build self-esteem.* It can be heartbreaking to see your little one struggle with same-sex friendships. Remember that children need reminders of what they do well often. For example, "You are awesome at riding your scooter!" Tell your child that he is a fun, likeable kid with lots of energy.

■ *Consider coaching a youth sports team.* If your kiddo loves soccer, why not volunteer to be the coach? Sure, it's added time and effort on your part, but you'll get to know the other children and their parents, and help *your* child at the same time. It may help develop lifelong friendships. The same goes for becoming a Girl Scout leader, den mother, or scoutmaster.

- *Help "coach" social situations.* You don't want to become known as a hovering parent, but if you stumble upon a potential social situation for your son or daughter (at the park, library, neighborhood), provide a few pointers before sending your child into the midst of it all. You may feel more comfortable doing it *with* your child (he'll see your model, and that is a good thing). For example, "Hi girls! This is Kate. Can she play with you?" Stay within earshot so you can help your child along if he gets stuck.

- *Encourage others to engage in active play.* If you are hosting a playdate or you see your child struggling with a group of friends, jump in and try to engage the other kids in the type of play where your child is more likely to shine.

- *Speaking of current kid culture,* you'll want to try extra hard to know what's in, what's out, and what's coming up. Your child may not know how to say some of the things that are cool (fads, foods, slang, toys, etc.). Learn what they are (ask other parents, teachers, or children's librarians) and practice with him. If it's "supersonic strawberry shakes" at Shakes R Us, then practice saying those words with him until he gets it just right. If the name of a current tween pop star is tough to say, practice that.

- *Get your child involved in same-sex sports.* Soccer, gymnastics, martial arts, baseball/softball, or T-ball just for girls or just for boys may be the ticket to help your child feel included and successful.

One mom in my "Small Talk: All About Apraxia" group mentioned that she didn't think she was ready for extracurricular activities, but her three-and-a-half-year-old daughter with CAS proved her wrong:

"I just wasn't 'there' yet. I had a lot of anxiety over having her in a gymnastics class, even though the class was designed for three-year-olds. I was afraid she wouldn't be able to communicate and would need me. But she did great. She had no problems whatsoever. No one even knew she had CAS. I should have done it sooner for Lila's sake."

Exercise and Extracurricular Activities

Since we've talked about kids with CAS needing vestibular stimulation to awaken the communication center (chapters 7 and 9), it should be no surprise that exercise has multiple benefits. Aside from ensuring that your child doesn't develop weight or health issues from inactivity, exercise boosts verbal skills and serves as a coping device.

What's a Parent to Do?

- *Encourage physical activity.* Sometimes you have to turn off the TV and say, "We're going outside and we're going to play catch." Your child might grumble, but soon you'll both be having a good time. While you're tossing the ball around, practice some target speech sounds or words.

- *Limit screen time.* I'm not just talking television but also computers, iPhones, and hand-held video games. Do what feels right for your family, but the American Academy of Pediatrics recommends no more than two hours a day of screen time for a child aged two to ten years.

- *Consider having your child* **earn** *screen time.* For every two minutes of outside/active time, you child can "earn" one minute of screen time. So, if your child rides his bike for thirty minutes, he can play a video game for fifteen minutes. See "Managing Your Child's Aggression" section, above, for ideas on behavior modification and sticker charts.

- *Get your child involved in a noncompetitive sport.* Not all sports need to be about peer competition. What about those that encourage self-directed competition and goal setting? Swimming, martial arts, gymnastics, and yoga are all examples your child may enjoy.

- *Check out your local park or community education department.* Many states and counties have a special recreation association. If your child has profound CAS and other special needs, there are likely services and programs designed especially for him. Many of these programs offer modifications and adaptations (adapted equipment, communication tools/aids, physical assistance, behavioral management, 1:1 staffing). Your park district may offer dance, soccer, gymnastics, cheerleading, golf, or tennis with accommodations. Refer to Appendix C for additional information.

- *Get involved with your child's physical life.* Consider becoming a coach for the team your child is on. Or sit on the sidelines and cheer him on. Learn the rules of the game. You could also join a program advisory committee and share thoughts, concerns, and ideas with coaches, staff, and folks in the community. Ask first at your park district or chamber of commerce.

- *Be a role model.* You know that kids learn what they see. If they see you actively engaged in physical exercise, they will be more likely to accept it as a normal, healthy, and smart choice for managing stress, weight, and maintaining a healthy lifestyle.

Balance It Out with Relaxation

Of course, life isn't all about running marathons and going to speech therapy. Kids need downtime too. In fact, in the study about the perceptions of children with speech and language concerns about their lives (Markham, 2009), relaxation was one important key for a "good" quality of life. Kids of all ages related to the notion of relaxation and discussed the ways in which they achieved it. Kids were asked which activities they did to relax that made their lives "better and happier." Here's a sampling of how these kids responded (all of the kids in this study had a speech/language/communication need; more than half—62 percent—had an "expressive language delay"):

- "Riding around in my [quad] bike."
- "My computer game calms me down."
- "I like listening to music . . . lying down . . . that's what makes me relax."
- "Coming home at the end of the day and being with my family . . . that relaxes me."

Parents Share

The Benefits of Yoga

We found that Kate responded well to yoga. Your child might too. Yoga helps calm the mind, strengthen muscles, improve flexibility and concentration, and manage feelings of frustration and anger. Plus, it's adorable to see your little one in a downward dog position! If you are looking for a program that fits your child, call around to local yoga studios and fitness centers. Ask if they have a kids' yoga class or a parent-child yoga class. Here are some other ways to fit yoga-like activities into your child's life:

- Wii Fit—yoga programs
- Balance boards and balancing games
- *Breathe Like a Bear* by Kira Willey is a beautifully illustrated collection of mindfulness exercises designed to teach kids techniques for managing their bodies, breath, and emotions and can be performed anytime, anywhere. (Rodale, 2017).
- *Listening to My Body* by Gabi Garcia is a delightfully interactive book that guides children through their bodily sensations and feelings, with added mindfulness (Skinned Knee Publications, 2017).
- *Yoga Bug: Simple Poses for Little Ones* by Sarah Jane Hinder. While this is technically a board book designed for young kids, it offers simple beginner poses in a fun, easy-to-understand way—you can even buzz like a bee or crawl like a caterpillar, which makes it more fun—and maybe vocal—for little ones. (Sounds True, 2017).

Say That Again?! Chapter Summary

As parents, we'll do just about anything to help our kids become happy, well-adjusted kids. Of course, there is no magic bullet or formula to ensure this happens, but there are things we can do to help. Kids with CAS may have a harder time fitting in with their peers, managing emotions, and navigating the often-harsh cultural climate of teenager-hood. There is hope—and skills you can equip your child with—the cornerstone being improved self-esteem and self-concept.

If problems arise and you feel as if you can't manage on your own, there are professionals who can assist you and your child. Please seek guidance when you feel you are stumbling. There is often nothing to lose by having a concern examined and evaluated in more detail. In the best case, you get skills and advice to manage the situation better than you did before. In the worst case, you get peace of mind. It's win-win, if you ask me. The bottom line is: kids with CAS just want to be accepted, to have friends, and not be labeled as "special."

Recommended Resources

- *Great Kids: Helping Your Baby and Child Develop the 10 Essential Qualities for a Healthy, Happy Life* by Stanley I. Greenspan, M.D. (DA Capo Press, 2007), as referenced earlier in this chapter.

- The Annie E. Casey Foundation produces the annual Kids Count report, which provides state-by-state data on key indicators of children's well-being. However, it is not specific to speech, language, and communication disorders. Available at https://datacenter.kidscount.org/.

- The Federal Interagency Forum on Child & Family Statistics releases an annual report entitled *America's Children: Key National Indicators of Well Being.* Visit their website at www.childstats.gov for more information.

- *What Is Friendship: Games & Activities to Help Children to Understand Friendship* by Pamela Day (Jessica Kingsley Publishers, 2009) is a nice resource with reproducible pages for teaching kids ages seven and up about friendship.

- If your child is dealing with sensory and cognitive processing concerns, you may find some help in *Fuzzy Buzzy Groups for Children with Developmental and Sensory Processing Difficulties* by Fiona Brownlee and Lindsay Munro. It's an easy-to-follow guide to helping kids interact with peers in a fun, relaxed way.

- The Social Thinking website (www.socialthinking.com) doesn't target CAS specifically but has books, products, and other resources you can use to help your kid consider the points-of-view of other people.

- *More Creative Coping Skills for Children: Emotional Support through Arts and Crafts Activities* by Bonnie Thomas (Jessica Kingsley Publishers, 2016) is a great resource for parents who want to help their children cope in fun, easy, and creative ways.

- *Helping Children Cope with Change, Stress and Anxiety: A Photocopiable Activities Book* by Deborah M. Plummer (Jessica Kingsley Publishers, 2010) is full of ideas and activities to use with kids.

- Consider *making your own story* about a child who struggles to fit in. A couple of tips: don't use your child's own name, keep the text simple, allow your child to participate in the "publication" of this title by illustrating or helping to write the text. For ideas and inspiration, read about *Social Stories* at www.carolgraysocialstories.com or in *The New Social Story Book* by Carol Gray (Future Horizons, 2015). The book has many examples of social situations children may need a little brushing up on. Note: Social Stories were first developed for use with kids on the autism spectrum. Autism and CAS are not the same thing! However, the concept of Social Stories can be applied to *all* children.

- If you are looking for *movies* that may subtly give your child the message that he's okay regardless of his abilities, consider these titles:

  - *The Trumpet of the Swan* (based on a book by E. B. White) depicts a swan with no voice. Out of desperation, the father steals a trumpet as an instrument for his son to express himself. It's a heartwarming approach to finding alternative ways of finding one's voice. Watch it first before showing it to your child.

  - Another E. B. White creation: *Charlotte's Web,* a kid-friendly movie (or book) that will show your child that it's not always easy to speak. It's especially touching when Wilbur finds his voice and begins singing and dancing to the song, "I can talk, I can talk!"

  - *The Tangerine Bear* presents a little bear whose smile is stamped on upside-down in a factory mishap. It's a heartwarming Christmas-themed story about appearances and appreciation.

  - *Annabelle's Wish* is a holiday book turned television special (released on DVD in 2000). Young Billy, who has been mute since being in a barn fire when he was younger, learns that Santa grants the animals the gift of voice on Christmas Eve. Includes a star-studded cast, including Rue McClanahan and Randy Travis, among others.

- For more ideas on how to create behavioral management programs and charts, as well as a good listing of prizes/rewards, read *How to Behave So Your Preschooler Will, Too* by Sal Severe (Penguin Books, 2004).

- Parents of physically aggressive or explosive children may find some good problem-solving techniques in these titles by Ross Greene: *The Explosive Child* (Harper, 2014) and *Treating the Explosive Child: The Collaborative Problem-Solving Approach*, with J. Stuart Ablon (Guilford Press, 2006).

- *The Anger Management Workbook for Kids* by Samantha Snowden and Andrew Hill (Althea Press, 2018) offers kid-friendly exercises and interactive activities to feel happier, calmer, and take control of anger.

- *SOS! Help for Parents* by Lynn Clark (S.O.S. Programs and Parents Press, 2017) offers great advice and problem-solving tips on dealing with behavior.

- *1–2–3 Magic: Effective Discipline for Children 2–12* by Thomas Phelan (Sourcebooks, 2017) was the "gold standard" when I was working as an RN in a child/adolescent treatment program. The message is simple, yet powerful and effective.

- Great children's books to read with your child on feelings, including anger:
  - *When Sofie Gets Really Really Angry* by Molly Bang (Scholastic, 1999). There are a few others in the series, too: **When Sofie Gets Her Feelings Hurt** (Blue Sky Press, 2015) and *When Sofie Thinks She Can't* (Blue Sky Press, 2018).
  - *Today I Feel Silly: And Other Moods That Make My Day* by Jamie Lee Curtis (Harper-Collins, 2007).
  - *No Hitting!* by Karen Katz (Grosset & Dunlap, 2004).
  - *Hands Are Not for Hitting* by Marine Agassi (Free Spirit Publishing, 2004).
  - *When I'm Feeling* series by Tracey Moroney (Mile Five, 2019). This series has a lot of titles/feelings from happy to scared and jealous.
  - *Let's Talk about Feeling Angry* by Joy Berry (Scholastic, 1996). Ms. Berry has a huge collection of books that may be of interest to you and your children, some with audio CDs.

- *Easing the Teasing: Helping Your Child Cope with Name-Calling, Ridicule, & Verbal Bullying* by Judy Freedman (Scholastic, 2002) is a great no-nonsense approach to dealing with teasing, building friendships, and developing self-esteem.

- For older kids who need some tips on staying safe online, read *Cyberbullying: Activities to Help Children and Teens to Stay Safe in a Texting, Twittering, Social Networking World,* by Vanessa Rogers (Jessica Kingsley Publishers, 2010).

- More help for girls who are being bullied: *Little Girls Can Be Mean: Four Steps to Bully Proof Girls in the Early Grades* (St. Martin's Press, 2010) by Michelle Anthony and Reyna Lindert.

- *Helping Your Angry Child: A Workbook for You and Your Family* by Darlyne Gaynor Nemeth, Kelly Paulk Ray, and Maydel Morin Schexnader (New Harbinger Publications, 2003) is packed with worksheets and engaging activities that may help you and your child understand and manage anger better.

- A resource for helping your kids relax during tense times: *Deeno's Dream Journeys in the Big Blue Bubble: A Relaxation Programme to Help Children Manage Their Emotions* by Julia Langensiepen (Jessica Kingsley Publishers, 2010).

Chapter 15

Resolving CAS

Where Do We Go from Here?

"In watching my son become more and more self-aware as he approaches adulthood, I no longer worry about his speech impeding his future. His own desire and persistence to overcome have added the final polish he needed to blast this issue right out of his life."

—Janice, mother of son with a history of CAS

I know you are asking, "Will my kid ever be able to talk?" For most children, the simple answer is *yes* (but we just can't predict when). Whether or not a child will be a talker depends on the severity of the CAS and whether she received appropriate, early, intense, and frequent speech therapy (ST), as well as any home programming and carry-over practice you might engage your child in. It also depends whether your child has any other diagnoses in addition to CAS (comorbidity). And then there's temperament and personality—some children are just more talkative and outgoing than others.

As parents of a child with CAS, we want to hear, "Your child will be an exceptional communicator! Just give her this magic pill every day and she will be spitting out oratories next year." The thing with CAS is that it is a dynamic disorder; it changes over time. Some say it will be with your child forever, but to a lesser degree—"once apraxic, always apraxic." Others say it goes away completely and you'd never be able to pick out the adult who had CAS as a youngster.

This chapter covers the idea of "resolving CAS" and shows you how a child with CAS might look and sound once she grows up. Believe it or not, most nonprofessionals won't be able to detect that your child once had a childhood speech disorder.

First, congratulations for having gotten this far on your CAS journey, or whatever made you crack open this chapter. Chances are if you've made it this far, you've made it through the thick of it. You've found hope. You're probably *hearing* hope from your child. It comes in bits and pieces. It comes in peaks and valleys. Give yourself a pat on the back and your child a big hug. You both deserve it.

Here's a little story I think you will appreciate. One weekend, my hugely supportive husband sent me away on a "writer's retreat"—a quick jaunt down the road to the hotel for which I had a Groupon. I checked in and began the invigorating task of writing some of the last chapters of this book. I called home around dinnertime to hear the chatter and clatter of my happy family. Yes, I said *chatter*. Kate had been diagnosed as "resolving" about six months prior. That summer-evening phone call made me smile through tears of pride. Why? I heard Kate shout from the background, "Mom sure has been working on that book for a long time!"

That's a twelve-word sentence about the book I was writing on the very motor-speech condition she had. Talk about coming full circle, so to speak! She can talk! She can talk! Which reminds me—watch *Charlotte's Web* and focus in on the part in which Wilbur "gets" his voice and can communicate with the other farmyard animals. I think this must be how our kids with CAS feel. Trust me, you'll get teary-eyed watching this movie, especially if your kiddo is parked on your lap.

The Nuts and Bolts of This Chapter

- Our personal experience with resolving CAS
- The debate over "resolving," "resolved," and "always apraxic"
- Why and when children have relapses, and what to do about them
- The *potential* ongoing academic and social struggles of a child/teen with CAS
- What to do when your child no longer wants to go to speech therapy
- Tips, advice, and suggestions on sending your child with resolving CAS to college
- Of course, lots of at-home tips for you to use right away

I so appreciate you coming along on our journey with CAS. Of course you're curious about Kate, and so I'll tell you: When Kate was a little over five years old, her SLP gently, kindly suggested that maybe something else was going on. I had suspected ADHD since she was a toddler. It's not within an SLP's scope to diagnose ADHD, and so we went to a specialist who did. Kate has both hyperactive and inattentive ADHD and we've treated it appropriately. This is a common accompanying diagnosis. And now she's fourteen and a freshman in high school. For five solid years, we dealt with CAS. For nine, we can honestly say CAS has been in our rearview mirror. Speech-wise, this girl won't stop talking. And sometimes, we tell her she needs to slow down because we can't catch everything. She's uber-creative and constantly inventing, making art, sewing, and producing her own iMovies. She's athletic and has participated in track, cross-country, and competitive tennis. Academically, Kate is above average and has been recommended for honors biology and history. Sometimes, she'll stumble on a new word—or even a familiar one—and will joke, "Hey—I had CAS as a kid." In all seriousness, no one would be able to tell she ever had a speech disorder.

Parents Share

One Christmas, Kate received a book, *Knuffle Bunny*, written by Mo Willems. I hated it. It was hard for me to read to her. In it, little Trixie misplaces her lovey and tries to tell her daddy where to find it. She uses words like "Aggle, flabble, klabble . . . wumpy, and flappy." I can see the pain in young Trixie's face just as I saw it in Kate's. Only Kate was much older than the character in the book. The story ends when Trixie says her first words, "Knuffle Bunny." I used to hope it was as simple as really wanting something badly enough (e.g., the lovey) to get those words out. Mo Willems actually wrote a sequel to this story, *Knuffle Bunny Too*. It begins with the words, "By now Trixie was really using her words. . . ." Again, I secretly hated the book. I wanted my child to be using her words. But she wasn't. Not like Trixie was, anyway.

Why am I telling you this story? Well, in the first book, you see how Trixie's daddy is working so hard to understand his little girl but can't. Everyone gets frustrated. In the sequel, Trixie is jabbering away, and you know . . . it's a little empowering. You can look at these two books as "CAS" (*Knuffle Bunny: A Cautionary Tale*) and "resolved CAS" (*Knuffle Bunny Too*). With appropriate treatment and support, your child will hopefully be jabbering up a storm by the time this tale is all said and done.

Families' Experiences with Resolving CAS

I can tell you all about our story, but that gets boring after a while. Plus, you want to know how other families got through the CAS journey as well. Every child is different. Every case of CAS is unique, and dynamic as well. Here are what some "apraxia parents" had to say about the experience of getting to the point where they could say, "She's talking!"

Amy, mother of son with a history of CAS, dismissed from speech therapy at five and a half and currently twelve years old, shares this: "People who meet my son are shocked to hear that he had almost four years of intensive speech therapy as a child. Only his teachers notice his fine motor skill planning problems—his handwriting is terrible! Most people see my son as a charismatic, loveable young man, as long as catching/hitting a ball or complex motor planning isn't involved. He's like the absent-minded professor—much to offer but quirky."

"My son Colton is resolved, and I believe it happened because he has a motor plan for all sounds. The last sound to come in for him was the *r* sound when he was in sixth grade. We are just working on articulation. He still has slight vowel distortions, but otherwise he is doing great!" says Lori regarding her twelve-year-old son with a history of CAS.

"Brooke [now 12] remained in speech therapy through our public school system until the end of fourth grade. There were definite sounds such as *r*, *w*, and *th* that she worked long and hard to achieve," says a St. Louis–based mom of her daughter who was in speech therapy for CAS and subsequent issues for about six years.

Toni Lee says of her son, "I wish I could say Drew's [CAS] is behind him, but it just isn't. We still struggle. He's a great kid, though, and recently made the seventh-grade track team, got an A+ on his Constitution test, and was awarded Student of the Month for perseverance, so we have a lot to be grateful for and to celebrate, but speech work is still in progress."

Jane, Abby's mom, says, "I really credit the speech therapy our daughter received between the ages of three and eight with her success. Now, at thirteen, no one would ever know she had difficulties with speech and learning to read. She's in all honors classes and receives straight As, except in Spanish, which is a bit of a challenge, but she still maintains a high B."

Learning a foreign language has also been a challenge for Kate. She's in her second year of Spanish and continues to struggle with pronunciation, prosody, and the new vocabulary of a second language. But she's persistent, and that's what matters.

One mom indicated that her son was in speech therapy for nearly two years before they saw any significant results, but her son was making progress (slowly). She felt that age five and a half was when he *really* made significant gains in speech. "At fifteen years old, he stutters when stressed," but for the most part, she indicates, no one would ever know.

Another mom, also of a teenager with a history of CAS, told me that her son speaks sloppily, mumbles, or talks in shortened phrases when he isn't "trying."

Aren't all teenagers—especially boys—like that? But seriously, when children go through significant growth spurts during adolescence, it may take some time, or perhaps some additional speech-language therapy, to help them reorganize their motor plans to match this significant change in structure.

The Differences between Resolved, Resolving, and "Always Apraxic"

As mentioned in the introduction, some professionals believe that CAS never completely goes away, even though the person may learn to talk so well that ordinary listeners do not detect anything wrong with her speech. Others use the term *resolved* to indicate that the symptoms of CAS have "worked themselves out" with ST and lots of work from the child and her family. Still others may talk about CAS "resolving," meaning "it's on the way out, but it's never really completely gone." Maybe something more along the lines of "managing" CAS?

Personally, I like the word *recovered* best. To me, it means there is no gray, no blurring, no nebulous blob hanging around you or your child anymore. It means CAS is gone. Done. Never coming back. It is very clear-cut. But not all kids with CAS may reach this stage. There is no magical age at which kids can be declared "resolved/ recovered," because that depends on the quality and amount of ST they receive, plus the severity of the disorder. For example, if a child with "mild CAS" was identified as "likely apraxic" at a very early age—say, two years—and she had quality 1:1 ST two or three times a week, she would "resolve" in a shorter amount of time than a child who was diagnosed with profound CAS at age three and received poor, intermittent ST.

While there really aren't any specific guidelines or criteria from the American Speech-Language-Hearing Association (ASHA) for determining who should receive the "resolved CAS" diagnosis, there are some general guidelines you can keep in mind:

- Consider the severity of the disorder. If your child was diagnosed with mild CAS, then it may be more likely that the disorder will resolve in less time and with less effort. Of course, there are various degrees of severity ranging from mild to moderate to severe to profound. You can ask your SLP where your child's diagnosis likely falls.

- CAS no longer interferes with your child's daily life or her functioning. This means your child can ask for what she needs intelligibly without the use of prompts, cues, or gestures.

- Others can understand what your child is saying to reasonable degree. Folks are no longer saying, "Huh? Can you say that again?"

- Most people cannot tell that she had a previous speech/language problem. In other words, they think little to nothing of a speech-related quirk your child may exhibit.

- Your child has learned and used coping and accommodation skills such as self-monitoring.

- The biggest and best indicator of recovery is that your child's articulation and speech are considered age appropriate. Your SLP will tell you when your child has reached that level. When you hear this, it's time to celebrate!

Keep in mind, though, that some SLPs won't say that your child's CAS has "resolved." Instead, they may say something like Rhonda Banford, MAT, CCC-SLP, does: "*Resolved* is not a term I use in my practice. Instead, I choose to say that the child no longer has difficulty with the motor aspects of forming words or sentences." Ms. Banford may sound like she is splitting hairs, but really she is not. Just because a child no longer struggles with the motor aspects of speaking does not necessarily mean that her speech and language skills are now normal. Remember how CAS is a motor-speech disorder? Well, it also affects other aspects of expressive language:

- syntax (grammar)
- morphology, or meaningful word segments—for example, "cats" has two morphemes or segments—*cat* + *s*

Both syntax and morphology have to do with the structure of the sentence, the length of utterance, and how complex it is. Problems with syntax and morphology are "language" disorders, whereas CAS is a "speech" disorder.

When you add in these characteristics of morphology and syntax, the whole equation gets more complicated. Your child may be able to initiate and imitate sounds, speak spontaneously, and even say multisyllabic words, but she still trips over syntax and morphology (involving the rules of language). Is that part of CAS? Some folks say yes; others don't. CAS is a motor-speech disorder, so why do children with CAS often have language disorders? Could it be that children with CAS have not had opportunities to practice morphology and syntax? Once children can *say* the words, they need to learn the rules of language by receiving feedback on their use of language.

Nanette Cote, MA, CCC-SLP, says, "I also like to treat struggles in phonemic awareness. This includes skills like identifying and naming rhymes, beginning and ending sound discrimination, blending two words into one to make a compound word, and identifying the final sound heard in a word." These are all important self-monitoring skills for older children and adults: knowing when something was said correctly and continuing to tweak errors.

How Motivated Is Your Child to Make Progress?

Children with CAS are motivated to improve their speech by various factors, including the following:

- the child's unique temperament and personality
- her intent and willingness to communicate
- her opportunities to practice at home
- how supportive the family environment is
- how engaged and proactive the parents are
- whether the child has other diagnoses in addition to CAS
- whether the child is given an effective carrot: a unique motivator she responds to. You'll learn what this is by trial and error. Examples may include verbal praise from parents (siblings or SLP), a sticker on a chart, a lollipop, extra video game time, a special time with mom or dad, or just feeling that her needs and feelings are getting heard.

Is Your Child "Resolving/Recovering?"

I picked my son up from a weeklong specialized comedy improv camp, and I don't think I've ever heard him speak so easily before. He was very well spoken, his grammar was excellent, and there were no "bumps" in his word finding whatsoever. On the way home, he told me that he purposefully chose workshops that were tougher for him speech-wise. He took on prominent positions in improv sketches—something he used to not do because he felt his speech would fail him at a crucial moment. However, he told me that not one person at the camp noticed any speech issues whatsoever. This gave him a lot of confidence.—Felix's mother

Hearing that your child's CAS is resolving is a fantastic stepping-stone to the "resolved/recovered" status. You're almost there. Now you know you will *both* get there.

Again, there are no hard-and-fast rules for declaring a child's CAS is "resolving," but here's a little cheat sheet:

- *Your child has started to mature in a social and emotional sense.* Try not to confuse this with physical maturity. Your child may still look like a child, but she can greet and connect with peers in an age-appropriate manner. She can control her emotions in a more "mature" way—fewer outbursts and temper tantrums because she can now communicate these in words. For example, Jane, mother of six-year-old Abby shares this: "Sometimes, I will try to hurry [my daughter] along by completing her sentence or prompting her as she struggles to find the 'right' word. But Abby, will come back and say, 'Mom, you are being rude. I haven't gotten all of my words out yet!'"

- *Mild issues may still remain.* Try not to scrutinize your child's speech so much. You may have been trained to look for perfection in her communication, but really—how many five-year-olds have absolutely perfect articulation? Many children are developing their speech sounds until around age eight.

- *CAS is "below the surface."* There will be times when your child stumbles or gropes for words. This happens to *all* of us. When you can see or hear your child struggling with speech just once or twice a day instead of *most* of the time, then it's likely that her CAS is resolving.

- *Your child is learning and beginning to use coping and accommodation skills.* Talk with your SLP about this. Is she teaching your child to self-monitor? What does your SLP suggest your child should be doing? For us, it was "Stop. Think. Slow down." However, your child must be ready to do this important step.

- *Your child's speech, or lack thereof, no longer stands out.* By the time your child reaches the "resolving" status, folks are no longer asking about or commenting on her speech.

- *Your child's CAS is no longer slowing her down or preventing her (or your family) from doing what you want to do.* Sign her up for a soccer team, allow her to attend a birthday party without a chaperone/translator, let her order her own food, place a drink order, or something similar, because she can do it!

- *You can look back at the journey and say, "We're really making progress!"* Think back to where you and your child began (I recommend journaling or marking small accomplishments on a calendar early on) and celebrating them together. When you can honestly say, "It's going to be okay," you know you've reached the resolving status. And if you're not there just yet, don't lose hope.

Right now, we are dealing with what remains, not apraxia [CAS] per se, but common co-morbid things like fine motor struggles and distractibility. I am not sure if any other struggles will be presented to us, but I do know that Allison is a smart, spunky little girl who can talk like any other kid and has a real future. For that, I am eternally thankful."
—Susan, mother of Ally, seven years old with resolving CAS

I followed up with Susan recently and learned so many wonderful things about Ally. She's a high school sophomore and very involved in the robotics team. She's eagerly counting down the days till she can start driving and hopes to get a part-time job. Her mother says, "Ally continues to do extremely well . . . her speech is truly excellent. I only occasionally notice that she has to put extra effort into producing a challenging word. We no longer worry about her speech!"

Like Kate, Ally was diagnosed with the inattentive subtype of ADHD, which is a common comorbidity of CAS. But Susan says, "Honestly, this hasn't stopped her; all of her teachers comment on what a hard worker she is; what they don't know is she has been working hard since she was a toddler."

What You Can Do at Home

When you are in the "resolving/recovering" mode, you might want a few pointers to boost your child's progress. Just keep in mind that it's not a race, and everyone develops at their own pace. Please don't push your child into something she's not yet ready to do.

Use simple and nonthreatening techniques. Find opportunities for success. The grocery store, school, the library, and the park all provide endless opportunities for your child to communicate with success. Look at chapter 9 for ideas. Remember to modify these ideas for your child's current communication level.

For example, when your daughter says something spontaneously, praise her. Saying a word or phrase she has heard dozens of times (but was previously unable to say) is a big step for a child with CAS. She has likely been mentally practicing and developing these neuropathways for quite some time. Now she spontaneously says the word(s) for the first time. Hooray! Acknowledge and honor this step.

Engage your child in play. When she's playing, get down to her level and talk to her about what's going on. You might say, "What's the superhero doing now? Who's the good one? Who's the bad guy?" If your child doesn't respond well to questions, you could make general statements: "Oh, look what the superhero is doing. He's flying fast." Just be a good verbal role model. Try making it more about play than about communication. You don't even have to make eye contact, if your child is not good at eye contact. You'd be surprised what might pop out of your child's mouth when she doesn't think you are quizzing her on speech sounds, words, or phrases.

> **Take a Two-Pronged Approach**
> Let's say your child's CAS is "resolving." The battle is half-over. Now it's time to start working on her phonological skills at the same time you continue to work on her motor-speech skills. See chapter 11 on phonological awareness to find some activities you and your child can do together at home.

"Once Apraxic, Always Apraxic"

I've repeated this comment several times, but what does it really mean? As you may recall, CAS may run in the family (immediate or close relatives may have a history of speech impairments or disorders). So, even if your child is considered "recovered" from CAS, she may still have the genetic predisposition for the disorder. And the bigger question is, "Will there be a relapse?" (We'll get to that later.) The short answer—and the good news—is *she will probably NOT always demonstrate CAS if she is recovered.*

According to Rhonda Banford, "If your child's apraxia [CAS] is mild enough, and her therapy is intensive and appropriate, then one can expect a child with CAS to become a proficient-enough speaker that no one would know her past struggles." She explains, however, that the situation is different if your child has another condition besides CAS: "We can't just tell a parent of a child who has CAS *and* autism, for example, that the child will speak just fine one day. If CAS is the child's *only* disorder, there's a good chance that with proper speech therapy, she will seem perfectly normal to everyone who knows her. If the child has CAS *and* other disorders, it is far less likely. Unfortunately, the other disorders affect how well the child will progress with the CAS therapy, so it is likely she will make progress, but she may never get to the same stage as the child without other disorders."

So why even bother with the label "resolving apraxia?" It helps to describe your child's progress in terms of her speech. It also helps you remember her recovery. And it helps you keep an eye on potential problems that may crop up in the future (see the section on "Remnants and Relapse" later in this chapter). You can say "resolving CAS" and have it mean "a child with a history of CAS who has fully intelligible—but not perfect—speech."

When should you let go of the label? Some folks hang on to the CAS label for years. What's the benefit, you wonder? First, the label can help the child/young adult get the services that may be needed at school or in a postsecondary institution. Some folks may like the secondary gain they receive from the attention or concern of others. Others may not have recovered enough to drop the label. Parents may still be working on a sense of closure from the intense parenting they went through during the "apraxic years"—shuffling therapy appointments, participating in home practice, and learning about the disorder. It may be hard for parents to let go of that identity even though they are happy CAS no longer plagues their child.

Can Childhood Apraxia of Speech Evolve into Something Else?

Some parents and SLPs will tell you that CAS doesn't really "resolve," meaning go away completely, but may *evolve* into something else.

You may hear something like I did: "We don't think Kate has apraxia anymore. In fact, I am not sure if she ever did. Who diagnosed her? She might have a slight phonological disorder, but that's all." I was taken aback when I heard this from the school IEP team. I was beyond certain that Kate had CAS. It was more likely that Kate was presenting—*at that time*—like a child with a phonological disorder.

Other parents have told me about hearing similar statements from professionals. These professionals indicated that the children who had previously had CAS had evolved into having moderate articulation disorders or mild phonological disorders or even auditory processing disorders.

If you are wondering if your child's CAS is evolving versus resolving, find an SLP who can help you sort this all out—preferably one who has been trained specifically in the treatment of motor-speech disorders.

Parents Ask

Are there tests to determine if CAS is resolving?

Many speech-language pathologists use more of a subjective interpretation to determine whether apraxia is resolving. For example, Diane Bahr, MS, CCC-SLP, uses a list of CAS characteristics to observe her clients' speech motor-planning concerns. The list is based on information found in the speech-language pathology literature. She assesses progress by looking at the percentage of change in her clients' skills over time. Ruth Stoeckel, PhD, CCC-SLP, indicates that sometimes the best way for families to determine whether their children are progressing is to look at data specific to what their child is working on and ask if the progress is significant to them. Doing so is going to help you look back on the experience of CAS and feel proud that your child has come as far as she has!

If you're really looking for some hard numbers, something more specific and tangible, you might want to ask your child's SLP about the Dynamic Evaluation of Motor Speech Skill (DEMSS), which can help identify and evaluate CAS for children over age three, including progress markers. It was cowritten by top CAS researchers and clinicians Edythe Strand PhD, CCC-SLP, and Rebecca McCauley, PhD, CCC-SLP.

Remnants, Relapse, and Resistant Residuals

Your child may have gotten to the point where she has intelligible speech and can pretty much communicate like any other Ivy, Vincent, and Elijah. But now you find yourself concerned about what might be "remnants" of apraxia. What are they? What do they mean? And, what can you do about them?

First, let's identify what the remnants *might* be:

- Fine motor delay (difficulties with handwriting, handling utensils or scissors), as *some* children with CAS also have limb apraxia

- Mild sensory symptoms (mouthing nonfood items, sensitivity to loud noise, touch, or smell, poor hand-eye coordination and tracking), as *some* children with CAS also have sensory processing disorders

- Lack of organization, especially in upper grades, as coursework becomes more difficult and students have multiple teachers and classrooms

- Inattention to detail, especially in instances in which your child is asked to describe objects or events in an open-ended way. Speech production requires great attention to detail and sequencing. For example, your child may have problems answering questions such as, "What did you do at day camp today?" You may have to ask very specific questions instead.

- The inability to verbally sequence information in a logical manner (e.g., "First we did some free play, and then had Circle Time, and after that we went on a hike and made a craft")

- Prosody issues—difficulties with speech rate, rhythm, inflection, syllable, and breath control

If these signs and symptoms are apraxia lingering, mention them to your child's SLP, teacher, or school psychologist. It's not the end of the world. All of these issues can improve with a little work and assistance. You may want to add an occupational therapist (OT) to the treatment team, if you haven't already. An OT can help your child with fine motor skills such as handling utensils and handwriting and can support sensory processing concerns. The OT can also assist with sequencing and organizational issues. An educational psychologist might also be a helpful resource. Check with your insurance company to find out what will and will not be paid by your insurance. (See Appendix B.)

The reasons children may have these remnants vary. Your child may still chew on toys, for example, because she has a sensory processing disorder, or perhaps the act of chewing helps her attend/focus/concentrate. Or maybe your child hasn't matured in some social or emotional sense. Could it be that she has found some unique way to compensate for her speech issues? For example, if chewing is a comfort to your child, it may be something you and your child learn to modify over time. You'll likely need to provide appropriate items to chew (gum, licorice, oral-motor toys). Be sure you also suggest a socially appropriate time to use them. If you need to find appropriate mouth toys for your child, try these sources:

- Ark Therapeutic (www.arktherapeutic.com)
- Therapy Shoppe (www.therapyshoppe.com)
- Pocketful of Therapy (www.pfot.com)
- Super Duper Publications (www.superduperinc.com)

Remember, CAS is an ever-changing, dynamic disorder that presents itself differently as it progresses. It looks different in every child.

Word Study: *Remnant, residual, lingering symptomology*, and *aftereffects* are all terms you may hear when professionals talk about your child's history of CAS. Just keep this in the back of your mind should you need to assess these concerns in greater detail someday.

Relapse and Backsliding

"Relapse," "backsliding," "slipping" or "downward spiral" might be ways to describe the phenomenon of CAS showing its ugly face after you thought everything was fine. It may happen once or twice or even more along your journey. Don't worry. Just get right back in the saddle and get the help you and your child need.

Here is our experience. Kate was doing great. She was in an intense preschool program five days per week. Her IEP had been discontinued because her testing and her classroom teacher indicated she was "doing well." We signed off and agreed to continue with private speech therapy. Three weeks later, her private SLP also thought her CAS was resolving. I ran out and purchased the scooter Kate had been wanting for months, and we all went out for dinner to celebrate. Six months later, we were back at the speech clinic. It's not that they were wrong. It's not that Kate stopped trying. It's just that something started to change. Here are some reasons a relapse might occur:

- *The motor plans/gestures/programs were never established to the extent they needed to be in the first place.* That is one of the hypotheses that SLP researchers have suggested to explain the "whys" of apraxia. What it may mean for your child at this point is simply *strengthening* those motor plans with increased speech practice.

- *The linguistic complexity of what the child is trying to say has increased beyond her capability, creating a greater linguistic load.* That is, when your child was saying simpler sentences, her speech skills seemed adequate, but now that her language skills have increased (knows more vocabulary, wants to express more complex thoughts) her speech skills simply "can't keep up." See the glossary for a fuller explanation.

- *She may have an incorrect underlying representation of the word.* Simply put, your child internalized the word wrong. Here are some examples from Rhonda

Banford: "A couple of kids with CAS really thought you read a 'boot' and not a 'book.' Another child insisted that the Star Wars character was 'Hand' Solo and not 'Han' Solo. Still another child was sure we ate 'state' and not 'steak' and insisted *I* was saying it incorrectly!"

■ ***She may also have actual muscle weakness.*** The fancy term for this is "dysarthria." That is, the child's speech suffers because she has some underlying muscle weakness.

As you are reading this, I know you have questions. First, of all—yes, it is possible that kids with CAS also have dysarthria. That is, children may have difficulty with motor programming and have difficulty with muscle weakness (dysarthria), which may include weak respiratory support and weak movements with reduced range of motion and reduced rate.

It is entirely possible to have both CAS and dysarthria at the same time. According to Edythe Strand, PhD, BC-ANCDS, "The co-occurrence of CAS and dysarthria is seen most often in the context of acquired disorders (like a traumatic brain injury or stroke). But it can also occur in the context of neurodevelopmental disorders, a variety of syndromes, etc. Children with no known cause of CAS (idiopathic) may sometimes show signs of dysarthria, which is typically mild."

Some people become a bit silly and incoherent in their speech when mentally exhausted. We all slip up when we are tired—some more than others—and it's actually pretty normal. When it comes to our kids with CAS, you can use this "slip-up method" as a gauge that your child is mentally taxed and would benefit from some downtime.

A mother in my Small Talk: All About Apraxia group described how her daughter relapsed when she became ill. She said: "When Lila got sick a few weeks ago, we noticed some major regression. It was then that I realized how much effort it takes for her to talk. This is hard work for these kiddos."

Here's your take-away message: If your child has trouble planning speech movements *and* her speech sounds slurred/distorted, then it's possible she has both CAS *and* dysarthria. Only your SLP can make that determination. If you have concerns, bring it up at your next therapy session.

Coping with Relapse

If you are concerned that your child is relapsing, try not to worry or blame the SLP, yourself, or your child. Sit back and reevaluate the situation. ***Try your best to be objective.*** You can start by documenting the behaviors/speech patterns you are seeing that lead you to question your child's progress. Again, I strongly recommend keeping track of successes and pitfalls on a daily calendar.

Give yourself a little time to think about what's going on (you might make a deadline and stick with it—say a week) and then take action. Call the speech clinic or the school and ask for a reevaluation or follow-up appointment. Tell them specifically why you are concerned. They will likely honor your request. Hopefully, with a little "brush-up" therapy, your child will be back on track. If you don't succeed with the speech clinic or school, consider getting a second opinion.

The Social Animal: Your Child's Social Group

As a parent, you know that at some point your child will connect more with her peers than with you. It's only normal and a part of growing up. Allow it. You may have been your child's translator, but eventually you'll want to start letting her learn and discover the world, even though she may struggle at times. Here are some tips for making the social experience for your child (and yourself!) a little easier:

- *Know your child's interests.* Find something your child is good at doing and enjoys. Sign her up and get her involved. Here are some activities your child may want to pursue: Suzuki violin, swim team, gymnastics, soccer, or band. These activities require concentration, practice, and persistence. Plus, it will place her in situations where she can interact with others where talking isn't always the focus. For example, a mother of a sixth grader with a history of CAS says this: "She competes regionally on a hip-hop dance team, and most people who meet her for the first time comment on how her smile and laughter light up the room. We are eternally grateful for the early intervention and speech services she received, and she now is considered typically developing."

- *Get to know your child's friends.* It sounds simple, but you'll need to make an effort to do this. There's a fine line between getting to know your child's friends and hovering. If they come to the house, greet them. Call them by name and learn at least one or two interesting things about each child. Then remember to ask them about their interests the next time you see them.

- *Get to know the parents of your child's friends.* Your child picks up behaviors and values from you (good or bad), right? This also happens with friends. If you have a sense of where these other children are "coming from" (their parents, their home), you'll have a better sense of the children with whom your child is associating. You don't have to become best friends with their parents, but get to know them in a social setting or two. Exchange periodic emails, or invite them to stay for a playdate.

- *Have some "cool" things at your house that other kids will enjoy and associate with your home.* It doesn't really matter what it is; just make sure it's safe and kid-friendly. Examples include a pet, a swing set, a nice assortment of Legos, or a popular book series. Of course, don't run out and buy something specifically for this purpose. Make sure it's something you and your family value and will use as well.

- *Your child may still stumble on certain words or phrases, or struggle to find the right word from time to time.* Other kids may find this funny. Some kids can be mean. Teach your child a few coping skills, just in case. For examples, please refer back to chapter 14.

- ▪ *Kids can be very patient.* They may take your child under their wing and help her out. They may prompt your child (they may not realize they're doing this) so your child can communicate more effectively. It's a sweet and touching blessing for your child to have a friend like this!

- ▪ *Let your child know what you think about her friends.* You don't have to draw any attention to this method. Just say something like, "I really like Leo. I think you two get along nicely. I like how he helps you out when you get stuck." Your child will begin to internalize that and will begin to seek out other like-minded friends. She will also see that you are paying attention to her friendships as well.

- ▪ *Finally, it's not important that your child have a ton of BFFs.* It's quality, not quantity that matters.

Please refer to chapter 14 for more ideas in helping your child cope with CAS.

Wanting to Quit Therapy

At some point, your little sweetie, who has been compliant in the speech therapy rigmarole, is likely to rebel. She won't want to go to speech anymore. You may have to poke, prod, and cajole her to get her into the car and to the clinic.

Kate once asked me in an exasperated voice, "Doesn't speech have a drive-through?" She was serious, but I died laughing.

Kids get tired of speech therapy, just as you get tired of driving them there, communicating with the SLP, paying the bill, and drilling your child at home. But you know your child needs to continue to receive the benefits of speech therapy. And sometimes, we have to continue to do things we aren't so keen on doing.

What's a Parent to Do?

- ▪ *Sympathize with her.* "I know you don't really want to go to speech today, but it's really important."

- ▪ *Remind her of her progress.* "But you have come so far. Just think, when we first started seeing Ms. Diane, you couldn't say all of the things you can say now. Isn't it fun to be able to talk?" You may even consider showing your child some old progress reports or charts if you have them.

- ▪ *Ask this tough question: "Are you okay if you aren't speaking as clearly—or as well—as some of your friends?"* This is a particularly important question to ask if you (and your child's SLP) really don't think your child is ready to end therapy but your child is. Often, kids will want to quit therapy when therapy is interfering with more fun and interesting activities. They may also want to quit when they perceive the work as "too hard." This is when you and your SLP simplify tasks so your child can feel successful.

- *Reward her with a treat.* Think of some positive reinforcement that will get your kiddo to therapy without struggle. It may work to have a prize box of trinkets stowed in your car. After therapy is over, offer her a choice from the box. Head over to the local park after a session or take her out for ice cream. It could even be as simple as allowing her to stay up a half hour later than usual on therapy days or providing extra video game time. You'll know what works best for your child and your family.

- *Talk to your child's SLP.* Maybe your child really *is* ready to stop therapy. Bring this up with your SLP; perhaps some readjustment can help. Some children participate more readily at a different time of day, a different day of the week, or in a shorter session. Perhaps group therapy with other socially and age- and diagnosis-matched kids would be more ideal. Your child may also do better if she assists in therapy planning—get her ideas for a more fun, effective session. Of course, your SLP must be willing to do this.

- *Go ahead, end ST (and other therapies, as indicated).* I am not saying this to be defiant. It really might be time, or your child may just need a break. After talking with your child's SLP, your child, and your partner, you may conclude that it's time to move on or take a break. It's not the end of the world if you end therapy for a time. You can always go back.

- *Go back to ST if you have to.* We were discharged from therapy at one point with the understanding that we monitor Kate's progress (or problems) for several months. We were encouraged to call and come back to the clinic if we had any concerns. And we did. Kate went right back once we saw a bit of regression. It was no big deal, and it was the appropriate thing to do.

> *We ended private speech therapy just after he turned ten when the therapist [SLP] told me she was having a hard time coming up with new goals.*
>
> —mother of Matt with autism and resolving CAS

How Does the End of Speech-Language Therapy Look?

Every situation and child is different, of course. So are speech clinics and SLPs, for that matter. Here's what you might expect:

- Your child's SLP will likely want to do a formal test to assess her progress. This will probably be done over the course of a couple of sessions. Your SLP will compare past assessment scores with "now" assessment scores too.

- You may have a sit-down results session with the SLP. If your child is speaking at "developmentally appropriate" levels, then it will likely be recommended that therapy end.

- Give yourself, your child, and the SLP a little bit of warning. After you have heard the good news, you might want to give your child one more session to bring things to closure. After all, she has likely developed a pretty close relationship with the SLP and needs some time to say goodbye. You might too.

- Mark your calendar and prepare for the final day. Kate's therapy sessions ended when she was entering full-day kindergarten. She would be in school until nearly 4:00 p.m. (after the bus ride home). We just couldn't imagine tacking on yet another "to-do" at the end of a long, busy day. Since she was speaking at "developmentally appropriate" levels at this point, it made the decision easier.

- Celebrate and recognize a job well done (for both your child and her SLP). Kate drew a picture of a kindergarten classroom, signed her name, and gave it to her SLP. I added a personal note, "Thanks for helping me prepare for school. I'm all ready because of you." I included a gift card to a coffee shop. We hugged our SLP and said "thank you." We were told to call or email with any questions whatsoever. Here are some other ideas:

  - Some clinics provide families and kids with a certificate of completion. If they don't, consider making your own. It really *is* a big accomplishment.
  - Take your child out for dinner at a special restaurant.
  - Bake cookies for your child's SLP.
  - Give the SLP a therapy-related toy, book, or game for his or her practice.
  - Donate a subscription to the speech clinic waiting room in your child's name.

Nanette Cote says, "In my practice, I slowly transition clients from speech if they are meeting most of their goals or needing more breaks. I like to reward accomplishments by reducing sessions from twice weekly to once. Parents like this transition better than abruptly ending services altogether." Another SLP said she likes to make paper chains with her clients, each link represents a speech goal. The chain starts off longer at the clinic. Once a particular goal is met, that link of the chain can go home with the child, where she adds it to her home chain. When the chain is longer at home than at the clinic, well, that is very telling to a child. This method is a very visual and tangible reminder of progress for everyone. If paper chains aren't for you, you can modify this idea by putting colored beads in a jar, or other items you may have handy.

Make sure that your child knows how proud and happy you are of her accomplishments!

Celebrating Your Child's Discharge from Speech Therapy

Kate Welder, a CAS parent, says this: "By all means, a small family celebration is in order. It could be something simple such as cooking your child's favorite meal or going to their favorite restaurant. We have always made home movies of our children since birth. With Josie, we often filmed her 'talking' in the movie, gathering these over a period of a few years. When we interviewed her for her graduation [from speech], it made a lasting tribute to her progress."

Another mother was less sentimental: "There was no big party or event to mark the end of this important and critical piece to [my son's] development . . . it just happened. Maybe to be compared to any kind of transition that just happens—from childhood to adolescence, from not reading to reading, from breastfeeding to not—it just comes to an end and you have to kind of squint to remember how that came about."

"I'm a card-maker, so I made the SLP a pack of greeting cards as a goodbye/thank-you," says one mom of a child who was dismissed from speech therapy at age ten. I love the personal touch of her thank-you for providing such a personal service: the gift of speech.

Finally, you will hear the emotional sentimentality as this mother shares her experience hearing from her child's long-time physician that things were okay: "I can distinctly remember the real 'end' moment for me. At her follow-up last year, we finally heard the words that we have been waiting years to hear. [The developmental pediatrician] said, 'Congratulations, [your daughter] presents as a typical child her age. She looks great.' I cried. Then I let it sink in. I really tried to be present in the moment. Then I cried some more. We hugged [our daughter] and told her we were so proud of her. At that moment, that was the perfect thing."

Parents Cope: Adjusting to the End of an Era

Now what? Your child isn't going to therapy several times a week and you have all of this free time. What are you going to do now? You have just spent a huge portion of your life trucking your kid to and from speech therapy. Your calendar was always booked on Monday afternoons and Thursday mornings for speech therapy. You'd think you'd be jumping for joy now that you have these "windows" of time open again. Instead, you may feel lost and directionless. Give yourself time to adjust. Slowly you can start adding in some new activities. If your child is not otherwise engaged, maybe you can use this time to enroll her in a class or sport. Maybe you can make this an opportunity to arrange a standing playdate for your child with a friend.

Just be prepared for an adjustment period for you and your child. While the end of therapy is something you both wanted, it can still be a time of transition.

One mother I spoke with talked about the transition from speech therapy to no speech therapy: "I did not find the adjustment hard at all. I was very proud of how far my daughter had come. It just seems like when time in my schedule opens up, something else comes in to fill it—it wasn't hard with three kids! It seems as kids grow, they have more opportunities for activities. [My daughter] did join Girl Scouts, so it is just a different kind of busy."

"I do remember feeling anxious about letting go and saying "Okay, this is over," commented Vicki on how it felt when her son, Evan, ended therapy.

A mother named Karyn relates: "I didn't think I would miss taking [my son] to therapy, but I did. [Speech Therapy] was also my therapeutic social hour with the other moms whose kids were there at the same time. I learned the most from those other moms, and together we got through all the drama that comes from being a mom of a child with special needs."

And just who do they tell? How does one share the "news" with others?

"I told my Mom. I told all my friends. I told my mother-in-law. They were so happy. While they have been supportive over the years, none of them really understood the enormity of the moment. Unless you have been there, you have no idea. My husband and I still cry when we think about it," relates Susan, after ending speech therapy for her daughter, now seven years old.

On a personal note, I made preschool graduation announcements for Kate and mailed them to our close friends and family. I started with something along the lines of "Preschool Graduation?! Really?!" I typed up a little blurb on the computer, complete with cute fonts and colors about Kate's struggle with CAS, along with information about the intense preschool she attended five days a week. I wasn't expecting anything in return—other than a sense of closure for me. But I was floored by the response Kate got—cards and small gifts came her way. It was a sweet way to end her "speech preschool" and send her on to mainstream kindergarten.

Middle Grades and Beyond

While I cannot say for certainty that your child will be speaking normally by middle school, note that childhood apraxia of speech is called a *childhood* speech disorder for a reason. It may be that you are really beginning to see that your child will overcome her CAS. Continue to keep an eye on your child's progress and look for any concerns that may crop up in the middle grades of elementary school, middle school, and into high school. If you do start to see concerns, you know there are resources available to help you and your child. Seek them out when it's appropriate. After a quick "refresher," your child may be back to performing at her top!

Some adolescents with a history of CAS really do not like the fact that the descriptor "childhood" is even part of the moniker. For example, you may hear your adolescent say something like "I don't have childhood apraxia of speech anymore. I am *not* a child!" This can become a touchy subject.

Instead, tweens and adolescents could explain their variable speech to friends or teachers like this: "I used to have a childhood speech disorder when I was younger. It's better now, but sometimes I still have trouble with certain words or phrases, especially when I am tired or stressed."

Amy, the mother of Brooke, age twelve, says: "She sounds like any other sixth grader. In fact, there are many times we have to tell her to slow down her speech so we can catch it all. She was not diagnosed with any other related conditions, but we do notice that she constantly has her 'motor' running and prefers to study while moving around the room."

Linda, the mother of a teenager previously diagnosed with CAS, described her daughter's lingering difficulties this way: "My daughter is sixteen and definitely has resolving CAS. She is easily understood by strangers. However, her CAS still has subtle impact. Last year, she was an honor roll student, yet we went round and round with her science teacher, who complained that my daughter raised her hand without having an answer ready. She could not understand that my daughter needed a few moments to figure out how to turn the words in her brain into spoken words with the unfamiliar science vocabulary."

Another mother mentioned this about her daughter's resolving CAS: "I also recognize that the end may not always be the end. I am confident in Avery's ability to communicate; her speech is perfect nowadays. I am confident that she has a bright future. I am incredibly optimistic, but I also know that with neurological differences, there may be additional surprises. She has come so very far, though, that I know that we can tackle anything that comes our way. Avery will have a great life. I believe that this experience has made her better, harder working, more empathetic."

Sending Your Young Adult to College

At this point, your child will probably be talking like any other college student (provided she had "pure" CAS, without any added disabilities). You may be able to detect slight variations in her speech because you've been there since the beginning. By the time your child reaches college age, she will have learned to accommodate and self-correct little errors in her speech. She will know that when she gets tired, she isn't as eloquent in her communication. She probably realizes that when she's stressed, she makes mistakes in her speech. Your child has come a long way and overcome some significant obstacles.

Be aware that if she still has disabilities that entitled her to special education or accommodations in high school, she may or may not qualify for accommodations in college. The Individuals with Disabilities Education Act (IDEA) discussed in chapter 11 does not cover college students. Your child may, however, qualify as a student with disabilities under Section 504 of the Rehabilitation Act of 1973 or the Americans with Disabilities Act (ADA). She will need to submit official reports of psychological and educational testing to the college after admittance (if she chooses to disclose her disability to the school). Students who qualify for Section 504 or ADA supports can receive extended time on tests, note-taking assistance, access to text-to-speech software, and other types of accommodations, depending on their needs. For more information on rights and supports for college-bound kids, you may want to start with the Wrightslaw flyer "Help for College Students with Disabilities" at: www.wrightslaw.com/flyers/college.504.pdf.

If your child is college-bound, read those college admission guides and help your child prepare for the ACT or SAT. Start thinking about scholarships. However, remember, *every child is different.* Not all children with CAS will go to college, based on many variables (academic ability, financial resources, interest, other co-occurring conditions, etc.). Like all young adults, your child will have her own hopes and dreams. There is nothing specific to CAS to stop her from joining the military, becoming an apprentice in a trade, graduating right into the world of work, trying a few online courses, or taking a "gap year" while she explores her options. Once your child does enter the workforce, she should be aware that the ADA also entitles her to necessary accommodations at work in the event any lingering effects of CAS or another disability make it difficult for her to perform one or more aspects of her job.

Say That Again?! Chapter Summary

This chapter covered resolving and recovering from CAS, shared some reasons for relapse and possible solutions, and then moved into the big question of when or if it's appropriate to end therapy, and how to determine when it's time to move on. We discussed potential problems and concerns as children move into higher grade levels at school (understanding and communicating complex multisyllabic words, among others). We briefly touched on the college years and beyond.

Please don't be overwhelmed. If you already are, then it's time to take a deep breath and remember *your child will likely get over her difficulty with verbal communication.* I know that at times, it feels doubtful. It may reassure you to look back at the beginning of this chapter, where parents commented on how well their children are doing or the "ah-ha" moments in which everything just fell into place.

Recommended Resources

- For information on the ***difference between an articulation disorder and a phonological disorder***, look at this page by Keri Spielvogle, MCD, CCC-SLP: www.superduperinc.com/handouts/pdf/45-ArticVSPhonology.pdf.

- You can find additional information on ***dysarthria*** from the American Speech-Language-Hearing Association (ASHA) at www.asha.org/public/speech/disorders/

dysarthria.htm or the Mayo Clinic at www.mayoclinic.com/health/dysarthria/DS01175.

■ If you want to **hear and see children with a history of CAS** speak (and sing!), go to www.Youtube.com and type "apraxia" or "CAS" or "childhood apraxia of speech" in the search field. You're sure to get several hits.

■ **What Color Is Your Parachute for Teens: Discovering Yourself, Defining Your Future**, by Carol Christen and Richard N. Bolles (Ten Speed Press, 2015) combines suggestions on finding one's passion with discussions of high-interest jobs in the twenty-first century.

■ For students with disabilities who are ready to **transition from high school to college**, check out the Department of Education's brochure, "Students with Disabilities Preparing for Postsecondary Education: Know Your Rights and Responsibilities": http://www2.ed.gov/about/offices/list/ocr/transition.html.

■ **The National Center for College Students with Disabilities Clearinghouse** is a wonderful resource for college-bound individuals loaded with resources about disability and higher education all in one place. For example, you can search "financial aid" or "speech disorders" and get several hits, including information for those who use communication devices, text-to-speech options, and how to become a confident speaker. https://www.nccsdclearinghouse.org/.

■ **The National Center for College Students with Disabilities** (NCCSD) is the only federally funded national center in the US for college and graduate students with *any* type of disability, chronic health condition, or mental or emotional illness. There is information for parents, faculty, and anyone working with college students. http://www.nccsdonline.org/.

■ **Careers: The Graphic Guide to Planning Your Career** by DK Children (2015) is just what it sounds like: a gorgeous, easy-to-navigate visual representation (including charts and tables) of over 400 career opportunities. It's never too early for your tween or teen to start getting ideas of what it's like to work in specific fields, from STEM to sports and from arts to administration.

■ **Teens' Guide to College and Career Planning** by Justin Ross Muchnick (Peterson's, 2016) is a valuable resource offering input from teens, parents, and experts on post–high school options. Whether your child is undecided or is heading to a two-year or four-year college, a technical school, an apprenticeship, the military, or directly into the workforce, this book has so much valuable advice.

Chapter 16

Shake Your Groove Thing

Networking, Advocating, and Resources

"There isn't a single book out there for parents on CAS," I complained to my daughter's SLP.

"I know," Ms. Jen replied. "There's not much out there."

I went on to explain that I just wanted a book, a *real-life* book, I could hold in my hands and read and go back to refer to if I needed. I wanted a comprehensive guide that would start at the beginning and cover the definition of childhood apraxia of speech, what caused it (even if it was just a bunch of theories—I didn't care—I wanted something, *anything),* and what I could do about it. Most of all, I wanted something I could relate to.

Ms. Jen listened like any good therapist or friend would do. When I was done with my wish list, another person chimed in, "Sounds like it's a job for you."

"What!" I shook my head in confusion and disbelief. I hadn't even noticed Sylvia— an SLP assistant—walk into the room.

"It sounds like the job is yours. Write a book about CAS," she repeated with utmost certainty.

I went home that evening and suggested the idea of writing a book about CAS to my husband.

"Why not?" he countered.

"I don't know anything about it, that's why. Remember, it's *me* who needs the book?"

"Well, make it a little research project," he suggested. "You'll learn something in the process."

After a few more rounds of rebuttals and excuses (I didn't have time, not to mention that I'd never written a book before), he convinced me to do it.

And so, the networking, advocating, and resource-getting began. I'm not going to fool you—it wasn't easy. There were days I wanted to claw my eyeballs out and delete everything about CAS from my computer. But I didn't. You are reading the fruits of my labor. I did it for you and for your little ones with CAS. I did it for me. And most of all, I did it for Kate. And you know what? I am so glad I did.

> ### The Nuts and Bolts of This Chapter
>
> - How to become an advocate for your child and why you are the best person to do the job
> - How you can network, advocate, and seek resources *all along* your child's journey with CAS; it doesn't have to come at the end of the journey
> - How to "navigate the field" to find your way out of the woods
> - Starting and establishing your own support group on CAS
> - National and local organizations devoted to CAS, as well as reputable online resources

What *You* Have to Offer

I know what a big job it is to raise kids. There's a lot to think about, take care of, organize, delegate, pay for, and understand. Not to mention the morals and values you hope to instill, the lessons you want to teach, and fun you so desire for your family. Why on earth would you want to add one more thing to your growing list of to-do's? Because you love your child. It's as simple as that. No one else can love and care for your child as much as you do. Not only do you *love* your child to the moon and back, but you also *know* your child inside and out. *You are the best, Mom and Dad.*

But you can't just hear that your child has CAS on Tuesday and then go out and tell everyone you know about it on Wednesday. You need time. You need understanding. You may need to shed a few tears. You may need to talk to a few trusted friends about it. You may need to do a little reading on CAS first. You may need to see your child make some progress in speech therapy (ST). Everyone has a different gauge as to what needs to happen before they are ready to move into the world of advocacy.

Think for a minute about what you might need before you reach out. Now jot it down.

Identifying Your Strengths and Weaknesses

Part of being a good advocate for your child is determining what you are good at doing. I bet you already have a good sense of your strengths and weaknesses. Think of things you naturally love to do, are particularly skilled at, have a strong interest in, or would like to learn more about. You'll know what you're weak at if it's something you often have to ask for assistance to complete, have failed at before, or hear complaints about (from friends, your spouse, or coworkers).

If you're honest with yourself, traits and skills will start to stand out. There might be something you might be able to apply to the world of CAS.

Networking, Advocating, and Seeking Resources

Besides helping your child, you will be helping others along their journeys when you advocate, network, and seek out resources. You say you aren't the "helping kind?" You are concerned that you don't have the time or knowledge to put into all of this "work?" Well, here are a few more reasons to convince you:

- You will recognize your own expertise.
- You will become more informed as a consumer.
- You will be able to ask the "right" professionals well-phrased questions.
- You will be able to give praise and credit to those in the field who deserve it.
- You will feel empowered.
- You will develop your own personal support team.
- You will be able to document your child's progress better.
- You will communicate more effectively with your child's SLP.
- You will control your emotions and feelings better when you understand more.
- ***You can teach your child to become his or her own advocate!***

Let's take a look at the grief cycle one last time. It may seem a stretch, but you actually need to work through these stages of grief in order to be an effective advocate for your child. Read on to see how this cycle can affect you as a parent and as an advocate.

Denial: You'll know you're here when you resist taking your child to the speech clinic or the pediatrician because you don't want to hear what you fear they'll say. You know you are here when you insist on a second opinion because "they don't know what they're talking about anyway."

Anger: You'll know you're here when you hate the sound of your neighbor's chatty two-year-old talking a mile a minute when your four-year-old is still grunting. You'll know you're here when your friend brings you this book and you feel like throwing it at her after shouting a few obscenities her way.

Bargaining: You'll know you're here when you say to your partner, "I suppose if you hadn't been late to talk, Gavin wouldn't have this problem either." You'll know you're here when you say, "Please—I'll give up coffee/shopping/Facebook if you just make my baby talk."

Depression: You'll know you're here when you can barely get out of bed because facing yet another day with your nonverbal kiddo makes you feel ill. You'll know you're here when you cry more than you smile, eat more (or less) than you should, or feel irritated most of the time.

Acceptance: You'll know you're here when you are ready to make a difference in the CAS world. You'll know you're here when you can smile and say, "My child has CAS too."

Moving from Denial and Bargaining to Acceptance

Vicki, whose son Evan is recovering from CAS, says this:

"I have had to let go of a lot of things in this journey—the early dreams, the expectations, the benchmarks I thought for sure we would make if only we worked hard enough. Letting go has allowed me to be quite okay with where my son is at and who he is. I am much freer to accept him and love him all the more for being so special. I try not to let myself be my own worst enemy wishing we had done more. . . .We did a lot, and he came a long ways from the frustrated little three-year-old who was so angry that he could not even get anyone to know he wanted a drink of water to a young man of twenty-one who shows great compassion for any small child or animal that seems to live out in the margin where he has so often found himself to be."

In looking over this list, it may appear as though the only time to be an advocate is when you are at the acceptance stage. Well, yes and no. Perhaps the acceptance stage is the best time to be a really effective and positive advocate. That doesn't mean that you can't do little things along the entire journey. Even when you are lounging in bed and crying yourself to sleep, you can be networking. Even when you are complaining to your spouse or partner that it was his or her "bad" gene that gave your child CAS, you can be looking for resources. Let's break it down with some hard-core suggestions.

Join a Support Group

I'm talking about a real live support group that offers face-to-face communication and support for you and other parents and caregivers of children with CAS. There may be one in your area. It's a great opportunity to get together with like-minded parents seeking support, education, and socialization. The benefit here is that you can form deep and meaningful relationships with parents who know *just where you are*—emotionally and psychologically.

Some of the parents may have been in your shoes a few years ago and can help you make sense of your child's newly diagnosed state; they can give you good "been-there-done-that" advice. Other members may be new to the game. You will be able to "repay" them with your expertise and advice. You may even find a lifelong friend in the group

If anything, membership in a group like this is validation that *you are not in this alone.*

How to Find a Group

Your child's speech clinic may have a name or contact information for a parent from their practice. If they don't and you still want the connection, you may consider starting your own group (see "Wanna Get Something Started" in this chapter). Head to the Apraxia Kids website (www.apraxiakids.org). From there, go to "Communities" and see if there is an official Apraxia Kids in-person or online support group for your area. Note that group facilitators need to register their group with Apraxia Kids, so not every available group in your area will appear here. You may have to get creative (keep reading).

By the way, a support group specifically on CAS may be a rare find. If you can't find something just for CAS in your area, consider joining a general support group for speech-language disorders.

What If Groups Aren't Your Thing?

If a support group isn't your style, or you're not into starting one of your own (it's a big task and not to be taken lightly), you can still make a difference and find a little understanding for yourself.

Create a Blog/Instagram or Pinterest Account: This may prove a worthwhile endeavor as you seek to make sense of your new normal. It did for me. In fact, I looked forward to jotting down the latest in our CAS journey and found this was a fabulous way to process the events of Kate's speech therapy and progress. Check out various free sites for starting your own blog such as www.wordpress.com or www.blogspot.com (just to mention a couple) and start blogging. You can control how you want the site set up (usually), how often you write, what you write about, and how it's distributed. Sure, it's a bit overwhelming at first, but you never know when someone might stumble upon your blog and find comfort and wisdom in your words.

If blogging (or writing) isn't your thing, you might want to consider other social media options. You might want something more visual with story-like captions such as Instagram, or maybe you'd just like to peruse speech ideas and tips—and post some of your own—on a site like Pinterest. Doing something like this might help others along their journey, but it can also give you a sense of progress when you look back on how far your child has grown.

One parent I spoke with said, "I don't think tweeting about my son's apraxia [CAS] will change the world, but it changes *my* world every day just to say a little something about Sawyer's progress."

Start a Website: The next step up from blogging is to start a website. Take a look at Site Build It—a build-your-own web business—at www.sitebuildit.com.

Dawn Villarreal of Naperville, Illinois, started an online special needs resource website, One Place for Special Needs (www.oneplaceforspecialneeds.com), after it dawned on her that her individual experiences as the mother of a child with autism were likely universal. Her site is comprehensive—not all about autism and not just about resources in Illinois, either. One Place for Special Needs covers many special needs, including childhood apraxia of speech.

Join Online Discussion Boards and Groups:

- **Apraxia Kids** is the leading nonprofit that strengthens the support of those vested in the lives of children with CAS by educating professionals and families; facilitating community engagement and outreach; and investing in the future through advocacy and evidence-based research. They offer official online support groups to ensure no family feels alone in their CAS journey. For more information or to join an online group, visit www.apraxiakids.org. Click "Community" from the drop-down menu, and select "support groups." Here, a variety of specialty groups are available—for example, one for Spanish-speaking families, those specifically for grandparents, others for profound CAS, and yet another tailored to parents of older kids (10+ years) with CAS. This is not an inclusive list, so if you think you might have a special interest need, pop over and see what Apraxia Kids can offer. Many of these are closed Facebook groups, so privacy and personal comfort have been carefully preserved.

- **The Apraxia Connection** was founded in 2012 by three Chicago-area mothers of children with varied degrees of CAS, global apraxia, and associated disorders. Through their online presence (Facebook) and face-to-face meetings in the Chicago area, the group provides great information and camaraderie on speech therapy approaches, IEPs, specialists, decreasing the costs of speech therapy, and raising a child with apraxia. For more information, visit the website at http://www.theapraxiaconnection.org/.

- **CHERAB** (Communication Help, Education, Research, Apraxia Base) is an organization on communication delays and disorders with neurological underpinnings. The group was founded by Lisa Geng, a mother of two late talkers. Lisa teamed up with Marilyn Agin and Malcolm J. Nicholl to pen the acclaimed book *The Late Talker: What to Do if Your Child Isn't Talking Yet* (Saint Martin's Press, 2004). Here you will find a plethora of links to websites: some have a more interactive approach, others more information-seeking. Visit www.cherab.org and click on "find support."

- **OPPEN CAS** is the Ontario Professionals & Parents Education Network of Childhood Apraxia of Speech. Founder and chair, Brooke Rea, was inspired to create her own organization in her home country of Canada after attending the 2014 Apraxia Kids training institute. The organization is ranked as the number one resource for Ontario professionals and parents interested in CAS. Their aim is to empower and connect individuals, sharing ideas, issues, and resources. For more information, see: www.oppencas.ca.

How They Got Connected with Other CAS Parents

Here's how it worked for one participant in Small Talk: All About Apraxia:

"I was just hanging out around my son's school when I casually mentioned that my son had a speech disorder. A woman overhead me and said hers did too. We got to talking and learned that both of our sons had CAS. I went home and 'friended' her on Facebook."

It worked this way for me: I was at the library when I bumped into a mom I had seen there before. We got to chatting about preschools, and I mentioned that Kate was attending the public school district's preschool. She cocked an eyebrow. I said, "She has a speech disorder," not wanting to get into the specifics of CAS. The other mother perked up: "Oh, really? We have apraxia." Needless to say, we've been friends ever since.

It's amazing how small the world really becomes when you start chatting and learning about others. So, look for excuses to strike up a conversation.

Wanna Get Something Started?

No support group? No problem. Start something of your own! Of course, every group starts small and grows bigger. It's up to you to determine where and how it happens. You may not even *want* a large group. But you *do* want something that matters to you and others who have a stake in CAS.

■ *Start small.* Gather a few CAS parents and meet at a coffee shop. Sip a cup of joe while you chat about CAS (I know, sounds kind of ironic). You may already know some parents from your child's speech clinic. Or post a note on a community bulletin board, "SEEKING: Individuals or families affected by Childhood Apraxia of Speech (CAS) to participate in small discussion/support group." Try posting something like that at your child's speech clinic or asking your SLP to help you connect with other like-minded parents.

■ *Grow a little bigger.* Once you have a few folks to meet with on a regular basis, consider expanding your circle. You can reach out to schools, speech clinics, physicians' offices, libraries, places of worship, online message boards, and local non-profit organizations. You'll want to market your group well. Send letters, make phone calls, connect online, and show up in person.

■ *Set some guidelines.* You'll likely want to have a set of bylaws or rules for your group. Determine how many participants you'd like, where you'll meet, how often you'll meet, how long the meetings will be, what the topics will be, if there will be a facilitator/leader (and how that person is chosen, what their duties are), and who will help organize and maintain the group. Confidentiality is important. Since everyone will likely be sharing private and potentially emotional information about a minor child, you'll want to keep your discussions just between the group participants.

- *Keep it warm, welcoming, and helpful.* Groups need to be supportive, while being educational and social. Make it an event folks *want* to attend. Have fun, provide snacks and encouragement. Let others know this group is about helping others cope with their CAS journey.

- *Know when it's time to let go.* Whether you're a participant or core leader, you'll want to gauge when it's the best time for you to move on. Leaders and facilitators get burned out just like the rest of us. It may be time to give control to another member. The worst thing you can do for yourself and your group is to continue when you are burned out.

- *Start a local nonprofit organization.* This is a huge task and certainly not for everyone. But you could do it if you really wanted to. Here's what Rebecca Christiansen, Executive Director of Celebrate Differences in Oswego, Illinois, did. Ms. Christiansen, a nurse who has a son with Down syndrome, was shocked to find that healthcare providers did not present children with special needs in a positive light. Celebrate Differences aims to help local parents through education workshops, information on local resources, and a library of resource materials. You can visit their website at www.celebratedifferences.com.

Tip: There are so many options and opportunities for connecting with others who may be walking the same path. You don't have to live in a large city or be especially outgoing, just resourceful. Joining Facebook groups for a specific demographic (I'm part of one for tweens and teens with CAS, for example) might work wonders. It'll give you connections, support, validation, advice, and a place to vent your frustrations.

My Road to Advocacy

As described above, I felt compelled to write this book because there wasn't anything specific enough out there for me. I joined a listserv or two—back when they were in fashion. Then I began blogging about parenting and CAS. I started a Small Talk: All About Apraxia education series, originally facilitated through the speech clinic where Kate received ST. My goal was to connect other parents and caregivers together once a week for five weeks. Each meeting had a specific topic and guided discussion. It was my hope these parents would continue to call upon one another for resources, support, and maybe even playdates! Even though many of our children have progressed from those early days of CAS, we are still in contact on Facebook. It's such a joy to see how these families—and children—have grown. Many are participating in CAS walks, fundraisers, school events and clubs, sports, and more. Some children still have remnants of CAS, and others you would never know once struggled with speech and language issues.

What Do Folks Want from a Support Group?

Here's what some of the participants in my Small Talk: All About Apraxia series had to say:

- "I found that I loved the session on resources and networking. Not only was there so much out there that I didn't know about, it was presented in such a fun, you-can-do-it manner that made me feel empowered."
- "I was really looking for support and to share my experiences with apraxia [CAS]. Talking with other women—moms of kids with CAS—was so helpful."
- "The group really met my expectations. I received so much information and knowledge that I otherwise would not have received."
- "Being with other parents struggling with CAS was a wonderful learning experience. We can all learn from others."
- "Support and friendship were big to me. I felt very isolated in this whole CAS thing. I didn't know anyone else with [apraxia] until this group."

The Leading Nonprofit Organization on CAS

As mentioned earlier in this chapter, Apraxia Kids is the leading nonprofit that strengthens the support systems in the lives of children with childhood apraxia of speech (CAS). They do this by educating professionals and families; facilitating community engagement and outreach; and investing in the future through advocacy and research. Apraxia Kids began as a virtual support group for parents looking for answers about apraxia, a relatively unknown motor speech disorder. Since that time, Apraxia Kids has grown to be the only national nonprofit in CAS education and support for both families and speech-language professionals not only in the United States, but worldwide.

Apraxia Kids continues to serve as the world's most trusted resource for CAS, offering help and hope for families and children. From understanding a new diagnosis—to becoming educated about CAS—to learning how to advocate, Apraxia Kids helps guide families along their personal journeys, as they strive for each child to find his or her voice.

Apraxia Kids was established in Pittsburgh in 2000 by founder Sharon Gretz after she experienced the confusion and isolation of parenting a child with CAS when there was relatively limited information available. As an attempt to help other parents working through the same issues, a listserv was developed to share what had been learned and to help others find appropriate care. In the early days of community building on the internet, supporters from across the country were asking similar questions—this became the start of Apraxia Kids. This backbone of parent-to-parent peer support still exists today as families new to a CAS diagnosis often go to the Apraxia Kids website or Facebook group first. Here they find a supportive community and evidence-based research.

Apraxia Kids is dedicated to the communities they serve by creating support through education, awareness, advocacy, and research. They are dedicated to:

- Cultivating **Hope** for families and children
- Curating high-quality, **Evidence-based** information about diagnosis and treatment
- Facilitating **Partnerships** among professionals and families to build a community of support
- Being responsible, **Trustworthy** stewards of charitable funds and resources to ensure a sustainable future for the organization
- Ensuring everyone has **Equal** access to resources and guidance to navigate the CAS journey
- Advancing **Innovation** through research and education
- Providing unwavering support of the whole person with **Compassion**, **Empathy**, and **Understanding**
- Fostering opportunities for our CAS **Communities** to come together

Apraxia Kids provides the following programs and services:

- Support groups
- Intensive professional education
- Online education/webinar library
- Article library
- Community workshops
- Innovative research
- Annual National Conference on Childhood Apraxia of Speech
- Social media
- Walk for Apraxia community events
- Print material and parent folder

(This official description of the organization is courtesy of Apraxia Kids.)

Do What's Right for You

Everyone copes and learns differently. Don't feel like you have to knock yourself out and write books and blogs or start a nonprofit after reading this chapter. You'll want to cherry-pick your favorite activities based on your skills, interest, time, and financial resources. But I encourage you to do something— big or small—it all makes a difference.

Final Bits of Wisdom

Maybe you are familiar with this early childhood jingle: "Smooth road, smooth road . . . bumpy road, bumpy road, rough road, rough road, whoops! Pothole!" When you play this game with a toddler, you seat him on your outstretched legs near your knees, usually facing you. You hold his hands and move your legs side to side during the "smooth road" part. When the road gets "bumpy," you wiggle your knees to give your child a little bounce, a little *more* for a "rough" patch, and then the grand finale is when you "pop" your child up in the air with extended arms for the "pothole" effect. Kids die with laughter and you see the twinkle in their eye as they ask for more.

Where am I going with this? Yep. It's an analogy for your journey with CAS. There will be smooth-sailing times. There will be bumps along the road. And it will be rough at times too. On really, really bad days, you will hit a pothole (or two).

But then, your child will look at you with bright, engaging eyes, he'll whisper or sign, "I love you," and it will renew your efforts to give him what he needs. Again. You'll do it because you love your child.

Say That Again?! Chapter Summary

This chapter is all about how you—mom, dad, or anyone else raising or caring for a child with CAS—can help. It is about empowering yourself and your child to be the best you can be and finding—or creating—the resources that matter to you. We covered in-person and online support groups, websites, blogs, and nonprofit organizations, but most of all, we talked about you. *You* are the best person to help *your* child. *Your little person depends on you for his or her success.*

Recommended Resources

- *The Parent You Want to Be: Who You Are Matters More Than What You Do* by Drs. Les and Leslie Parrott (Zondervan, 2007) is a very readable book that explains how to cultivate the traits you most desire for your children.

- *Know Your Parenting Personality: How to Use the Enneagram to Become the Best Parent You Can Be* by Janet Levine (Wiley, 2003) is another book that may help you determine your strengths and weaknesses as you look at ways you can help advocate for your child.

- *MotherStyles: Using Personality Type to Discover Your Parenting Strengths* by Janet Penley and Diane Eble (Da Capo Press, 2006) may be of interest to mothers who want to identify their strengths when navigating the road of advocacy.

- Otto Kroger and David Goldstein teamed up to write *Creative You: Using Your Personality Type to Thrive*, a book about finding practical ways to fuel your passion based on personality traits. (Atria Books, 2013).

- *Special Needs Advocacy Resource Book: What You Can Do Now to Advocate for Your Exceptional Child's Education* by Rich Weinfeld and Michelle Davis (Prufock Press, 2008) covers how to work with schools to achieve optimal learning situations and accommodations for children with disabilities, from IEPs to 504 plans.

- Your local community may hold a *special education community services fair* offering speakers, services, and exhibitors. Ask at your school district or speech clinic for more information.

- *"How You Can Help Your Child Learn to Be a Good Self Advocate"* is available on the website of the Pacer Center at www.pacer.org/parent/php/PHP-c95.pdf. Also check out the publications on topics such as dispute resolution and parent engagement/student success available for free download (click on the "Resources and Workshops" tab at www.pacer.org).

- You and your older child may want to check out *Kids as Self-Advocates* for articles, resources, and a forum where kids and young adults with a variety of special needs meet in cyber space to discuss their concerns: www.fvkasa.org.

References

Chapter 1

Goddard, Sally. *Reflexes, Learning, and Behavior: A Window into the Child's Mind, a Non-Invasive Approach to Solving Learning and Behavior Problems.* Eugene, Oregon: Fern Ridge Press, 2002.

Hall, Penny, Jordan, Linda, and Robin, Donald. *Developmental Apraxia of Speech: Theory and Clinical Practice.* 2nd ed. Austin, TX: Pro-Ed, 2007.

Hamaguchi, Patricia. *Childhood Speech, Language, and Listening Problems: What Every Parent Should Know.* New York, NY: John Wiley and Sons, 2010.

Koballa, Joyce. "Conference Held to Discuss Speech Disorder." *Herald Standard*, August 26, 2010.

Lewis, B. A., Freebairin, L. A., Hansen, A. J., Iyengar, S. K., and Taylor, H. G. (2004). "School-age Follow-up of Children with Childhood Apraxia of Speech". *Language, Speech, and Hearing Services in Schools* 35:122–40.

McCauley, Rebecca. "Childhood Apraxia of Speech: An Overview and Assessment Considerations." Accessed July 27, 2011. http://www.speechpathology.com.

Vossbeck, Kelli and Meredith, Amy. "Diagnostic Criteria for CAS: A Survey Study." 2008 ASHA convention handout. http://www.asha.org.

Weitzman, Elaine. "A Closer Look at the Late Talker Study: Why Parents Should Beware of a 'Wait and See' Approach." Accessed Feb. 25, 2020. http://www.hanen.org.

Chapter 2

American Psychiatric Association. *Diagnostic and Statistical Manual of Mental Disorders*, 5th ed. Washington, DC: American Psychiatric Association, 2013.

Caruso, Anthony, and Strand, Edythe. *Clinical Management of Motor Speech Disorders in Children.* New York, NY: Thieme, 1999.

Doughtery, Dorothy. *Teach Me How to Say It Right: Helping Your Child with Articulation Disorders.* Oakland, CA: New Harbinger, 2005.

Eliot, Lise. *What's Going on in There? How the Brain and Mind Develop in the First Five Years of Life.* Minneapolis: Bantam, 1999.

Feit, Debbie. *A Parent's Guide to Speech and Language Problems.* New York, NY: McGraw-Hill, 2007.

Hamaguchi, Patricia McAleer. *Childhood Speech, Language & Listening Problems: What Every Parent Should Know.* 3rd ed. Hoboken, NJ: Wiley, 2010.

Owens, Robert E., Jr. *Language Development: An Introduction.* 8th ed. Upper Saddle River, NJ: Allyn & Bacon, 2011.

Pulvermuller, F., and Fadiga, L. "Active Perception: Sensorimotor Circuits as a Cortical Basis for Language." *Nature Reviews in Neuroscience 11* (May 2010).

Rousey, Carol G. *A Practical Guide to Helping Children with Speech and Language Problems: For Parents and Teachers Only.* Springfield, IL: Charles G. Thomas, 1984.

Schetz, Katherine, and Cassell, Stuart Kent. *Talking Together: A Parent's Guide to the Development, Enrichment and Problems of Speech and Language.* Blacksburg, VA: Pocahontas Press, 1994.

Chapter 3
Feit, Debbie. *A Parent's Guide to Speech and Language Problems.* New York, NY: McGraw-Hill, 2007.

Hamaguchi, Patricia McAleer. *Childhood Speech, Language & Listening Problems: What Every Parent Should Know.* 3rd ed. Hoboken, NJ: Wiley, 2010.

Chapter 4
Feit, Debbie. *A Parent's Guide to Speech and Language Problems.* New York, NY: McGraw-Hill, 2007.

Kumin, Libby. "You Said It Just Yesterday, Why Not Now? Developmental Apraxia of Speech in Children and Adults with Down Syndrome." *Disability Solutions 2,* no. 2 (Nov./Dec.2002).

McCauley, Rebecca J. *Assessment of Language Disorders in Children.* Hillsdale, NJ: Lawrence Erlbaum Associates, 2001.

Chapter 5
Boh, Andrea, Csiacsek, Emily, Duginske, Rachel, Meath, Theresa (student researchers), and Carpenter, Linda, PhD (faculty collaborator and mentor). "Counseling Parents of Children with CAS." Poster presentation at ASHA Conference, 2008.

"Dr. Muriel Morley." Craniofacial Society of Great Britain and Ireland. Accessed March 4, 2020. http://craniofacialsociety.co.uk/dr-muriel-morley.

Duffy, J. *Motor Speech Disorders.* St. Louis: Mosby, 1995.

Hall, Penelope K., Jordan, Linda, and Robin, Donald. *Developmental Apraxia of Speech: Theory and Clinical Practice,* 2nd ed. Austin, TX: Pro-Ed Publishers, 2007.

Hickman, Lori. "Prognosis for Apraxia: What Does the Future Hold?" Accessed Feb. 25, 2020. http://www.apraxiakids.org/apraxia_kids_library/prognosis for-apraxia-what-does-the-future-hold/.

Morley, Muriel. *The Development and Disorders of Speech in Childhood.* London: E & S Livingstone, Ltd., 1957.

Strand, E. A. "Assessment and Treatment of Childhood Apraxia of Speech." Presentation at CASANA conference, February 19–20, 2010.

Strand, E. A., and McCauley, R. J. "Differential Diagnosis of Severe Speech Impairment in Young Children." *The ASHA Leader 13,* no. 10 (Aug. 12, 2008): 10–13.

Strohm, Kate. *Being the Other One: Growing Up with a Brother or Sister Who Has Special Needs.* Boston: Shambhala, 2005.

Velleman, Shelley. *Childhood Apraxia of Speech Resource Guide.* Albany, NY: Delmar Publishing, 2003.

Chapter 6

"About Potocki-Lupski Syndrome." NIH: Genetic and Rare Diseases Information Center. Accessed Feb. 25, 2020. https://rarediseases.info.nih.gov/ diseases/10145/potocki-lupski-syndrome.

American Speech-Language-Hearing Association. "Childhood Apraxia of Speech."

Bridgeman, Elizabeth, and Snowling, Maggie. "The Perception of Phoneme Sequence: A Comparison of Dyspraxic and Normal Children." *British Journal of Disorders of Communication 23* (1988): 245–52.

Fish, Margaret. *Here's How to Treat Childhood Apraxia of Speech.* San Diego, CA: Plural Publishing, 2015.

Horsthemke, B., and Wagstaff, J. "Mechanisms of Imprinting of the Prader–Willi/ Angelman Region." American Journal of Medical Genetics, Part A (2008): 2041–2052.

Guenther, Frank H. "Cortical Interactions Underlying the Production of Speech Sounds." *Journal of Communication Disorders 39* (2006): 350–65.

Hurst, J. A., Baraitser, M., Auger, E., Graham, F., and Norell, S. "An Extended Family with a Dominantly Inherited Speech Disorder." *Developmental Medical Child Neurology 32,* no. 4 (April 1990): 352–5.

Kumin, Libby. *Early Communication Skills for Children with Down Syndrome: A Guide for Parents and Professionals.* Bethesda, MD: Woodbine House, 2012.

Kumin, Libby. "You Said it Just Yesterday, Why Not Now: Developmental Apraxia of Speech in Children and Adults with Down Syndrome." *Disability Solutions 2,* no. 2 (Nov./Dec. 2002).

Lewis, Barbara, Freebarin, Lisa A., Hansen, Amy, Taylor, Gerry, Ivengar, Sudha, and Shriberg, Lawrence. "Family Pedigrees of Children with Suspected Childhood Apraxia of Speech." *Journal of Communication Disorders 37,* no. 2 (March/ April 2004): 157–75.

Maassen, Ben. "Issues Contrasting Adult Acquired versus Developmental Apraxia of Speech." *Seminars in Speech and Language 23* (2002): 257–66.

Nelson, C. et al. "Verbal Dyspraxia in Treated Galactosemia." *Pediatrics, 88,* no. 2 (1991): 346–50.

Rosenbek J., and Wertz, R. "A Review of Fifty Cases of Developmental Apraxia of Speech." *Language, Speech, and Hearing Services in Schools 5* (1972): 207–24.

Shriberg, Lawrence. "What Do Researchers Know about Genetics and CAS?" Apraxia Kids library. Accessed August 7, 2011. https://www.apraxia-kids.org.

Strand, E. A. *Childhood Apraxia of Speech: Description, Definitions, and Underlying Neurologic Factors.* Paper presented at the Childhood Apraxia of Speech Association of North America (CASANA) National Conference on Childhood Apraxia of Speech, July 2009.

Chapter 7

Bahr, Diane. *Nobody Ever Told Me (or My Mother) That: Everything from Bottles to Breastfeeding to Healthy Speech Development.* Arlington, TX: Sensory World, 2010.

Cole, Kevin, Maddox, Mary, Notari-Syverson, A., and Lim, Y. S. *Language Is the Key: Video Programs for Building Language and Literacy in Early Childhood.* Seattle, WA: Washington Learning Systems, 2006.

Drake, Martha. *Just for Kids: Apraxia.* East Moline, IL: LinguiSystems, 1999.

George, Karen. "Treatment of Childhood Apraxia of Speech by Chicago Therapy." Accessed Feb. 15, 2020. http:// www.chicagospeechtherapy.com/ treatment-of-childhood-apraxia-of-speech-by-chicago-speech-therapy.

Hall, Penelope K., Jordan, Linda, and Robin, Donald. *Developmental Apraxia of Speech: Theory and Clinical Practice.* 2nd ed. Austin, TX: Pro-Ed, 2007.

Helfrich-Miller, Kathleen. Information on Melodic Intonation Therapy (MIT) acquired from email correspondence on Sept. 13, 2011.

Hammer, David. *Treatment Strategies for Childhood Apraxia of Speech with David Hammer.* Pittsburgh, PA: Children's Hospital of Pittsburgh, 2006.

Kent, Ray D. "Theory in the Balance." *Perspectives on Speech Science and Orofacial Disorders 18* (July 2008): 15–21.

Marshalla, Pam. *Becoming Verbal with Childhood Apraxia: New Insights on Piaget for Today's Therapy.* Kirkland, WA: Marshalla Speech and Language, 2007.

McCauley, Rebecca J., and Fey, Marc E. *Treatment of Language Disorders in Children.* Baltimore, MD: Paul H. Brookes Publishing, 2016.

Strand, Edythe, and Caruso, Anthony. *Clinical Management of Motor Speech Disorders in Children.* New York, NY: Thieme, 1999.

Strode, Robin, and Chamberlin, Catherine. *Easy Does It for Apraxia-Preschool.* East Moline, IL: LinguiSystems, 1994

Velleman, Shelley. *Childhood Apraxia of Speech Resource Guide.* Clifton Park, NY: Delmar Publishing, 2003.

Chapter 8

American Music Therapy Association. "What Is Music Therapy?" Accessed Feb. 26, 2020. https://www.musictherapy.org/about/musictherapy/.

American Speech-Language-Hearing Association, Working Group in AIT. "Auditory Integration Training." Accessed March 9, 2020. https://www.asha.org/policy/PS2004–00218/.

Cuthbert, S. C., and Barras, M. "Developmental Delay Syndromes: Psychometric Testing Before and After Chiropractic Treatment of 157 Children. *Journal of Manipulative Physiological Therapy 32,* no. 8 (2009): 660–9.

Feit, Debbie. *Parent's Guide to Understanding Speech and Language Disorders.* New York, NY: McGraw-Hill, 2007.

Fish, Dee. *Here's How to Treat Childhood Apraxia of Speech.* San Diego: Plural Publishing, 2010.

Goddard, Sally. *Reflexes, Learning, and Behavior: A Window into the Child's Mind: A Non-Invasive Approach to Solving Learning and Behavior Problems.* Eugene, OR: Fern Ridge Press, 2002.

Kranowitz, Carol Stock, and Miller, Lucy Jane. *The Out-of-Sync Child.* Rev. ed. New York, NY: Perigee Trade, 2006.

Kaplan, Melvin. *Seeing through New Eyes: Changing the Lives of Children with Autism, Asperger's Syndrome, and Other Developmental Disabilities through Vision Therapy.* Philadelphia: Jessica Kingsley Publishers, 2008.

Morris, Claudia, MD, Oakland Children's Hospital. Interview and quote from email reprinted with permission granted on April 23, 2011.

Morris, Claudia R., and Agin, Marilyn C. "Syndrome of Allergy, Apraxia, and Malabsorption: Characterization of a Neurodevelopmental Phenotype That Responds to Omega 3 and Vitamin E Supplementation." *Alternative Therapies,* Volume 15, no. 4 (July/August 2009).

Rutek, Donna. "Animal-Friendly Therapy: Contact with Horses Has Profound Effect on Kids with Disabilities." *Chicago Tribune,* June 2, 1999.

Sena Moore, Kimberly. "Music, Rhythm, and Their Potential Benefits for Childhood Apraxia of Speech." PediaStaff. May 28, 2010. www.pediastaff.com/blog/music-rhythm-and-their-potential-benefits-for-childhood-apraxia-of-speech-647.

Chapter 9

American Academy of Pediatrics. "Children and Media Tips from the American Academy of Pediatrics." May 1, 2018. https://www.aap.org/en-us/about-the-aap/aap-press-room/news-features-and-safety-tips/Pages/Children-and-Media-Tips.aspx.

Bahr, Diane. *Oral Motor Assessment and Treatment: Ages and Stages.* Upper Saddle River, NJ: Allyn and Bacon, 2001.

DeThorne, Laura S. et al. "When 'Simon Says' Doesn't Work: Alternatives to Imitation for Facilitating Early Speech Development." *American Journal of Speech-Language Pathology 18,* no. 2 (May 1, 2009): 133–45.

Doughtery, Dorothy, P. *Teach Me How to Say It Right: Helping Your Child with Articulation Disorders.* Oakland, CA: New Harbinger Publications, 2005.

Fish, Margaret. *Here's How to Treat Childhood Apraxia of Speech.* San Diego, CA: Plural Publishing, 2015.

Osby, Jasmine. "Company Helps Students Learn by Playing Games." *St. Louis Post-Dispatch,* August 20, 2010.

Schetz, Katherine, and Cassell, Stuart Kent. *Talking Together: A Parent's Guide to the Development, Enrichment, and Problems of Speech and Language.* Blacksburg, VA: Pocahontas Press, 1994.

Schwartz, Sue. *The New Language of Toys: Teaching Communication Skills to Children with Special Needs, a Guide for Parents.* 3rd ed. Bethesda, MD: Woodbine House, 2004.

Chapter 10

Caspari, Susan S., Strand, Edythe A., Kotagal, Suresh, and Bergqvist, Christina. "Obstructive Sleep Apnea, Seizures, and Childhood Apraxia of Speech." *Pediatric Neurology: Science Direct.* Vol. 38, Issue 6, pp. 422–25.

Doheny, Kathleen. "Can't Sleep? Adjust the Temperature." *WebMD.* Accessed March 9, 2020. www.webmd.com/a-to-z-guides/features/cant-sleep-adjust--the-temperature.

Haiken, Melanie. "5 Foods to Help You Sleep." *Yahoo Health.* Accessed Feb. 3, 2011. http://health.yahoo.net/caring/5-foods-that-help-you-sleep.

Hiss, Tony. *The Experience of Place: A New Way of Looking at and Dealing with Our Radically Changing Cities and Countryside.* New York, NY: Vintage, 1991.

Mindell, Jodi, PhD. Quote from personal correspondence used with permission.

Mosheim, Jason. "Apraxia and Obstructive Sleep Apnea: Is There a Link?" *Advance for Speech-Language Pathologists and Audiologists.* Vol. 18, no. 10.

Chapter 11

Anderson, Winifred, Chitwood, Stephen, Hayden, Deirdre, and Takemoto, Cheri. *Negotiating the Special Education Maze: A Guide for Parents and Teachers.* 4th ed. Bethesda, MD: Woodbine House, 2008.

Encyclopedia on Early Childhood Development. www.child-encyclopedia.com/en-ca/home.html.

Morin, Amanda. "8 Steps to Kicking Off Your Child's IEP the Right Way." Greatschools.org. July 11, 2019.

Wrightslaw. "Do You Know Who Is Providing Your Child's Speech Language Therapy?" Wright's Law Blog. www.wrightslaw.com/blog/?p=129. Jan. 29, 2009.

Chapter 12

Al Otaiba, S., Puranik, C., Ziolkowski, R., and Montgomery, T. "Effectiveness of Early Phonological Awareness Interventions for Students with Speech or Language Impairments." *Journal of Special Education 43* (2009): 107–28.

Bourdreau, D. M., and Hedberg, N. L. "A Comparison of Early Literacy Skills in Children with Specific Speech Language Impairment and Their Typically Developing Peers." *American Journal of Speech-Language Pathology 8* (1999): 249–60.

Catts, H. W. "The Relationship between Speech-Language Impairments and Reading Disabilities." *Journal of Speech & Hearing Research 36* (1993): 948–58.

Catts, H. W., Fey, M. E., Zhang, X. Y., and Tomblin, J. B. "Estimating the Risk of Future Reading Difficulties in Kindergarten Children: A Research-based Model and Its Clinical Implementation." *Language, Speech and Hearing Services in Schools 32* (2001): 38–50.

Catts, H. W., Fey, M. E., Zhang, X., and Tomblin, J. B. "Language Basis of Reading and Reading Disabilities: Evidence from a Longitudinal Investigation." *Scientific Studies of Reading 3* (1999): 331–62.

Gillon, Gail. *Phonological Awareness: From Research to Practice.* New York, NY: Guilford Press, 2004.

Larrivee, L., and Catts, H. "Early Reading Achievement in Children with Expressive Phonological Disorders." *American Journal of Speech-Language Pathology 8* (1999): 118–28.

Liberman, Alvin M., Cooper, Franklin S., Shankweiler, Donald P., and Studdert-Kennedy, Michael. "Perception and the Speech Code." *Psychological Review 74,* (1967): 431–61.

Lewis, B. A., Freebairn, L. A., and Taylor, H. G. "Academic Outcomes in Children with Histories of Speech Sound Disorders. *Journal of Communication Disorders 33,* no. 1 (2000): 11–30.

McNeill, Brigid, Gillon, Gail, and Dodd, Barbara. "Effectiveness of an Integrated Phonological Awareness Approach for Children with Childhood Apraxia of Speech (CAS)." *International Journal of Language & Communication Disorders 44,* no. 2 (2009): 175–92.

Meier, Daniel R. *The Young Child's Memory for Words.* New York, NY: Teachers College Press, 2004.

Rvachew, Susan. "Phonological Processing and Reading in Children with Speech-Sound Disorders." *American Journal of Speech-Language Pathology 16* (2007): 260–70.

Stackhouse, Joy. *Persisting Speech Difficulties in Children: Children's Speech and Literacy Difficulties.* Hoboken, NJ: Wiley and Sons, 2006.

Chapter 13

Baskin, Amy, and Fawcett, Heather. *More Than a Mom: Living a Full and Balanced Life When Your Child Has Special Needs.* Bethesda, MD: Woodbine House, 2006.

Feit, Debbie. *The Parent's Guide to Speech and Language Problems.* New York, NY: McGraw-Hill, 2007.

Marshak, Laura E., and Prezant, Fran. *Married with Special Needs Children: A Couples' Guide to Keeping Connected.* Bethesda, MD: Woodbine House, 2007.

Michael, Rudolph, Rosanowski, Frank, Eysholdt, Ulrich, and Kummer, Peter. "Anxiety and Depression in Mothers of Speech Impaired Children." *International Journal of Pediatric Otorhinolaryngology 67* (2003): 1337–41.

Murphy, Ann Pleshette. *The Seven Stages of Motherhood: Making the Most of Your Life as Mom.* New York, NY: Knopf, 2004.

Chapter 14

Freedman, Judy. *Easing the Teasing: Helping Your Child Cope with Name-Calling, Ridicule, & Verbal Bullying.* Chicago: Contemporary Books, 2002.

Markham, C., van Laar, D., Gibbard, D., and Dean, T. "Children with Speech, Language, and Communication Needs: Their Perceptions of Their Quality of Life." *International Journal of Language and Communication Disorders 44,* no. 5 (Sept./Oct. 2009): 748–68.

Nixon, Robin. "Studies Reveal Why Children Get Bullied and Rejected." LiveScience. com. February 2, 2010.

Sparrow, Joshua. "When Children Hit." *Scholastic Parent and Child.* October 2008.

Chapter 15

Ashmore, Jean. "Transitioning from High School to College—Students with Disabilities." Sept. 23, 2010. https://blog.bookshare.org/tag/planning-for-college/.

Bahr, Diane. *Oral Motor Assessment and Treatment: Ages and Stages:* Upper Saddle River, NJ: Allyn & Bacon, 2000.

Jakielski, Kathy J. "Will My Child with CAS Ever Achieve Normal Speech?" Accessed Feb. 26, 2020. www.apraxia-kids.org/apraxia_kids_library/prognosis-for-apraxia-what-does-the-future-hold/.

McCauley, Rebecca, and Strand, Edythe. "A Review of Standardized Tests of Nonverbal Oral and Speech Motor Performance in Children." *American Journal of Speech-Pathology 17* (February 2008): 81–91.

Wright, Pam, and Wright, Pete. *From Emotions to Advocacy: The Special Education Survival Guide.* Hartfield, VA: Harbor House Law Press, 2004.

Chapter 16

Apraxia Kids. Permission to quote information on history and mission of Apraxia Kids granted by Angela Grimm, Oct. 17, 2019. https://www.apraxia-kids.org/about-apraxia-kids/.

Appendices

"Apraxia a Common Occurrence in Autism, Study Finds." *ASHA Wire.* September 2015. https://leader.pubs.asha.org/doi/full/10.1044/leader.RIB1.20092015.18.

Blume, Gina, and Murray, Donna. "Recognizing and Treating Apraxia of Speech in Children with Autism." July 31, 2015. https://www.autismspeaks.org/.

Eliot, Lisa. *What's Going on in There: How the Brain and Mind Develop in the First Five Years of Life.* New York, NY: Bantam, 2000.

"Facts for Families: The Depressed Child." The American Academy of Child & Adolescent Psychiatry. July 2013. https://www.aacap.org/App_Themes/AACAP/docs/facts_for_families/04_the_depressed_child.pdf

Feit, Debbie. *A Parent's Guide to Speech and Language Problems.* New York, NY: McGraw-Hill, 2007.

Hamaguchi, Patricia McAleer. *Childhood Speech, Language & Listening Problems: What Every Parent Should Know.* Hoboken, NJ: Wiley, 2010.

Mahoneab, E. et al. "A Preliminary Neuroimaging Study of Preschool Children with ADHD." *The Clinical Neuropsychologist* (June 9, 2011): 1009–1028.

Newmeyer, Amy et al. "Results of the Sensory Profile in Children with Suspected Childhood Apraxia of Speech." *Physical & Occupational Therapy in Pediatrics 29,* no. 2 (2009): 205–20.

Nijland, Lian. "Speech Perception in Children with Speech Output Disorders." *Clinical Linguistics & Phonetics 23*, no. 3 (2009): 222–239.

STAR Institute for Sensory Processing Disorder. Online articles on SPD. Accessed Feb. 27, 2020. http://www.spdstar.org/.

Sharma, M., Purdy, S., and Kelly, A. "Comorbidity of Auditory Processing, Language, and Reading Disorders." *Journal of Speech, Language, and Hearing Research 52* (2009): 706–22.

Squires, Jane, Bricker, Diane et al. *Ages & Stages Questionnaire (ASQ)*. 3rd ed. Baltimore, MD: Paul Brookes Publishing, 2009.

A Guide to the Most-Asked-About Conditions in Relation to CAS

Because of its neurological underpinnings, childhood apraxia of speech is rarely found alone. This question-and-answer guide provides an overview of some of the most common conditions associated with CAS. *Your child may or may not have these conditions or symptoms.* Bear in mind, however, that many of them become more apparent over time, as conditions and demands on the child increase or change. Refer back to this appendix if you begin to have concerns.

Auditory Processing Disorder (APD)

APD, which is also known as central auditory processing disorder (CAPD), is not well-defined just yet. In fact, the jury is still out on whether it is a *central* (nervous system) issue, or "just" an auditory processing issue. Some folks refer to it as "central deafness." Others compare it to dyslexia, calling it "dyslexia of the ear." Still others wonder if it really exists. Generally, auditory processing is what we do with the sounds we hear. Kids who struggle with APD have a hard time organizing the information they hear, so their speech is often affected. Think of it this way: your child's brain doesn't "know" how to listen. Why APD *may* be associated with CAS: In a 2009 study on the sensory profile, the group of children with suspected apraxia had significant differences from same-age peers in auditory processing, as well as visual processing and multisensory processing.

In a basic sense, kids with APD hear sounds, but they can't make sense of what they are hearing (it may look like a receptive language disorder). Clinicians and practitioners indicate that there may be subtypes of APD. According to the authors of *The Mislabeled Child* (see references at the end of this chapter) the seven subtypes are: background noise, discrimination, prosody, localization, delayed processing, memory, and hypersensitivity.

Causes: The number one theory is that there is a familial tendency. Another theory is that chronic ear infections as a young child may be a contributing factor. If kids are missing sounds due to an ear infection(s), then that may lead to a processing problem like APD. Another theory is that it has to do with neuromaturational development—that is, the child's auditory perception is somehow delayed or immature.

Red flags that a child may have (C)APD:

- At around eighteen months, your child has delayed gibberish speech patterns (is not making the normal singsong sounds mimicking speech).

- Your older child has difficulty with rhyming words and articulation and frequently says "huh?" or "what?" or asks speakers to slow down.

- Your child has a decreased attention span, inability to concentrate, difficulty following directions, and is easily distracted. Of course, these symptoms overlap with ADHD and childhood in general.

- Your child is sensitive to sound or has a sensory integration disorder (SID).

- Your child has poor prereading skills (difficulty matching sounds with letters or rhyming).

- Your child has relatively poor social skills.

Bear in mind that APD has nothing to do with IQ, although some kids with APD have some other developmental disability that *may* affect overall intelligence.

Diagnosis: Only an audiologist trained in APD can diagnose this condition. The SCAN test is the "gold standard" screening tool for APD in children.

Treatment: Based on various diagnostic tests (electrophysiologic and behavioral measures done in a sound room with earphones and an audiometer), the audiologist will determine which treatment(s) is right for your child. Therapy treatments and tools may include

- Auditory Training (AT)
- Auditory-based computer programs such as *Fast ForWord Learning Programs* and *Earobics*
- FM trainers
- Multisensory reading programs like Lindamood-Bell and the Orton-Gillingham methods
- Modified listening programs such as Auditory Integration Program (AIT)
- Speech therapy and occupational therapy, with a focus on sounds/words, rhymes, and body language awareness

How can I help a child with APD?

- Make sure the child is seated close to the speaker/teacher so he can see and hear well.

- Minimize background noise (turn off fans and heaters, attempt to control road noise and classmate chatter, consider asking the teacher to use a microphone).
- Decrease visual distractions (streamline the space so there is less chance of verbal confusion).
- Improve acoustics (carpeting and wall hangings help).
- Simplify language you use around your child—avoid metaphors and abstract references.

For more information on APD

- American Speech-Language-Hearing Association: www.asha.org/public/hearing/disorders/understand-apd-child.htm
- "Auditory Processing Disorders: Classroom Accommodations and Modifications Checklist for APD": http://aitinstitute.org/auditory_processing_classroom_modifications.htm
- Dr. Maxine Young's website: www.maxineyoungcentral.com
- Karen Foli's book, *Like Sound through Water: A Mother's Journey through Auditory Processing Disorder* (Pocket Books, 2003)
- *The Sound of Hope* by Rosie O'Donnell and Lois Lam Heyman (Ballantine, 2010)

ADHD/ADD

Attention deficit disorder, with or without hyperactivity, is a common syndrome that can result in a variety of academic, social, and behavioral problems. Parents often notice these problems beginning in early childhood and continuing into teen and adult years. Kids with attention concerns can have difficulty working up to their academic potential, as well as trouble with follow-through, distractibility, impulsivity, and/or forgetfulness. Why it *may* be associated with CAS: Researchers from the Kennedy Krieger Institute in Baltimore found that the region of the brain responsible for cognitive and motor control was smaller in preschool children with symptoms of ADHD. Since CAS is a motor-neurological speech disorder, this *may* account for the correlation.

Red flags that a child may have ADHD:

- Challenges with following through and completing schoolwork or chores
- Difficulty organizing himself, tasks, paperwork, and materials
- Making careless mistakes: lack of attention to details
- Easily distracted
- Forgetful
- Blurting out answers, interrupting others often

- Restless/fidgety, acting as if "driven by a motor"
- Difficulty carrying out simple three-step directions, even ones that are part of the household routine
- Difficulties working up to academic potential
- Interpersonal clashes due to inability to meet expectations
- Impulsive

This list is not exhaustive, nor is it diagnostic! Many of these "red flags" are common in young children anyway. A trained professional (see below) can help tease out what is due to ADHD or ADD or just "typical kid" behavior.

Diagnosis: A neuropsychological evaluation needs to be conducted. This battery of tests includes a medical history, structured questionnaires, and tests to assess attention, concentration, learning, processing speed, perceptual organizational skills, and encoding of rote input, among others. *The Vanderbilt Attention Deficit/ Hyperactivity Disorder Parent Rating Scale* (VADPRS)—also a teacher version of this test, the *Vanderbilt Teacher-Behavior Evaluation Scale* (VTBES)—and the *Conners 3* rating scales are the most commonly used screening tests.

Many factors must converge before a formal diagnosis can be made (not usually before age six). There is not one magic assessment tool that will tell you, "Yes, your child has ADD (ADHD)." You'll want to complete testing if you have strong concerns, a teacher (or other service provider such as your child's SLP) has concerns, or if ADHD runs in your family. The earlier ADD/ADHD is confirmed, the better your child's chances of school success.

Any of these professionals are considered qualified to diagnosis ADHD:

- Child/adolescent psychiatrist—an MD who can prescribe medication
- Child/adolescent psychologist (a PhD or PsyD)—can't prescribe medication, but can provide counseling and may be less expensive than psychiatrists
- Pediatrician—an MD who is familiar with childhood illnesses and development but may lack the skills and specific knowledge to make a formal ADHD diagnosis
- Pediatric neurologist—an MD who specializes in disorders of the nervous system in children
- Psychiatric nurse practitioner (an RN with advanced training who can prescribe medication under a doctor's supervision and often works in collaboration with a medical practice)

Treatment: The MTA study (multimodal treatment of ADHD, funded by the NIMH) indicated that the best treatment is stimulant medication. Medication helps control symptoms—but is not a cure. Children and adolescents on stimulant medications need careful monitoring by a physician. The "best" treatment is often a combination (medication plus therapy) approach. Some parents supplement their child's treatment with behavioral modification programs (designed with a psychologist), social skills training, or occupational therapy.

How can I help a child with ADD or ADHD?

- Model good time and organizational management yourself.
- Develop and stick with household/school routines.
- Establish clear and reasonable expectations.
- Improve your communication style so that kids are clear as to what is expected.
- Use clocks and timers to create tangible parameters for completing a task.
- Design a place for quiet reflection at home and school.
- Pursue a 504 plan or IEP at school if your child could benefit from accommodations such as extended time, small group testing, use of a calculator, note-taking assistance, etc.

For more information on ADHD:

- CHADD (formerly Children and Adolescents with ADD): www.chadd.org
- *Identifying and Treating ADHD: A Resource for Home and School:* http://www2.ed.gov/teachers/needs/speced/adhd/adhd-resource-pt1.pdf
- *ADDitude Magazine*: www.ADDitudeMag.com
- *Raising Your Spirited Child* by Mary Sheedy Kurcinka
- *Understanding Girls with AD/HD* by Kathleen Nadeau, Ellen Littman, and Patricia Quinn
- You and your child may enjoy reading *The ADHD Kid* by Tobias Stumpf, who wrote the book as a teen to explain the pros and cons of having ADHD to other young people
- Drs. Gregory Stasi and Peter Dodzik of North Shore Pediatric Therapy offer a free e-book that covers ADHD—*Neuro-Development of Children: 4 Common Childhood Disorders* (go to https://NSPT4kids.com, select "Resources & Downloads, and then under e-books, select Neuropsychology)

Autism Spectrum Disorder (ASD)

Autism and apraxia are both neurological disorders, but they are completely different in nature. However, the same child can have both autism and CAS. Just as with CAS, autism runs on a continuum (spectrum). Therefore, kids can have mild to profound symptoms. Kids with autism have impaired communication, social, and emotional skills, whereas kids with CAS have impaired speech skills and may have impairments in gross and fine motor skills. Why ASD *may* be associated with CAS: Because of their neurological underpinnings, ASD and apraxia are sometimes found together. Children with ASD have difficulties with social and communication skills that sometimes overlap into the apraxia diagnosis.

Red flags that a child may have ASD:

- Facial expressions tend to be unanimated; smiles often not related to social interactions
- Not readily making eye contact and seeming to look beyond others
- Not responding to name when called
- Delayed or nonexistent waving, pointing, or other basic communicative gestures
- Using another person's hand as a tool (e.g., taking his mother's hand to open a door)
- Delays in speech or using speech for noncommunicative purposes (repeating dialog from a TV show to himself); sometimes speech develops on a normal timetable but the child talks excessively about his special interests without noticing others' cues that they are bored
- Difficulty imitating others' actions
- Not playing in a typical manner (performing the same action over and over, such as spinning the wheels on toy cars or placing toys in a line)
- Having little or no interest in reciprocal play with others

Diagnosis: The "best" diagnosis for an autism spectrum disorder (autism) is given by a child/adolescent psychiatrist or pediatric neurologist. Some child/adolescent psychologists specialize in autism spectrum disorders and may be involved with assessment.

Your pediatrician may give you a screening tool. Examples of such screening tools are *M-CHAT-R (Modified Checklist of Autism in Toddlers, Revised)*, the *STAT (Screening Tool for Autism in Toddlers & Young Children)*, or the *SCQ (Social Communication Questionnaire)*. After a series of screenings, a child who is considered a "concern" for autism should be given a complete evaluation by a multidisciplinary team.

Treatment: There is no one treatment that is "best" for ASD, although it is essential to begin early intervention once the disorder has been properly identified. Parents often advocate for intensive ABA (applied behavior analysis) treatment, which involves breaking tasks down into small steps, "errorless learning," and frequently reinforcing or rewarding the child for progress. Therapies that can help include behavioral, communication, occupational, and physical therapies, and social play. In elementary school and beyond, most children with ASD benefit from special education services and accommodations provided either in the regular classroom or in a specialized setting that allows the child to best learn up to his abilities. Medication may help a child with ASD for symptomatic treatment. For example, a child who is aggressive may benefit from an antipsychotic, and kids who have difficulty with inattention and hyperactivity may benefit from a stimulant. Children with ASD may not respond to medications in the same manner as a "typically developing" child. Medication administration should be carefully monitored by a treating physician.

How can I help a child with ASD?

Allow your child to select the type of play he engages in. Do not insist that he try to talk. Give him a slow introduction to sounds, events, and experiences, and gentle encouragement to verbalize. Educate yourself about how to reinforce the behaviors you want to see, as well as the optimal methods and placements for educating children with autism.

Where can I learn more?

- Autism Society of America: www.autism-society.org
- *Autism and Childhood Apraxia of Speech: From Preverbal to Sentences* by Karen Massey
- *Not My Boy: A Father, a Son, and One Family's Journey with Autism*, a memoir about raising a son with autism written by former NFL quarterback Rodney Peete
- *The Everyday Advocate: Standing Up for Your Child with Autism* by Areva Martin, a step-by-step guidebook with lots of personal stories
- *Dancing with Max: A Mother and Son Who Broke Free* by Emily Colson, a nice resource to turn to for hope and thought-provoking insight
- Woodbine House, which publishes books on a variety of issues related to raising children with autism, including *Visual Supports for Children with Autism*, *Activity Schedules for People with Autism*, and others

Anxiety Disorders

Anxiety is a broad umbrella covering many specific disorders, such as generalized anxiety disorder (GAD), separation anxiety disorder, specific phobias, selective mutism, and obsessive-compulsive disorder (OCD). Different types of anxiety disorders have different symptoms, but generally these kids worry excessively over a variety of events—their health, academics, athletics, friends, world events, what will happen if they do/don't do something, or family matters. Why it *may* be associated with CAS: Sometimes kids with CAS can become anxious or unsure in situations in which speaking and socializing is a large part of the event.

Red flags that a child may have an anxiety disorder:

- Constant feeling of being "keyed up" or "on edge"
- Restlessness
- Easily fatigued
- Decreased concentration

- Increased irritability
- Muscular tension
- Poor sleep/sleep concern
- In the case of OCD, repeated actions that seem senseless or excessive to an outside observer (such as frequent hand washing or needing to arrange items "just so")

Diagnosis: It is best to have a full assessment and evaluation conducted by a child/adolescent psychologist (PhD or PsyD) or child/adolescent psychiatrist (MD). It's difficult to diagnose kids with an anxiety disorder because it is often accompanied with disruptive behavior, which may overlap with symptoms consistent with ADHD or oppositional defiant disorder (ODD). In addition, childhood anxiety shares some characteristics with some autism spectrum disorders, learning disorders, bipolar disorder, and depression. Mental health specialists are likely to administer a screening tool such as the *Hamilton Anxiety Rating Scale* or the *Beck Anxiety Inventory* to help determine cause, type, and severity.

Treatment: Several different approaches to therapy may be used for childhood anxiety. Exposure response prevention treatment is highly evidence-based, especially in cases of OCD. Cognitive behavioral therapy (CBT) can be effective for children. In addition, it is helpful to teach children about anxiety, its symptoms, and nonmedical ways of managing it. In some cases, medication may help manage symptoms.

How can I help a child with an anxiety disorder?

Both parents and teachers can help children recognize symptoms of impending anxiety, as well as ways to change those anxious thoughts into more positive ones (reframing). In addition, teachers and parents ought to provide positive reinforcement for kid's continued success in school and home matters.

For more information about childhood anxiety

- *Freeing Your Child from Anxiety: Powerful, Practical Solutions to Overcome Your Child's Fears, Worries, and Phobias* by Tamar Ellsas Chansky
- *Helping Your Anxious Child: A Step-by-Step Guide for Parents* by Ronald M. Rapee, Ann Wignall, Susan H. Spence, and Vanessa Cobham
- *Childhood Anxiety Network:* www.childanxiety.net/index.htm
- Childhood anxiety disorders are covered in the free e-book, *Neuro-Development of Children: 4 Common Childhood Disorders,* by Drs. Stasi and Dodzik: www.NSPT4kids.com

Childhood Depression

Depression is a disorder involving several neurotransmitters within the brain. Although it is a real concern, affecting 5 percent of children and adolescents, it is very treatable. It tends to run in families, so if there is a tendency for depression in your family, be aware that it *could* affect your child. Significant life events (loss, stress) can contribute to depression, as can chronic illness. Why it *may* be associated with CAS: Kids who lack social connections may be more likely to be depressed than their more socially connected peers.

Red flags that a child may have depression:

- Sadness, tearfulness, crying
- Decreased interest in typical activities
- Feelings of hopelessness and helplessness
- Decreased energy
- Social isolation
- Irritability, anger
- Decreased self-esteem
- Psychosomatic complaints (frequent complaints of headaches or tummy aches when there is nothing physically wrong)
- Major change in eating or sleeping behavior (increased or decreased weight)
- Destructive behavior or acting out

Be aware that this list is not exhaustive, nor is it diagnostic!

Diagnosis: A qualified mental health professional makes the official diagnosis of childhood depression. An evaluation by a child/adolescent psychiatrist (MD) is imperative. Psychologists (PhD or PsyD) can provide counseling. Generally, children who have five or more of the above "red flags" for two or more weeks are considered depressed. If you are concerned about your child and depression, early intervention by a qualified professional is needed. They will provide screening tools (such as the *Beck Depression Inventory*) to determine cause and severity, and to develop a treatment plan.

Treatment: Comprehensive family and/or individual therapy in conjunction with an antidepressant is often the treatment for childhood depression. Talk with your prescribing physician for guidance and supervision of a medication regimen.

How can I help with childhood depression?

It may not be apparent to you that your child is struggling with depression since it is often masked by other symptoms such as anger, irritability, or destructive behavior. Ask your child if he is sad or unhappy. Doing so will often give you additional insight if he is exhibiting these non-typical symptoms of depression. Providing emotional support, building self-esteem, and assisting with medication monitoring are important ways others can help a child with depression.

For more information on depression:

■ *KidsHealth,* a comprehensive site on various topics, including depression, for parents, kids, and teens: http://kidshealth.org/parent/emotions/feelings/understanding_depression.html#

■ The American Academy of Child & Adolescent Psychiatry has a nice "for parents page": https://www.aacap.org/aacap/families_and_youth/facts_for_families/fff-guide/the-depressed-child-004.aspx

■ Childhood depression is covered in Drs. Stasi's and Dodzik's free e-book, *Neurodevelopment of Children: 4 Common Childhood Disorders:* www.NSPT4kids.com

■ *Helping Your Depressed Child: A Step-by-Step Guide for Parents* by Martha Underwood Barnard

Neurodevelopmental Delay (NDD)

A neurodevelopmental delay is an umbrella term for various disabilities and delays that overlap with one another. A neurodevelopmental delay is an omission or arrest of an early developmental stage of a child. It is difficult to pinpoint any one cause but may be due to a combination of developmental and environmental factors that delay the neurodevelopment of the child. Many of the symptoms of NDD overlap with the diagnostic categories of dyslexia, (dys)apraxia, and ADD, as well as a dysfunction of attention, motor, and perception (DAMP). For example, 80 percent of kids with dyslexia have some symptoms of (dys)apraxia, and up to 80 percent of kids with (dys)apraxia have some problems in common with dyslexia (especially difficulties with balance, orientation, and motor skills). Why it *may* be associated with CAS: If a child is delayed in a variety of neurological areas, speech and language may be affected as well, including the possibility of having CAS.

Red flags that a child may have NDD:

■ Attention and focus problems on a specific task

■ Poor balance, orientation, and motor skills (difficulty learning to ride a bicycle)

■ Poor body awareness (proprioception)

■ Poor hand-eye coordination, inability to sit still and remain silent

■ Mixed laterality (no true preference for handedness, foot, eye, or ear beyond the age of eight years)

■ Difficulty learning to read and write

■ Poor speech and articulation problems

■ Travel sickness beyond puberty

This list is not exhaustive, nor is it diagnostic!

Diagnosis: If you are concerned that your child has a neurodevelopmental delay (NDD), then chances are, your child's pediatrician has seen some red flags as well. Concerns are often noticed during a well-child exam. Visiting a developmental pediatrician, pediatric neurologist, or a pediatric psychiatrist may be the next step in a diagnosis.

Children need a full neurological assessment and evaluation, testing for reflexes, balance skills, and central nervous system (CNS) maturity levels, in addition to other recommended testing. A free screening tool developed by the Institute for Neuro-Physiological Psychology can be found at www.inpp.org.uk/questions/index.php. According to the research (*British Journal of Occupational Therapy,* October 1998), a score of 7 or more "yes" answers indicates the need for further evaluation for underlying neuromotor immaturity for kids over age seven.

Treatment: Generally, the treatment for neurodevelopmental delay(s) is geared toward the underlying cause of the delay. If you are concerned about the possibility that your child has an NDD, please consult your physician, who can advise you on professionals to consult about diagnosis and treatment.

How can I help with NDD?

Parents and teachers need to support these children academically and emotionally by monitoring homework, helping to increase the child's self-esteem, helping the child identify and implement rewards that are motivating to him, and participating in social and academic areas of the child's life. Depending on the diagnosis, you may also need to educate yourself on appropriate educational supports for your child and seek out an IEP or 504 plan to help him succeed in school.

For more information on NDD:

- Institute for Neuro-Physiological Psychology: https://www.inpp.org.uk/intervention-adults-children/more-information/about-ndd/causes-of-ndd/
- Brain and Behavior Enhancement website: www.brainandbehaviour.ie/en/understanding-neuro-developmental-delay.html
- *Comprehensive Intervention for Children with Developmental Delays: Program Manual and Checklists* by Prathibha Karanth and Priya James
- Other books you may find helpful in your journey: *A Parent's Guide to Developmental Delays* by Laurie LeComer and *How to Detect Developmental Delays and What to Do Next: A Practical Intervention for Home and School* by Mary Mountstephen

Sensory Processing Disorder (SPD)

In the recent past, this disorder was referred to as sensory integration disorder. In a general sense, SPD occurs when the nervous system doesn't recognize and organize input from the senses in an appropriate and meaningful way. According to the Star Institute for Sensory Processing Disorder, at least 1 in 20 children's daily lives are affected by SPD. Another research study suggests that 1 in every 6 children experiences sensory symptoms that may be significant enough to affect aspects of everyday life functions. As with ADHD, CAS, and autism spectrum disorders, researchers propose that SPD falls along a spectrum of severity. Why it *may* be connected to CAS: According to a 2007 study headed up by Amy Newmeyer, children with CAS had significant differences from same-age peers in a number of areas, including sensory seeking (particularly oral stimulation), emotional reactivity, and academic skills. Also, the 2007 ASHA technical document on CAS suggests that CAS may be motoric *and* sensory in nature.

Red flags that a child may have SPD:

- Overly sensitive to physical touch (e.g., clothing tags are very bothersome)
- Problems eating or sleeping
- Difficulty coping; prone to temper tantrums
- Very clumsy; "floppy"
- Little reaction to extreme temperatures
- In constant motion
- Often these children are referred to as being "in your face"

   This list is not exhaustive, nor is it diagnostic!

Diagnosis: A multidisciplinary team (MD, child psychologist, nurse practitioner, etc.) may diagnose a sensory processing disorder, but not necessarily so. An occupational therapist (OT) is also qualified to make the diagnosis. Often, kids who are suspected of having SPD are screened in a pediatrician's office, at school, or at a private clinic. Screening tools that may be used include the following:

- Sensory Integration & Praxis Test (SIPT, ages 4–8 years)
- Miller Function and Participation Scales (MFUN)
- Bruinicks-Oseretsky Test of Motor Proficiency
- Movement Assessment Battery for Children
- Miller Assessment for Preschoolers (MAP)
- Goal-Oriented Assessment of Life Skills (GOAL)

Based on the results of the screening test, a more in-depth evaluation may be conducted.

Treatment: It's often recommended that children with SPD work closely with an occupational therapist (OT) who has training in and uses a sensory integration approach in his or her practice. Medication typically does not help.

How Can I Help with SPD?

Help build these kids' self-esteem, as they are often referred to as "klutzes," and may not make friends as easily as their typically developing peers. Good modeling of social skills may also be helpful. Parents can ask their child's OT about a possible "sensory diet," which is an individualized plan to provide the child with the types of sensations throughout the day that can help him stay focused and organized and control his behavior.

For more information on SPD:

- The Star Institute for Sensory Processing, an organization designed for parents, pediatric professionals, and educators: https://www.spdstar.org/
- Tips, hints, and activities on creating a sensory diet at Sensory Smarts: http://sensorysmarts.com/sensory_diet_activities.html
- *The Sensory Processing Disorder Answer Book: Practical Answers to the Top 250 Questions Parents Ask* by Tara Delaney
- *The Everything Parent's Guide to Sensory Processing Disorder: The Information and Treatment Options You Need to Help Your Child with SPD* by Terri Mauro and Jenni L. Clark

General Resources and Recommended Reading:

- *The Well-Balanced Child: Movement and Early Learning* by Sally Goddard Blythe (Hawthorn Press Early Years, 2006).
- *The Mislabeled Child: How Understanding Your Child's Unique Learning Style Can Open the Door to Success* by Brock Eide and Fernette Eide (Hyperion, 2006).
- *Different Learners: Identifying, Preventing, and Treating Your Child's Learning Problems* by Jane Healy, PhD (Simon and Schuster, 2010).

Appendix B

Health Insurance

Early in our CAS journey, I phoned our insurance company. We lived in a small Minnesota town at the time, and I made the call on my cell phone, fearful I would lose coverage during this fateful phone call. Yes, "coverage" has multiple meanings here.

After the usual interminable hold, I got through. "I'm calling to see if speech therapy is covered for my daughter. She isn't talking much. I don't know what to do. My doctor thinks she needs to see a speech-language pathologist. Are we covered?"

"What is your policy number?"

"Uh . . . um," I stammered. I had no idea what my policy number was.

The member services representative sighed, "Ma'am, is the policy in your name or your husband's?"

"Uh, it's in my husband's," I responded.

"And what is his social security number?" As if I knew that off the top of my head! Somehow, I managed to muster up his social security number and provide it to the woman on the other end of the phone.

"I see your policy does cover speech therapy by a qualified speech-language pathologist if the child is found to be moderately to severely impaired in their communication, also if there is a distinct neurological or medical necessity."

"So I can take her to see this person recommended by our doctor?" I asked cautiously.

After giving the member services representative the clinic and SLP's name, I got the green light to head to the speech clinic the next week.

I hung up the phone, biting the side of my cheek in an effort to hold back tears. I called my husband. I reiterated the part about moderate to severe impairment and medical or neurological necessity. He sighed. I heard his office chair squeak. Hot tears rolled down my face.

"Honey, you don't need to cry," he reassured me. "It's covered. She'll be okay."

And she *is* okay. Speech therapy *was* covered. But it hasn't always been smooth sailing.

I know this process—the speech therapy and paying for it—can leave you feeling emotional, drained, and overwhelmed. Coverage for speech and language disorders can be tricky, to say the least. Each policy has its own set of rules and parameters, and it's helpful to know early on what they are. Here are a few pointers to keep in mind:

- *Understand your policy.* Get your hands on a copy of your policy. If you can't find it at home, check with your HR contact at work, call your insurance company directly for an extra copy, or see if you can access it from an online portal.
- *Find the section on speech and language therapy.* It may be listed under headings such as "rehabilitative services," "physical and occupational therapy," "other medically necessary services," or "therapies." Read it and be sure to note any "exclusions."
- If you *are* covered, consider yourself lucky, but realize this is not the end of the game.

Here are the top five questions to ask:

1. *Are both the evaluation and ongoing therapy covered?* You'd assume they *would* be, but stranger things have happened. Be sure you know ahead of time.

2. *Is therapy covered for CAS?* You will want to know what diagnostic code (ICD-10) your speech clinic is using when they submit to insurance. The ICD-10 code for CAS is R48.2. Know this early on to avoid a bill because the clinic coded for something that your insurance company doesn't cover. If you are interested in more ICD-10 codes, refer to this website: https://www.icd-10data.com/ICD10CM/Codes. You may also find ASHA's website helpful if you run into snags: https://www.asha.org/practice/reimbursement/coding/icd-10-cm-coding-faqs-for-audiologists-and-slps/#slpApraxia.

3. *"Do you need to choose a SLP who is in network?"* Some insurance plans require that you see providers who are in network, others allow you to see out-of-network providers but may pay less per visit (more dollars out-of-pocket for you and often with a high deductible). Some others will allow you to go wherever you want. It depends on the plan you have.

4. *Is there a deductible or copay?* In our case, we had a $1,500 deductible to meet for the calendar year. "Deposits" toward this $1,500 accrued each time we took Kate to ST. For example, ST cost $140/hour. We paid that amount toward our $1,500 deductible each time until we hit the deductible. Afterward, insurance was billed, and we were responsible for a copay for each visit. Other plans may not be as generous, with family deductibles often ranging in cost from $3,000–$6,000 or even higher. Each plan is different; find out how yours works.

5. *Is there a maximum number of visits per year/dollar amount paid?* I can't overemphasize how important it is to know this! Some insurance companies only allow a set number of visits per year (e.g., ten or a hundred). Others have a yearly maximum of a predetermined dollar amount, such as $5,000. Ask how your policy operates. Ask if there are allowances for more ST if your SLP recommends it. Ask, too, if speech therapy falls under the same umbrella as occupational and physical therapy. We were lucky—each therapy had a $5,000 max/year.

> **Help! We maxed out our yearly dollar coverage!**
> Kate had been making lots of new speech sounds. Her SLP recommended we consider feeding therapy for her eating issues (overstuffing, "forgetting" to chew, etc.), so we added "feeding therapy" to our already busy therapy schedule. She was going to the clinic three or four times a week. We didn't think much of it until a bill came in the mail for over $1,000. I was shocked! The year wasn't over yet! I called the insurance company after I simmered down. We had reached our $5,000 max on these therapies, they told us. (Feeding and speech therapy came out of the same "pot," in our case). I was dumbfounded. Sure, I was responsible for knowing and managing our insurance, but you would think that when we got close to that $5,000 max, our insurance company would have given us a heads-up. Or that the speech clinic might have said, "Oh, by the way, a claim was denied. It may be time to cut back on therapy or check your insurance." None of that happened, nor does it typically. Learn from my mistake: keep careful track of your insurance dollars!

If you're not covered for ST at all, there are a few things you can do:

- *Talk to your employer's HR person or department and see if they can offer another plan that has coverage.* It's your employer's choice which insurance plan they offer employees. They may have no idea that your child needs speech therapy if you don't speak up. If you present a compelling enough case, they may back you up by finding a better-suited plan, but don't bank on this.

- *For help persuading your employer to switch insurance plans,* request an "Employer Insurance Packet," by visiting ASHA (www.asha.org) or calling 800–498-2071. The packet suggests ways to talk with your employer's HR person, make the case for more speech coverage, and hold a meeting with your HR department.

- *Look for free or reduced cost speech therapy at a local college or university.* This was the number one suggestion we received when our insurance was maxed out and Kate still needed services. It didn't work out for us, but it may for you. Call the college's communication disorders department or program and inquire. You can also place an ad at the college indicating you are seeking the services of a student to come to your home and work with your child on speech-language concerns. Pay him or her a small fee, just as you would a tutor or babysitter. A college student isn't likely to turn down quick cash and useful experience. Plus, you won't have to drive to and from the clinic, and your child has additional interaction with someone who cares.

- *Early intervention programs and public school–based preschools offer free or very low-cost speech services.* Early intervention programs often provide therapy (including ST) free of charge or based on a sliding scale. Generally, EI will help you get your foot in the public preschool door as well. Providing your child meets criteria set forth by the evaluation and treatment team, your child may be eligible to attend a public preschool with speech services at no additional cost to you.

- *Apply for financial assistance such as Medicaid.* According to Debbie Feit, author of *The Parent's Guide to Speech and Language Problems,* the Medicaid program allows for direct reimbursement to speech-language pathologists. Each state's eligibility rules vary, so do your homework by checking www.cms.hhs.gov.

- *You may even qualify for a grant through United Healthcare Children's Foundation (UHCCF).* These grants can help families pay for children's medical expenses that are not covered, or partially covered by a commercial healthcare plan. Qualifying families may receive up to $5,000 for services and equipment such as physical, occupational, and speech therapy and counseling services, surgeries, prescriptions, and the like. Parents or legal guardians can apply for grants at www.uhccf.org.

- **Look for other organizations that offer financial assistance.** Go to ASHA's website (www.asha.org) and head to "Advocacy" in the menu bar. From there, you will see "Tools for Consumers & Employers." If you're happy there, great. Otherwise, you can try clicking on "Latest Developments in Billing and Reimbursement." After you've done that, look at the maroon-colored box on the right-hand corner, then click on "The Public." You will find many organizations listed offering funding for speech-language therapy (Easter Seals, March of Dimes, Scottish Rite/ RiteCare, to name a few). Each organization requires an application process, and eligibility varies, so be sure to look into each one carefully. You may also try contacting those organizations directly.

Parents Ask

Can I deduct therapy costs on my income tax?
Generally speaking, if (1) you itemize deductions on your tax return, *and* (2) your medical expenses for the year exceed 10 percent of your adjusted gross income (AGI), then you can deduct the amount over and above that 10 percent. Let's say your income is $50,000. $5,000 is 10 percent of your AGI. If all of your medical and therapy costs for the year top out at $6,000 for the year, then $1,000 would be deductible (6,000 – 5,000). If those therapy costs go up to $7,500 (and your AGI is still $50,000) then you might be able to write off $2,500 (7,500 –5,000). (You can only take a medical deduction if you itemize deductions, however.) It's a bit mind-boggling, but it can be done. For more information on deducting medical expenses, call 800–829-1040 and ask for Publication 502, or go to www.irs.gov/taxtopics/tc502.html.

As you can see, there are many ways to seek financial assistance to pay for your child's speech-language treatment. Please do not let money stop you from giving your child what she needs most to overcome CAS: frequent and intense ST provided by a qualified speech-language pathologist.

Summer Speech Camps and Enrichment Programs

School's out! As a parent reading this, you may have mixed feelings about summer "vacation." While having months of not having to deal with the morning rush or nagging your child(ren) to complete their homework *is* a break, you still have things to think about, especially when it comes to your child's speech and language goals.

Your child may or may not qualify for extended school year (ESY), depending on his age and severity of CAS. Even if he does, it's not a bad idea to supplement your child's summer with some additional speech enrichment. Keep in mind, your speech clinic *may* offer summer social skills classes or day camps as well, so be sure to ask.

An ideal summer program will offer

- a balanced program with daily opportunities for enrichment of a variety of skills, including recreation;
- engaging, kid-friendly activities;
- a safe and structured program with positive, caring, and professional role models;
- low camper-to-staff ratio.

You may have to select a summer program months in advance to secure your child's spot. Consider asking these questions to help you winnow down your decisions for your child's needs, abilities, and interests:

1. Does the program have a mission? What is it?
2. How is a typical day/week organized? How will children spend their time?
3. What are the program hours and dates?
4. How does the program assess or track each child's progress? What evidence does the program have to show past results?
5. What is the typical experience of the staff members who will work with my child? Are any of them SLPs, OTs, or PTs?
6. Does the staff receive any special training?

7. What type of communication can families expect?

8. Is financial aid available? Does insurance cover any of the costs?

For more information about what makes a summer learning program successful, visit the National Summer Learning Association at www.summerlearning.org. Apraxia Kids has a very comprehensive state-by-state (and province-by-province) guide listing summer programs in the United States and Canada that may be of interest to you: https://www.apraxia-kids.org/apraxia_kids_library/summer-speech-language-camps-for-apraxia/.

Speech and Language Milestones

I don't want to make you feel worse by introducing you to the "typically speaking child." But I do want to present you with some facts. Read over these charts quickly, without putting much thought into it. Make a little tick mark next to the milestones your child has reached. Look at this as a quick assessment tool from your own perspective.

Keep in mind, these charts are just guidelines to development. Please don't get too hung up on the idea that these are the absolute way things must go. No two children develop at the same rate. The charts are here for your reference, so you can see where your child meets, exceeds, or falls behind in terms of what typically developing kiddos often experience.

Birth to 3 months

- Reacts to sudden noises by crying or jerking limbs (Moro reflex)
- "Knows" familiar objects (pacifier, bottle, breast) and people (parents & siblings)
- Watches objects with great interest
- Has a different type of cry for hunger vs. pain vs. boredom
- Begins to coo and make prolonged vowel sounds ("ahh")

3–6 months

- Babbles: "ba-ba-ba"
- Laughs and shows pleasure, especially when favorite things are presented
- Looks for source of sound(s) by turning head
- Knows own name and will react when she hears it
- Voice is now louder for crying and babbling

Babbling and cooing are the same thing, right? Not quite. When an infant coos, she is practicing open-throat consonants—*h*, *k*, *g*, and vowel sounds such as *ah* and *oo*. When she starts to babble, at around four months, she will add consonants made with her palate and lips (*ta, na, da, ma, pa*).

6–9 months

- Understands simple words such as *yes* and *no*
- Will look at family members upon hearing them named
- Babbling becomes singsong in nature
- Sometimes sounds as though she is saying "mama" but doesn't understand the label yet
- Reacts to facial expressions of others; will attempt to mimic them
- Attempts peekaboo and bye-bye gestures
- Shakes head to indicate *no*
- Uses more sounds when babbling—*da, ba, ka, pa, ma, and wa*

Babbling gets more complicated the older the baby. "Complicated" can be defined in terms of more complex syllable structure and faster consonant-vowel transitions. Complex babbling is a direct result, according to one study, of direct nonverbal contact (smiles, kisses, and touches) from those who care for the baby (2003 study at Franklin & Marshall College). For more information about infant babbling, see www.vocaldevelopment.com (provides good information and audio clips).

9–12 months

- Enjoys imitating simple sounds
- Begins to say *mama* and *dada* with meaning
- Understands that words stand for objects
- May "dance" to music
- Imitates common animal sounds
- Will find a toy or object when asked
- Watches and imitates others

By twelve months, the typically developing baby is mixing consonants and vowels together and is able to say *dada, baba, mama, nana, and papa.* She can pronounce most of the vowel sounds and about half of the consonants of her native language. Keep in mind that babies are captivated by the people in their life and their names. That is why first words are often *mama* and *dada.* Secondly, babies find the actions that their caregivers do especially enthralling—these may very well become their next spoken words.

12–18 months

- Understands 50–75 words
- Uses 3–20 real words consistently, even if not said clearly
- Will accurately point to the right place when asked where something is located

- Points to a few body parts when asked (eyes, nose, ears)
- Will babble and use nonsense words while pointing to something of interest
- Follows simple commands: "Put this in the toy basket."
- Uses words such as *all-gone, more, down, done, mine, no, mama, daddy, gimme*

Around fifteen months, children understand more and more words. They are most interested (and able to say) the words that are important and meaningful, such as family members' or pets' names and the words for familiar objects like cup and ball. They may be able to use some modifiers such as *hot* and *mine*. Keep in mind that a typically developing child won't be able to say much more than one word at a time. When she says "cup," she is trying to communicate a more complex idea such as "I want my cup," "Take my cup," or "Where is my cup?"

18 months–2 years

- Understands about 300 words
- Uses about 50 words, mostly nouns
- Uses real words most of the time; occasionally babbles and uses jargon
- Shakes head yes/no to questions
- Will show a change in tone when asking a question: *"More?"*
- Follows two-step commands: "Go to the laundry room and get your shoes."
- Begins to use some verbs (e.g., *go*) and adjectives (e.g., *little*)
- Use two related words to make one word (*allgone*)
- Speech often difficult to understand
- Tells her name when asked (but may not be very clear)
- May start to ask, "What's that?" ("What 'at?")
- Wants to hear same stories over and over; may join in when singing or reading

At this point, the typically developing child can make many speech sounds, but not always use them in the correct context. She might be able to say "shh" to her stuffed animals or while singing "The Wheels on the Bus" (the mommy on the bus goes "shh, shh, shh"), but is unable to say *shoe*. Why is this? It's easier to produce strings of the same sound than it is to make a quick change from *sh-* to *-oe* to form *shoe*. She may even substitute a *t* sound for the *sh-* simply because it's easier.

2–3 years

- Understands about 900 words
- Can say about 500 words
- Speech is understandable about half the time (maybe as much as 70 percent)
- Uses eye contact appropriately

- Voices frustrations more with words and less with whining and crying
- Wants to show you everything: "Look, Mommy!"
- Will correctly answer questions beginning with *who, where, what* ("What goes meow?")
- Understands prepositions (e.g., *in, on, under, on top of*)
- Begins to ask yes/no questions ("Is it night-night?")
- Talks to self aloud when playing
- Begins to use function words such as *the* and *is*
- May use past tense verbs (e.g., *walked, jumped*), but will use some incorrectly (e.g., "runned," "sleeped")
- May stutter when especially excited
- Consistently pronounces sounds of *m, n, p, d, b, f, h, y*

3–4 years

- Understands about 1,200 words
- Uses about 800 words
- Speech is understandable about 70–80 percent of the time
- Begins to use *Is* at the beginning of a question
- Asks lots of questions: "Why?" "Who is . . . ?"
- Often will ask the same question many times in a row
- Understands time concepts such as *now, later, morning, lunchtime*
- Uses plurals consistently: *books, plates, blocks*
- Uses the words *are* and *and* (The boys *are* playing; Davin *and* Rhys are here)
- Initiates conversations by making comments and observations
- Consistent eye contact during conversations
- Produces beginning, middle, and ending sounds in words
- Consonant blends are still difficult (*bl, st, fr, cr*)
- Uses *k* and *g* sounds correctly
- May lisp on *s* sounds and distort the *r* sound

4–5 years

- Understands 2,500–2,800 words
- Uses 1,500–2,000 words
- Understandable about 80–90 percent of the time
- Uses pronouns correctly (e.g., I, he, she, you, them)

- Uses past, present, and future tenses of verbs correctly (run, runs, running, ran, will run)
- Uses irregular verbs (sleep = slept, eat = ate) and irregular nouns (child = children, woman = women)
- Explains events from the past in detail
- Can describe pictures with complete sentences
- Understands common opposite terms: *yummy/yucky*, *big/little*, *quiet/loud*
- Consonant blends still difficult
- May mispronounce *s, r, v, l,* and *j* sounds

5–7 years: Refinement

- Increases vocabulary by adding new words into spontaneous speech
- Refines pronunciation, sentence structure, attention span for listening
- Retells experiences in cohesive, sequential manner
- Participates in group discussion; knows when it's her turn to speak
- Begins to learn language relationships: opposites, synonyms, classifications/categories, and associations (e.g., *peanut butter/jelly, pen/paper*)

7 years to Adolescence

- Language system is functional and abstract
- Reading, writing, speaking, and listening skills are age-appropriate
- Understands and uses idioms (e.g., pain in the neck, cut it out, wear me out)
- Can pronounce multisyllabic words after practice
- Language of a child at this stage will mimic an adult's, but with greater simplicity
- Masters word relationships

Charts adapted from *A Parent's Guide to Speech and Language Problems* by Debbie Feit (McGraw-Hill, 2007) and *Childhood Speech, Language & Listening Problems: What Every Parent Should Know* by Patricia McAleer Hamaguchi (Wiley, 2010).

For more insight into where your child is developmentally, check with your SLP or child's school for "HELP . . . at Home" handouts by VORT Corporation. They are useful little guides with checklists that will give you an idea of where your child's abilities are, developmentally speaking. They'll also give you lots of ideas on how you can move the process along at home. They are not meant to be diagnostic in nature.

Please remember that any given child may be at a different level on the communication skills continuum. For example, you may have a three-year-old who is not doing the things she is "supposed" to be doing at that age. If so, find out where she really is, and work from there. Trying to force your child to perform at the level where experts say she should be is just frustrating for you both. See chapter 9 for activities you can do at home.

Appendix E

Glossary

Accommodation: A change made in the learning environment to help a student compensate for the effects of a disability, thereby leveling the playing field. Examples include extra time to complete a test or seating closer to the teacher. Accommodations do not change the content of what the student is expected to learn, in contrast to *modifications*.

ADHD: **A**ttention **d**eficit **h**yperactivity **d**isorder. A common childhood neurological disorder in which a child has difficulty with attention, impulsivity, distractibility, and sometimes hyperactivity. When the disorder occurs without hyperactivity, may be referred to as ADD.

Anxiety: As a psychological condition, an anxiety disorder is an overwhelming sense of dread or worry that affects daily life. *Some* anxiety in life is normal and should not be confused with an anxiety disorder. Children with CAS may experience heightened levels of anxiety when asked to speak in uncertain or new situations, or when a phrase is too demanding.

Apraxia: See Childhood Apraxia of Speech (CAS)

Articulation: The ability to form speech sounds correctly and clearly. Sometimes abbreviated as "artic."

Articulators: The articulators for speech production are primarily the jaw, lips, and tongue.

Autism Spectrum Disorder (ASD): A developmental disorder that appears in the first three years of life and results in difficulties in social and communication skills and unusual or restricted interests.

Babbling: Can be referred to as pre-speech. It consists of relatively long strings of syllables such as *ba-ba-ba*, *ah-ah-ah*, or *ee-ee-ee*, or combinations of these sounds that may be used communicatively, or as solo sound-play. *See also* Conversational Babble.

Broca's Area: A part of the brain named for Pierre Paul Broca, a French physician who reported language impairments in two of his patients after an injury to their posterior inferior frontal gyrus of the brain. These two patients lost the ability to speak after their injuries, leading researchers to conclude that this area is likely responsible for speech production.

CAS: A disorder characterized by difficulties planning movements. Someone with apraxia of speech has difficulties planning the movements needed for speech. In the US, the most accepted term for apraxia of speech in children is childhood apraxia of speech.

(C)APD: An acronym that stands for *central auditory processing disorder*. Kids who struggle with APD have a hard time organizing the information they hear receptively, and their speech is often affected. The jury is still out as to whether the condition affects the central nervous system. Sometimes you will find that the disorder is referred to as "just" auditory processing disorder (APD).

CCC: Certificate of Clinical Competence, certification from the American Speech-Language-Hearing Association that a speech-language pathologist has completed a rigorous professional program including master's degree work from an accredited program and extensive supervised practice and has also passed a national certification examination.

Comorbid, Co-occurring, or Concomitant: Two or more medical or educational conditions that exist together, although typically independent of one another.

Conversational Babble: Speech sounds produced by a young child in which tone, eye contact, and gesture strongly resemble those used in adult conversational interactions but no identifiable words are used. *See also* Babbling and Expressive Jargon.

Critical Period: A period in development during which certain events must take place if they are to take place at all.

Cued Speech: A mode of communication in which hand shapes placed on the face are used to represent the sounds of a spoken language. Cueing allows users who are deaf, hard of hearing, or who have language/communication disorders to access the basic, fundamental properties of spoken languages through the use of sight.

Dysarthria: Refers to a group of motor speech disorders that are caused by central or peripheral nervous system damage. This damage results in muscle tone differences that cause weakness, paralysis, or incoordination of the speech muscles. Dysarthria may affect respiration, phonation/voicing, articulation, and resonance.

Dyspraxia: An older term that may be used in place of *apraxia*. Dyspraxia can be translated to mean "difficult" (dys) "planned motor movement" (praxis).

Executive Function (and self-regulation skills): are the mental processes that enable one to plan, focus attention, remember instructions, and juggle multiple tasks successfully.

Expressive Jargon: Babbling consisting of strings of sounds uttered with a variety of stress and intonation patterns. *See also* Conversational Babble.

Expressive Language: The use of speech, gestures, text, or other communication systems to communicate with others.

IDEA: The Individuals with Disabilities Education Act, a federal law in the United States that governs the provision of special education to qualifying children with disabilities, ages birth to 21. The law requires the provision of a free, appropriate public education in the *least restrictive environment.*

IEP: Individualized Education Program, the document setting out prescribed goals, services, educational setting, and other details related to the education of students with disabilities ages 3 to 21 under *IDEA.* The IEP document is jointly developed by teachers, therapists, teachers at an IEP meeting and revised at least annually.

IFSP: Individualized Family Service Plan, the document setting out agreed-upon objectives, goals, and services for infants and toddlers with disabilities (ages birth through age two) who are receiving early intervention.

Itinerant services: In a public school setting, children with mild to moderate disabilities may be provided educational support or therapy by therapists or teachers who move from school to school or classroom to classroom.

Jargon: Strings of unintelligible speech sounds produced with the intonation pattern of adult speech.

Language: A system of symbols (spoken and/or written words, gestures) and rules for using those symbols to communicate. Languages are specific to particular cultures or groups of people. For example, English and Spanish are spoken languages used within the United States, and ASL is a gestural language used by some deaf people in the US.

Learning Disability: A condition that results in difficulties learning in one or more specific areas (such as reading or math) that would not be expected based on the individual's overall intellectual abilities. That is, the child's performance in one or more areas of learning is notably lower than in other areas of learning.

Least Restrictive Environment: The requirement under IDEA that a child who is receiving special education services must be educated to the maximum extent possible in the regular education environment while still achieving the goals in his IEP.

Linguistic Load: The complexity of what is being communicated verbally. This includes the difficulty of movements of the articulators (tongue, palate, jaw, teeth, lips) from one place to the next and how much planning/programming is required to get the thoughts out verbally. Tongue twisters, for example, have a high linguistic load.

Loudness: The volume of our voice from quiet to loud. You've no doubt noticed voices that "carry well." That would be an example of loudness combined with good articulation resulting in projection.

Motor Cortex: The portion of the brain's frontal cortex that plans, controls, and executes voluntary motor movements.

Motor Planning/Programming: In a speech-language pathology sense, motor planning/programming refers to the formation of a spatial (space) and temporal (time) strategy for producing a sequence of speech sounds. The "space" is within the brain, which orchestrates where the *articulators* need to be in order to sequence a desired string of sounds. Children with CAS have a disruption in learning and controlling the motor planning/programming process of speech.

Multidisciplinary Treatment Team: A group of professionals such as a speech-language pathologist (SLP), an occupational therapist (OT), a physical therapist (PT), an educator, a psychologist, and perhaps a doctor or nurse who pool their expertise to arrive at a diagnosis or treatment plan for a child. An evaluation completed by such a team can result in a more complete understanding and diagnosis of a child's strengths, weaknesses, and needs.

Neurobehavioral disorders: Conditions caused by differences in the brain that result in behavioral challenges.

Neuromuscular: Pertaining to the brain, nerves, and muscles.

Phonics: The correspondence between letters and the sounds they make. For example, in English, the sound /k/ can be represented by *c*, *k*, *ck*, *ch*, or *q* spellings. Phonics also involves teaching the blending of sounds to produce approximate pronunciations of unknown words.

Phonological: Relating to the scientific study of phonology, which is concerned with the sound structures of languages.

Phonological Disorder: A range of developmental communication disorders in which sound production is affected. *See also* Speech Sound Disorder.

Phonology: The language rules that control speech sound use.

Pitch: The highness or lowness of a voice (or musical tone).

Pragmatics: The rules for the use of language in social context (such as when greeting others or making a request) and in conversation, or the study of these rules.

Prosody (intonation): "The melody of speech," including syllable stress, intonation, inflection.

"Pull-out" services: When a therapist or special educator removes a child for a short time from the typical classroom to work on a particular skill or to focus on a specific area of concern. This may be accomplished in a peer group setting, or one on one.

"Push-in" services: When a therapist or special educator comes into the general education classroom to provide services and works with the classroom teacher on a specific skill or area of concern.

Rate: Refers to the overall speed at which someone speaks.

Receptive Language: Language comprehension; the ability to understand others' spoken or written messages or gestures.

Resolved CAS: A term applied to a child whose previous concerns regarding childhood apraxia of speech have improved to the point that they no longer affect learning, social relationships, and general functioning. Also known as "recovering apraxia [CAS]" or "resolving apraxia [CAS]."

Response to Intervention (RTI): A procedure used by school staff to identify students who need additional support to learn and then provide that support. RTI is tried before a student is referred for special education evaluation.

Retention: The ability to maintain a skill or information over time. *Grade retention* refers to "being held back" in a grade level due to difficulties mastering key academic skills.

Semantics: A Greek word meaning "the study of meaning." This scientific discipline is often concerned with studying the meaning of words, phrases, signs, and symbols.

Speech: The neuromuscular process of producing voice and sounds and combining them in words to communicate.

Speech or Language Impairment: One of the disability categories listed in IDEA as qualifying a child for special education services such as speech therapy (ST). It is defined as "a communication disorder such as stuttering, impaired articulation, language impairment, or a voice impairment that adversely affects a child's educational performance."

Speech Sound Disorder: Some professionals prefer to use the term *speech sound disorder* over *phonological disorder*. The reason is that the word *phonological* is so closely linked with language and reading. Calling it a *speech sound disorder* helps distinguish the two. *See also* Phonological Disorder.

Stress: Refers to the emphasis (stress) placed on certain syllables of words.

Syntactic: Relating to the rules of syntax or grammar, including the grammatical arrangement of words and phrases into sentences.

Transfer: The ability to generalize a skill to other contexts; to use a skill learned in one setting or situation in another setting or situation.

Vocal Quality: Refers to the "smoothness" of voice—whether it is harsh or hoarse, smooth or gravelly. Resonance also affects vocal quality (e.g., *nasal*, if too much sound comes from the nose, or *denasal*, if the person sounds "stuffed up" as if he has a cold).

Wernicke's Area: Originally identified by the Polish-German neurologist/psychiatrist Carl Wernicke, this is the area of the brain necessary for speech comprehension. It is located in the posterior (back) section of the superior temporal gyrus in the left (dominant) cerebral hemisphere.

Advisory Board

Much heartfelt gratitude to these amazing individuals who lent their time, talents, and expertise to read and review portions of this book.

Nanette Cote, MA, CCC-SLP, is a certified speech-language pathologist and private practice owner of Naperville Therapediatrics in Illinois. She is trained in PECS, PROMPT, and DTTC with specialties in treating children with apraxia and stuttering. During the summer, you can find her singing and laughing with pediatric clients in the pool during her innovative speech and language group sessions at the Rush Copley Healthplex. In June 2019, she launched her guidebook *We Talk on Water: Guide for Developing and Orchestrating Successful Group Social Communication* on Amazon. In addition to her private practice work, Nanette authors Speech2me, an educational speech and language blog for families and colleagues. She has been featured in her industry's monthly magazine, *The ASHA Leader*; appeared on local television news channels; and presented a poster session at a national ASHA convention. You can connect with Nanette via social media on Facebook and Instagram through her speech2me accounts or email her at: nanettecote@gmail.com. Her website is https://napervilletherapediatrics.com.

Renee Mindy, MSED, is an educator with twenty-five years of experience working as a special education teacher and reading specialist. She teaches at Thomas Jefferson Junior High School in Woodridge, Illinois, where she serves as a district mentor and department chair. Additionally, she serves on numerous committees involving school improvement initiatives, teacher evaluation, RTI, and special education reform. Renee supports students within their general education classrooms and provides intensive reading interventions to students who have IEPs with eligibilities in speech, SLD, ED, OHI, and autism. She can be reached at mindyr@woodridge68.org or on LinkedIn at http://linkedin.com/in/renee-mindy-48b87865.

Erik X. Raj, PhD, CCC-SLP, holds a Certificate of Clinical Competence from the American Speech-Language-Hearing Association and is a practicing speech-language pathologist who works with school-age children and adolescents with various communication difficulties. He regularly presents interactive workshops demonstrating how speech-language pathologists can use mobile and internet-based technologies to educate and motivate school-age children and adolescents. In addition to developing over twenty-five mobile apps for children with communication difficulties, he is the creator of Your Face Learning, an educational app for the iPhone and iPad that was named Creative Child Magazine's 2019 Children's App of the Year. You can connect with him at his website: www.erikxraj.com.

Index

About the Author

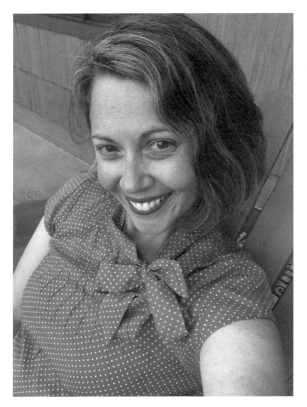

Leslie Lindsay is the award-winning author of ***Speaking of Apraxia***, originally published in 2012 following her daughter's 2007 diagnosis of childhood apraxia of speech (CAS). Leslie's writing and photography have appeared in various literary journals; she has been recognized as one of the most influential book reviewers, interviewing hundreds of bestselling and debut authors at www.leslielindsay.com. Leslie is a former Child and Adolescent Psychiatric R.N. at the Mayo Clinic and is at work on a memoir. She and her family, including a basset hound, reside in suburban Chicago.

Also published by Woodbine House:

A Picture's Worth
PECS and Other Visual Communication Strategies
Andy Bondy, Ph.D. & Lori Frost, M.S., CCC-SLP

Early Communication Skills for Children with Down Syndrome
A Guide for Parents and Professionals
Libby Kumin, Ph.D., CCC-SLP

Getting from Me to We
How to Help Young Children Fit In and Make Friends
Shonna L. Tuck, M.A., SLP

Going Solo While Raising Children with Disabilities
Laura E. Marshak, Ph.D.

Late, Lost, and Unprepared
A Parents' Guide to Helping Children with Executive Functioning
Joyce Cooper-Kahn, Ph.D. & Laurie Dietzel, Ph.D.

Views from Our Shoes
Growing Up with a Brother or Sister with Special Needs
Edited by Donald J. Meyer

Visual Supports for People with Autism
A Guide for Parents and Professionals
Marlene J. Cohen, Ed.D., BCBA & Peter F. Gerhardt, Ed.D.

For a FREE catalog featuring these and all our titles, contact us by mail, phone, or email.

WOODBINE HOUSE · 6510 Bells Mill Road · Bethesda, MD 20817
800-843-7323 (toll-free) · 301-897-3570 · 301-897-5838 (fax)
info@woodbinehouse.com · www.woodbinehouse.com